The SAGES Manual of Quality, Outcomes and Patient Safety

The SAGES Manual of Quality, Outcomes and Patient Safety

David S. Tichansky, MD, FACS
Thomas Jefferson University, Philadelphia, PA, USA

John Morton, MD, MPH, FACS
Stanford School of Medicine, Stanford, CA, USA

Daniel B. Jones, MD, MS, FACS
Harvard Medical School, Boston, MA, USA

Editors

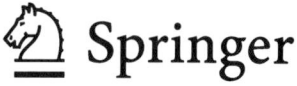

Springer

Editors

David S. Tichansky, MD, FACS
Minimally Invasive and
Bariatric Surgery
Thomas Jefferson University
1100 Walnut Street
Philadelphia, PA 19107, USA
david.tichansky@jefferson.edu

John Morton, MD, MPH, FACS
Minimally Invasive Surgery
Stanford School of Medicine
300 Pasteur Drive, H3680
Stanford, CA 94305, USA
morton@stanford.edu

Daniel B. Jones, MD, MS, FACS
Professor in Surgery
Harvard Medical School
Vice Chair of Surgery
Office of Technology and Innovation
Chief, Minimally Invasive
Surgical Services
Beth Israel Deaconess Medical Center
330 Brookline Avenue
Boston, MA 02215, USA
djones1@bidmc.harvard.edu

ISBN 978-1-4419-7900-1   e-ISBN 978-1-4419-7901-8
DOI 10.1007/978-1-4419-7901-8
Springer New York Dordrecht Heidelberg London

Library of Congress Control Number: 2011936966

Springer is part of Springer Science+Business Media (www.springer.com)

Preface

Sages Manual QOS

The *SAGES Manual on the Quality, Outcomes and Safety* is the first easy-to-read paperback book to outline best practices in the operating theatre. Experts in the field drill down on quality measures, and the use of the SAGES-AORN MIS Safety Checklist, Surgical Time out, and clinical pathways to improve quality. Administrative databases, such as NSQIP, track and benchmark surgeon outcomes. The *SAGES Manual on QOS* helps us to better understand adverse events and near misses, disclose error to patients, and how to develop a culture of safety first. Preoperative risk assessment, common complications, and management are discussed in detail for minimally invasive surgery, endoscopy, robotic surgery, and NOTES.

Many organizations have been developing safer surgery through education and training, and the contributions of the American College of Surgeons, American Board of Surgery, American Society of Metabolic and Bariatric Surgery, Association for Surgical Education, and Society for Gastrointestinal and Endoscopic Surgeons have been highlighted. Medical–legal considerations are addressed from informed consent, off-label use of devices to liability and tort issues.

The use of simulation and team training is thoroughly reviewed. "See one, do one, teach one" is not in the best interest of patient safety. Instead, trainees and staff surgeons can hone their technical and communication skills in the Skills Lab. The Fundamentals of Laparoscopic Surgery (FLS), the Fundamentals of Endoscopic Surgery (FES), and the Fundamental Use of Surgical Energy (FUSE) assess proficiency and promote safe practices. Teamwork improves with practicing closed loop communication, speaking up, and use of checklists. In a culture of safety, the new adage must be "perfect practice makes perfect."

Boston, MA, USA   Daniel B. Jones, MD, MS, FACS

Foreword

In this time and in this place, surgeons find themselves in a new age of accountability. A demand is heard from payor and patient alike that we deliver care that is safe and effective. This is not a refrain that is new to the field of surgery. Quality and safety are bywords for the profession of surgery. As a profession, it is critical that surgeons seize the initiative to lead quality improvement and patient safety efforts. A cornerstone to surgical professionalism is our collective ability to hold ourselves accountable.

The time for advancing the quality of science is now. We are able to draw from vast mounds of data, perform precise analysis, and interest and demand are high now. The consumer revolution that has affected other fields of endeavor has arrived to surgery where patients are able to research publicly available outcomes reporting. Payors are insisting on quality outcomes so better care is provided.

Surgeons are well equipped to meet this challenge. Quality is a surgeon's birthright. Surgeons initiated cancer registries, advanced trauma life support, and minimally invasive surgery. The Joint Commission was actually founded by surgeons. Thousands of times a day, surgeons enter into an explicit contract of risk and benefit of surgery with patients as we have done for centuries. Surgery is based on attention to detail and constant, unremitting evaluation of our results as we demonstrate through the first iteration of quality improvement, the morbidity and mortality conference. While we have led efforts in quality, surgeons must not rest upon prior accomplishments. There are many questions we must ask ourselves before others answer it for us.

Why have we always done it this way? To be frank, surgery is a high-risk field: many opportunities for harm and a small handful of avenues for success. Surgical complications actually account for 10% of the overall disease burden with 50% of those complications being potentially preventable. If your mentor was able to accomplish a quality surgical outcome, then it is eminently logical that you will emulate that mentor to achieve the same results. This emphasis on tradition has tremendous benefit but can limit innovation for new approaches. An example of where a traditional paradigm was supplanted by a new innovation is open surgery and minimally invasive surgery. SAGES surgeons answered calls for evidence with carefully planned and executed trials demonstrating the superiority of a laparoscopic approach in many circumstances. Quality was promoted through technology and innovation. With demands on accountability and cost, can these advances occur in the future? Surgeons must find a way.

Can we do it better? This is a question that we must pose to ourselves on a daily basis. Quality is the residue of design, inquiry, reflection, and action. Comparative effectiveness is based upon the head-to-head evaluation of competing therapies that must prove their worth. The philosophy for continuous, persistent examination of quality and outcomes is best exemplified by this quote from Franklin Roosevelt when faced with the crisis of the Great Depression: "Take a method and try it. If it fails, admit it frankly, and try another. But by all means, try something."

Should we do it? This a core question for surgeons because it addresses appropriateness. Appropriateness is a "meta" value because it incorporates polar values of effectiveness, cost, and safety all at once. For many years, a surgeon's judgment was unquestioned and there was clear consensus for a surgical approach. Currently, we are asked by patient and payor alike if a surgery is necessary. Even in times of economic plenty, surgery is a scarce resource limited by available surgeons and attendant resources. If we are to invest the scarce resource of surgery, a reliable and robust return on investment is required. Outcomes must be proven and complications avoided. Surgeons must practice preventive care heeding the concept that it is better to prevent than repair. Complications consume resources that will inhibit our future ability to provide more care. It is for these reasons that payors are demanding that complications be avoided or they will withhold payment. Although the goal of adverse event reduction is laudable and desired, we must engage this process as professionals to best determine what should be measured and rewarded.

Who should do it? We all realize that surgery has become increasingly more specialized and that there is a clear indication that volume may improve outcomes. Has the time come for regional referral for complex procedures or disease treatment like we see for either bariatric or trauma surgery? While it may be highly advantageous to have patients go to highly experienced centers and surgeons, will patients have enough access to care? How do centers and surgeons become experienced if they are not certified as such? These are health policy questions that must be informed and led by surgeons who will maintain the best interests of the public and profession alike.

Education for quality care is even more critical now given that it takes over 17 years to implement best practices and we have limited time to teach quality to surgeons in training given work hour restrictions. This book is an effort to reach out to the past, present, and next generations of surgeons to inspire them to do better than before.

Quality improvement and patient safety research and practice are new fields of endeavor providing enormous opportunity for surgeons to discover how to better care. As we have before, surgeons will continue to practice quality by selecting the right patients, placing them in right hands, and doing the right things at the right time.

Stanford, CA, USA   John Morton, MD, MPH, FACS

Contents

PART IX   CONCLUSIONS

Contributors

Kate Atchley, PhD
Center for Executive Education, College of Business Administration,
University of Tennessee, 608 Stokely Management Center, Knoxville,
TN 37996-0562, USA

Robert W. Bailey, MD, JD, FACS
Clinical Professor of Surgery, Department of Surgery, Mount Sinai
Medical Center, Florida International University College of Medicine,
200 Crandon Boulevard, Suite 360, Miami, FL 33149, USA

Limaris Barrios, MD
Instructor in Surgery, Department of Surgery, Harvard Medical School,
Cambridge Health Alliance, 1493 Cambridge Street, Cambridge,
MA 02139, USA

Renée Bernard, JD
Director, Department of Risk Management, Stanford University
Medical Center, 300 Pasteur Drive, MC 5713, Stanford,
CA 94304, USA

Tracy Palmer Berns, JD
Vice President, Chief Compliance and Regulatory Counsel, Covidien,
15 Hampshire Street, Mansfield, MA 02048, USA

L. Michael Brunt, MD
Professor of Surgery, Department of Surgery, Barnes Jewish Hospital,
660 South Euclid Avenue, St. Louis, MO 63110, USA

Jo Buyske, MD
Associate Executive Director, American Board of Surgery,
1617 John F. Kennedy Boulevard, Suite 860, Philadelphia,
PA 19103, USA

Ian Choy, MD
Department of Surgery, Centre for Minimal Access Surgery,
St Joseph's Healthcare Hamilton, 50 Charlton Ave E, Hamilton,
ON, Canada, L8N 4A6

Cybil Corning, MD
Clinical Resident, Department of Colon and Rectal Surgery,
Cleveland Clinic Florida, 2950 Cleveland Clinic Boulevard, Weston,
FL 33331, USA

Chirag A. Dholakia, MD
Clinical Instructor, Department of Surgery, Irvine Medical Center,
University of California, 333 City Boulevard West, Suite 850, Orange,
CA 92868, USA

Justin B. Dimick, MD, MPH
Assistant Professor, Department of Surgery, University of Michigan,
211 North Fourth Avenue, Suites 2A & 2B, Ann Arbor, MI 48104, USA

Jeffrey Driver, JD, MBA, DFASHRM
Chief Risk Officer, Department of Risk Management,
Stanford University Medical Center, 300 Pasteur Drive, MC 5713,
Stanford, CA 94304, USA

Brian J. Dunkin, MD
Head, Section of Endoscopic Surgery, Department of Surgery,
The Methodist Hospital, 6550 Fannin Street, Suite 1661, Houston,
TX 77031, USA

David Earle, MD
Director of Minimally Invasive Surgery, Baystate Medical Center,
759 Chestnut Street, Springfield, MA 01199, USA

Assistant Professor of Surgery, Tufts University Medical Center,
Boston, MA, USA

Jonathan E. Efron, MD
Chief of Ravitch Division, Department of Surgery,
Johns Hopkins Medicine, 600 North Wolfe Street, Blalock 656,
Baltimore, MD 21287, USA

Nestor F. Esnaola, MD, MPH, MBA
Department of Surgery, Medical University of South Carolina,
25 Courtenay Drive, Suite 7018, MSC 295, Charleston,
SC 29425, USA

Nathaniel Evans, MD
Department of Surgery, Jefferson University Hospital, 1100 Walnut St,
5th Floor, Philadelphia, PA 19107, USA

Liane S. Feldman, MD
Department of Surgery, McGill University Health Care,
1650 Cedar Avenue, L9-412, Montreal, QC, Canada, H3G 1A4

Edward Felix, MD
Director, Department of Surgery, Bariatric Surgery, Clovis Hospital,
7060 N. Recreation, Suite 108, Fresno, CA 93720, USA

Josef E. Fischer, MD
William V. McDermott Professor of Surgery, Harvard Medical School,
1135 Tremont Street, Suite 512, Boston, MA 02120, USA

Dennis L. Fowler, MD, MPH
Department of Surgery, Columbia University College of Physicians
and Surgeons, 161 Fort Washington Avenue, HIP 805, New York,
NY 10032, USA

Pascal Fuchshuber, MD, PhD, FACS
Department of Surgery, The Permanente Medical Group,
Kaiser Medical Center, 1425 South Main, Walnut Creek,
CA 94596, USA

Associate Clinical Professor of Surgery, University of California,
San Francisco, CA, USA

Denise W. Gee, MD
Minimally Invasive Surgeon, Division of General and Gastrointestinal
Surgery, Massachusetts General Hospital, 15 Parkman Street,
WACC460, Boston, MA 02459, USA

Philip M. Gerson, JD
Gerson & Schwartz, PA, 1980 Coral Way, Coral Gables,
FL 33145-2624, USA

Alexander J. Greenstein, MD, MPH
Department of Surgery, Mount Sinai Medical Center, 5 East 98th St,
15th floor New York, NY 10029, USA

William Greif, MD
Department of Surgery, The Permanente Medical Group,
Kaiser Medical Center, 1425 South Main Street, Walnut Creek, CA
94596, USA

Jeffrey Hazey, MD
Department of Surgery, Ohio State University, 410 West 10th Avenue,
N 724 Doan Hall, Columbus, OH 43210, USA

Tina Hernandez-Broussard, PhD, MPH
Co-Director, Department of Surgery, SCORE, Stanford Medical Center,
300 Pasteur Drive, Stanford, CA 94306, USA

Santiago Horgan, MD
Department of Minimally Invasive Surgery, UC San Diego Medical
Center, 200 West Arbor Drive, 3rd Floor, San Diego, CA 92103, USA

David B. Hoyt, MD, FACS
Executive Director, American College of Surgeons, 633 N Saint Clair
Street, Chicago, IL 60611, USA

John G. Hunter, MD
Mackenzie Professor and Chair, Department of Surgery, Oregon Health
and Sciences University, 3181 SW Sam Jackson Park Road, Portland,
OR 97239, USA

Matthew M. Hutter, MD, MPH
Associate Visiting Surgeon, Harvard Medical School, Massachusetts
General Hospital, 55 Fruit Street, Boston, MA 02114, USA

Gretchen Purcell Jackson, MD, PhD
Assistant Professor of Surgery and Biomedical Informatics,
Department of Pediatric Surgery, Monroe Carell Jr. Children's
Hospital at Vanderbilt, 2200 Children's Way, Doctor's Office Tower,
Suite 7100, Nashville, TN 37232, USA

Michael R. St. Jean, MD, FACS, COL MC US Army
Chief, Department of Surgery, Northeast Surgery of Maine,
417 State Street, Suite 330 Bangor, ME 04401, USA

Stephanie B. Jones, MD
Associate Professor, Harvard Medical School, Vice Chair
for Education, Department of Anesthesia, Critical Care
and Pain Medicine, Beth Israel Deaconess Medical Center,
1 Deaconess Rd, CC470, Boston, MA 02215, USA

Daniel B. Jones, MD, MS, FACS
Professor in Surgery, Harvard Medical School, Vice Chair of Surgery,
Office of Technology and Innovation, Chief, Minimally Invasive
Surgical Services, Beth Israel Deaconess Medical Center 330
Brookline Avenue Boston, MA 02215, USA

John J. Kelly, MD
Chief, General Surgery, Department of General Surgery,
UMass Memorial Medical Center, Associate Professor of Surgery,
UMass Medical School, 55 Lake Avenue North, Worcester,
MA 01655, USA

Jadd Koury, MD
Department of Surgery, Monmouth Medical Center,
300 Second Avenue, Long Branch, NJ 07740, USA

James N. Lau, MD, FACS
Clinical Associate Professor of Surgery, Department of Surgery,
Stanford School of Medicine, 300 Pasteur DriveStanford,
CA 94305, USA

Michael J. Lee, MD
Resident, Department of Surgery, University of Texas Southwestern
Medical Center, 5323 Harry Hines Boulevard, Dallas, TX 75390, USA

Anne Lidor, MD, MPH
Assistant Professor, Department of Surgery, Director, Minimally
Invasive Surgery Fellowship, Johns Hopkins Hospital, 600 N. Wolfe
Street, Blalock 656, Baltimore, MD 21287, USA

Robert B. Lim, MD, LTC
Chief of Bariatric and Metabolic Surgery, Department of Surgery,
Tripler Army Medical Center, 1 Jarrett White Road, Honolulu,
HI 96734, USA

Atul K. Madan, MD, FACS
Medical Director, New Life Surgery Center, LLC, Bariatric Surgery,
9001 Wilshire Boulevard, Suite 106, Beverly Hills, CA 90211, USA

John Marks, MD
Chief of Colorectal Surgery, Department of Colorectal Surgery,
The Lankenau Hospital & Institute for Medical Research,
100 East Lancaster Avenue, MOB W, Suite 330, Wynnewood,
PA 19096, USA

Kimberly A. Matzie, MD
Clinical Fellow, Department of Colorectal Surgery, Cleveland Clinic
Florida, 2950 Cleveland Clinic Blvd, Weston, FL 33331, USA

Pinckney J. Maxwell IV, MD
Assistant Professor of Surgery, Division of Colon and Rectal Surgery,
Department of Surgery, Thomas Jefferson University, 1100 Walnut
Street, Suite 500, Philadelphia, PA 19107, USA

Andrew Jay McClurg, JD
Herbert Herff Chair of Excellence in Law, & Associate Dean
for Faculty Development, University of Memphis Cecil C. Humphreys
School of Law, 1 Front Street, Memphis, TN 38103, USA

Kathryn McDonald, MM
Executive Director and Senior Scholar, Center for Health Policy,
Center for Primary Care and Outcomes Research, Stanford University,
117 Encina Commons, Stanford, CA 94305, USA

Scott Melvin, MD
Professor of Surgery, Department of Surgery, Ohio State University,
410 West 10th Avenue, N 724 Doan Hall, Columbus, OH 43210, USA

John Morton, MD, MPH, FACS
Associate Professor of Surgery, Section Chief, Minimally Invasive
Surgery, Director of Quality, Surgery and Surgical Sub-Specialties,
Director of Bariatric Surgery, Stanford School of Medicine,
300 Pasteur Drive, H3680, Stanford, CA 94305, USA

Sharon Muret-Wagstaff, PhD, MD
Department of Anesthesia, Critical Care, and Pain Medicine,
Beth Israel Deaconess Medical Center, 330 Brookline Avenue,
Yamins 219, Boston, MA 02215, USA

Harvard Medical School, 25 Shattuck Street, Boston, MA 02115, USA

Allan Okrainec, MD
Advanced Medicine and Surgery, University Health Network,
190 Elizabeth Street, Toronto, ON, Canada, M5M 1M1

David Olson
Vice President of Regulatory Affairs, Covidien, 15 Hampshire Street,
Mansfield, MA 02048, USA

Julian Omidi, MD
Plastic and Reconstructive Surgery, 9001 Wilshire Boulevard,
Suite 106, Beverly Hills, CA 90211, USA

Philip Omotosho, MD
Department of General Surgery, Duke University Medical Center,
407 Crutchfield Street, Durham, NC 27704, USA

Rocco Orlando III, MD
Senior Vice President and Chief Medical Officer, Hartford Hospital,
Professor of Clinical Surgery, University of Connecticut School
of Medicine, 80 Seymour Street, Hartford, CT 06106, USA

Adrian Park, MD
Campbell and Jeannette Plugge Professor, Head, Division of General
Surgery, Vice Chair, Department of Surgery, University of Maryland,
22 South Greene Street, Baltimore, MD 21201, USA

John Pawlowski, MD, PhD
Director of Thoracic Anesthesia, Beth Israel Deaconess Medical
Center, Assistant Professor in Anesthesia, Harvard Medical School,
1 Deaconess Road, Boston, MA 02215, USA

Timothy Plerhoples, MD, MPH
Resident, Department of General Surgery, Stanford University,
300 Pasteur Drive, Stanford, CA 94305, USA

Dana D. Portenier, MD
Assistant Professor of Surgery, Department of General Surgery,
Laparoscopic – Bariatric and General Surgery, Duke University
Medical Center, 407 Crutchfield Street, Durham, NC 27704, USA

Bernadette C. Profeta, MD, FACS
Assistant Professor, Department of Surgery, Thomas Jefferson
University, 1100 Walnut Street, Suite 500, Philadelphia, PA 19107, USA

David W. Rattner, MD
Chief, Division of Gastrointestinal and General Surgery, Massachusetts
General Hospital, 55 Fruit Street, Boston, MA 02114, USA

Kevin M. Reavis, MD
Assistant Professor of Clinical Surgery, Department Surgery,
Irvine Medical Center, University of California, 333 City Boulevard
West, Suite 850, Orange, CA 92868, USA

Homero Rivas, MD, MBA, FACS
Assistant Professor of Surgery, Department of Surgery,
Director of Innovative Surgery, 300 Pasteur Drive, Stanford,
CA 94305, USA

Ernest Rosato, MD
Department of Surgery, Jefferson University Hospital, 1100 Walnut St,
5th Floor, Philadelphia, PA 19107, USA

Francis Rosato, MD
Department of Surgery, Jefferson University Hospital, 1100 Walnut St,
5th Floor, Philadelphia, PA 19107, USA

Ajit K. Sachdeva, MD, FACS, FRCSC
Adjunct Professor in Surgery, Department of Surgery, Northwestern University, 251 East Huron Avenue, Chicago, IL 60611, USA

Bryan J. Sandler, MD
Department of Minimally Invasive Surgery, UC San Diego Medical Center, 200 West Arbor Drive, 3rd Floor, San Diego, CA 92103, USA

B. Fernando Santos, MD
General Surgery Resident, Department of Surgery, Northwestern University, 251 East Huron Avenue, Chicago, IL 60611, USA

Joe Sapiente
Vice President of Global Quality Assurance, Covidien, 195 McDermott Road, North Haven, CT 06473, USA

Bruce Schirmer, MD
Stephen H. Watts Professor of Surgery, Department of Surgery, University of Virginia Health System, Charlottesville, VA 22908, USA

Benjamin E. Schneider, MD
Instructor in Surgery, Department of Surgery, Beth Israel Deaconess Medical Center, Harvard Medical School, 330 Brookline Avenue, Boston, MA 02215, USA

Steven D. Schwaitzberg, MD
Chief of Surgery, Associate Professor of Surgery, Department of Surgery, Harvard Medical School, Cambridge Health Alliance, 1493 Cambridge Street, Cambridge, MA 02139, USA

Daniel J. Scott, MD
Associate Professor, Frank H. Kidd, Jr. MD Distinguished Professorship in Surgery, Department of Surgery, Director, Southwestern Center for Minimally Invasive Surgery, University of Texas Southwestern Medical Center, 5323 Harry Hines Boulevard, Dallas, TX 75390, USA

Neal E. Seymour, MD
Department of Surgery, Baystate Medical Center, 759 Chestnut Street, Springfield, MA 01199, USA

Brett A. Simon, MD, PhD
Department of Anesthesia, Critical Care, and Pain Medicine,
Beth Israel Deaconess Medical Center, 330 Brookline Avenue,
Yamins 219, Boston, MA 02215, USA

Harvard Medical School, 25 Shattuck Street, Boston, MA 02115, USA

Carter Smith, MD
Surgical Resident, Department of Surgery, University of Wisconsin
Hospital and Clinics, University of Wisconsin Clinical Science Center,
600 Highland Avenue, Madison, WI 53792, USA

Nathaniel J. Soper, MD
Chair, Department of Surgery, Northwestern University Feinberg
School of Medicine, 251 East Huron Street, Galter 3-150, Chicago,
IL 60611, USA

Erica Sutton, MD
Department of Surgery, University of Maryland, 22 South Greene Street,
Baltimore, MD 21201, USA

Michael Tarnoff, MD
Assistant Professor of Surgery, Tufts University School of Medicine,
800 Washington Street, South Building, 4th Floor, Boston,
MA 02111, USA

David S. Tichansky, MD, FACS
Associate Professor of Surgery, Director, Minimally Invasive
and Bariatric Surgery, Thomas Jefferson University, 1100 Walnut Street,
Philadelphia, PA 19107, USA

Shawn Tsuda, MD
Assistant Professor of Surgery, Division of Minimally Invasive
and Bariatric Surgery, Department of Surgery, University of Nevada
School of Medicine, 2040 West Charleston Avenue, Suite 601,
Las Vegas, NV 89102, USA

Kevin Tymitz, MD
MIS Fellow, Department of Surgery, Johns Hopkins Hospital,
600 N. Wolfe Street, Blalock 610, Baltimore, MD 21287, USA

Esteban Varela, MD
Associate Professor, Department of Surgery, Barnes Jewish Hospital,
660 South Euclid Avenue, St. Louis, MO 63110, USA

Elsa B. Valsdottir, MD
Lankenau Hospital, 100 E Lancaster Ave # 361, Wynnewood,
PA 19096, USA

Vic Velanovich, MD
Professor of Surgery (Clinician Educator), Wayne State University,
Division Head, General Surgery, Henry Ford Hospital,
Department of Surgery, 2799 West Grand Boulevard, Detroit,
MI 48202, USA

Eric Weiss, MD, FACS, FASCRS, FACG
Vice Chairman of Colorectal Surgery, Department of Colorectal
Surgery, Cleveland Clinic Florida, 2950 Cleveland Clinic Road,
Weston, FL 33331, USA

Steven D. Wexner, MD, FACS, FRCS, FRCSEd., FASCRS, FACG
Chief Academic Officer, Professor and Chairman,
Department of Colorectal Surgery, Associate Dean for Academic
Affairs, Florida Atlantic University, 2950 Cleveland Clinic Blvd,
Weston, FL 33331, USA

Associate Dean for Clinical Education, Department of Colorectal
Surgery, Florida International University, Cleveland Clinic Florida,
2950 Cleveland Clinic Road, Weston, FL 33331, USA

Brandon Williams, MD
Assistant Professor of Surgery, Department of Surgery,
Vanderbilt University Hospital, 1211 Medical Center Drive, Nashville,
TN 37232, USA

Bruce M. Wolfe, MD
Professor of Surgery, Department of Surgery,
Division of General Surgery, Oregon Health and Science University,
3181 SW Sam Jackson Park Road, Portland, OR 97239, USA

Grant R. Young, MD
Clinical Fellow in Anesthesia, Department of Anesthesia,
Critical Care and Pain Medicine, Beth Israel Deaconess Medical Center,
Harvard Medical School, 1 Deaconess Road, CC 470, Boston,
MA 02215, USA

Minhao Zhou, MD
MIS Fellow, Department of Surgery, UMass Medical,
55 Lake Avenue North, Worcester, MA 01655, USA

Part I

Patient Safety Is Quality

1. Defining Quality in Surgery

Justin B. Dimick

Introduction

With growing recognition of wide variations in surgical performance, demand for information on surgical quality is at an all time high. Patients and families are turning to their physicians, hospital report cards, and the Internet to identify the safest hospitals for surgery [1]. Payers and purchasers of health care are ramping up efforts to reward high quality (e.g., pay for performance) or steer patients toward the highest quality providers (e.g., selective referral) [2]. In addition to responding to these external demands, providers are becoming more involved in creating their own quality measurement platforms, such as the National Surgical Quality Improvement Program (NSQIP) [3]. Finally, professional organizations are now accrediting hospitals for some surgical services, including bariatric surgery [4].

Despite the need for good measures of quality in surgery, there is very little agreement about how to best assess surgical performance. According to the widely used Donabedian paradigm, quality can be measured using various aspects of structure, process, or outcome [5]. Recently, there is growing enthusiasm for composite, or "global," measures of quality, which combine one or more elements of structure, process, and outcome [6]. In this chapter, we consider the advantages and disadvantages of each type of quality measure. We close by making recommendations for choosing among these different approaches.

Structure

Structure refers to measurable attributes of a hospital (e.g., volume) or surgeon (e.g., specialty training) (Table 1.1). Because they are relatively easy to ascertain, measures of health care structure are widely

D.S. Tichansky, J. Morton, and D.B. Jones (eds.), *The SAGES Manual of Quality, Outcomes and Patient Safety*, DOI 10.1007/978-1-4419-7901-8_1, © Springer Science+Business Media, LLC 2012

Table 1.1. Approaches to measuring the quality of care for aortic surgery with advantages and disadvantages of each approach.

Type of measure	Example	Advantages	Disadvantages
Structure	Hospital or surgeon volume	Inexpensive and readily available Good proxy for outcomes	Not actionable for quality improvement Not good for discriminating among individual providers
Process	Prophylactic antibiotics given on time Adherence to venous thromboembolism prevention guidelines	Actionable as targets for improvement Less influenced by patient risk and random errors	Known processes relate to unimportant or rare surgical outcomes Very few "high leverage" process of care are known
Outcome	Anastomotic leak rates with bariatric surgery Wound infection with ventral hernia repair	Seen as the bottom line of patient care Enjoy good "buy in" from surgeons	Sample sizes often too small at individual hospitals Need for detailed data for risk adjustment
Composite	Leapfrog Group's "Survival Predictor"	Addresses problems with small sample size Makes sense of multiple conflicting measures	Not granular enough to identify specific clinical areas that need improvement

used in health care. The American College of Surgeons (ACS) and the American Society of Metabolic and Bariatric Surgeons (ASMBS) are now accrediting hospitals for bariatric surgery based largely on measures of structure, including hospital volume, surgeon volume, and other structural elements necessary for providing multidisciplinary care for the morbidly obese [4].

Structural elements have several key strengths as quality measures. First, they are relatively easy to ascertain. Often, structural elements (e.g., volume) can be obtained from readily available administrative data. Second, many structural measures are strong predictors of hospital and surgeon outcomes. For example, with high-risk gastrointestinal surgery, such as pancreatic and esophageal resection, there are up to fivefold differences in mortality between high- and low-volume surgeons [7].

However, there are certain limitations of using structural quality measures. Most importantly, they are proxies for quality rather than direct measures. As a result, they only hold true on average. For example, while high-volume surgeons are better than low-volume surgeons on average, there are likely to be some high-volume surgeons with bad outcomes and low-volume surgeons with good outcomes [5]. Structural measures are also not actionable for quality improvement. Further, it is unclear how low-volume hospitals can change to replicate the excellent results of high-volume surgeons. Despite decades of research on the volume-outcome relationship, there is very little information about the details of care that differs between high-volume and low-volume hospitals [7].

Process

Processes of care refer to those details of care that lead to good (or bad) outcomes. Using processes of care to measure quality is extremely common in ambulatory and inpatient medical care, but is not as widely used in surgery. Although processes of care in surgery can represent details of care in the preoperative, intraoperative, and postoperative phases of patient care, most existing process measures focus on details of preoperative patient care. For example, the Center for Medicare and Medicaid Services (CMS) Surgical Care Improvement Project (SCIP) measures focus on processes of care related to the prevention of complications, such as surgical site infection and venous thromboembolism.

Process measures have several strengths as quality measures (Table 1.1). First, processes of care are extremely actionable in quality improvement. When hospitals and surgeon are "low outliers" for process compliance (e.g., patients not getting timely antibiotic prophylaxis), they know exactly where to target improvement. Second, in contrast to risk-adjusted outcomes measurement, processes of care do not need to be adjusted for differences in patient risk, which limits the need for data collection from the medical chart and saves valuable time and effort.

But using processes of care has several significant limitations in surgery. First, most existing process measures are not strongly related to important outcomes. For example, the SCIP measures, which are by far the most widely used process measure in surgery, are not related to surgical mortality, infections, or thromboembolism [8]. The lack of a relationship between SCIP measures and surgical mortality is easily explained by the fact that the complications they aim to prevent are secondary (e.g., superficial wound infection) or extremely rare (e.g., pulmonary embolism). However, there is also a very weak relationship between process measures and the outcome they are supposed to prevent (e.g., timely administration of prophylactic antibiotics and wound infection) [9]. This finding is more difficult to explain. It is possible that there are simply multiple other processes (many unmeasured or unmeasurable) that contribute to good surgical outcomes. As a result, it is likely that adherence to SCIP processes is necessary but not sufficient for good surgical outcomes.

Outcome

Outcomes represent the end results of care. In surgery, the focus is often on operative mortality and morbidity. For example, the NSQIP, the largest clinical registry focusing on surgery, reports risk-adjusted morbidity and mortality rates to participating hospitals [3]. While morbidity and mortality have long been the "gold standard" in surgery, there is a growing focus on patient-oriented outcomes, such as functional status and quality of life.

Directly outcome measures have several strengths (Table 1.1). First, everyone agrees that outcomes are important. Measuring the end results of care makes intuitive sense to surgeons and other stakeholders. For example, the NSQIP has been enthusiastically championed by surgeons and other clinical leaders [10]. Second, outcomes feedback alone may improve quality. This so-called "Hawthorne effect" is seen whenever outcomes are measured and reported back to providers. For example, the

NSQIP in the Veterans Affairs (VA) hospitals and private sector has documented improvements over time that cannot be attributed to any specific efforts to improve outcomes [11].

However, outcome measures have key limitations. First, when the event rate is low (numerator) or the number of cases is small (denominator) outcomes cannot be reliably measured. Small sample size and low event rates conspire to limit the statistical power of hospital outcomes comparisons. For most operations, surgical mortality is too rare to be used as a reliable quality measure [12]. For example, a recent study evaluated seven operations for which mortality was advocated as a surgical quality measure by the Agency for Healthcare Research and Quality (AHRQ). The authors found that only one operation, coronary artery bypass surgery, had high enough caseloads to reliably measure quality with surgical mortality [13].

Another limitation of measuring outcomes is the need to collect detailed clinical data for risk adjustment [14]. Because patient differences can confound hospital quality measurement, it is important to adjust hospital comparisons for these differences in baseline risk. For example, the NSQIP presently collects more than 80 patient variables from the medical chart for this purpose [11]. This data collection is labor-intensive and expensive. Each NSQIP hospital employs a trained nurse clinician to collect this data.

Composite

Composite measures are created by combining one or more structure, process, and outcome measures [6]. Composite measures offer several advantages over the individual measures discussed above (Table 1.1). By combining multiple measures, it is possible to overcome problems with small sample size discussed above. Composite measures also provide a "global" measure of quality. This type of measure is increasingly used for quality for value-based purchasing or other efforts that require an overall or summary measure of quality.

One key limitation with composite measures is that there is no "gold standard" approach for weighting input measures. Perhaps the most common approach is to weight each input measure equally. For example, in the ongoing Premier/CMS pay for performance demonstration project, Medicare payment bonuses are based on a composite score of process and outcome variables which are equally weighted. However, this approach is severely flawed. Recent data show that variation in these composite measures is entirely driven by the process measures [15]. Newer approaches for empirically weighting individual measures will be discussed later.

Another limitation with composite measures is that they are not always actionable for quality improvement. By combining information on multiple measures and/or clinical conditions, there is often not enough "granularity" for clinicians to use the information for quality improvement. To target quality improvement efforts, it will often be necessary to deconstruct the composite into its component measures and find out where the problem lies (e.g., the specific procedure or complication).

Choosing the Right Measurement Approach

No approach to quality measurement is perfect. Each type of measure – structure, process, and outcome – has its own strengths and limitations. In general, selecting the right approach to measure quality depends on characteristics of the procedure and the specific policy application [5].

Certain characteristics of the surgical procedure should be considered when selecting a quality measure (Fig. 1.1). Specifically, one should consider (1) how common adverse outcomes are and (2) how often an operation is performed. For procedures that are both common and relatively high risk (e.g., colectomy and gastric bypass), outcomes are reliable enough to be used as measures of quality (Fig. 1.1, Quadrant I). For procedures that are common but low risk (e.g., inguinal hernia repair), measures of process of care or functional outcomes are the best approach (Fig. 1.1, Quadrant II). For procedures that are high risk but uncommon (e.g., pancreatic and esophageal resection), structural measures such as hospital volume are likely the best approach (Fig. 1.1, Quadrant IV). In fact, empirical data suggests that structural measures such as hospital volume are better predictors of future performance than direct outcome measures for these uncommon, high-risk operations [16]. Finally, for operations that are both uncommon and low risk (e.g., Spigelian hernia repair), it is probably best to focus quality measurement efforts on other, more high leverage procedures.

When choosing an approach to quality measurement, the specific policy application should also be considered. In particular, it is important to distinguish between policy efforts aimed at selective referral and

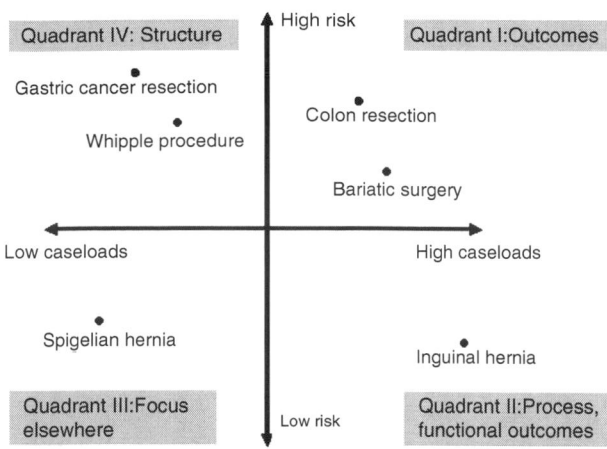

Fig. 1.1. Choosing among measures of structure, process, and outcomes. For high risk, high caseload operations (e.g., colectomy and bariatric procedures), outcomes are useful quality measures. For low risk, common procedures (e.g., inguinal hernia repair), processes of care or functional outcomes are appropriate measures. For high risk, uncommon operations (e.g., gastric and pancreatic cancer resection), measures of structure, such as hospital volume are most appropriate. For low risk, low caseload operations (e.g., spigelian hernia repair), it would be best to focus measurement efforts elsewhere. Figure modified by Birkmeyer et al. [5].

quality improvement. For selective referral, the main goal is to redirect patients to the highest quality providers. Structural measures, such as hospital volume, are particularly good for this purpose. Hospital volume tends to be strongly related to outcomes and large gains in outcomes could be achieved by concentrating patients in high-volume hospitals. In contrast, structural measures are not directly actionable and, therefore, do not make good measures for quality improvement. For improving quality, process, and outcome measures are better because they provide actionable targets. Surgeons and hospitals can improve by addressing problems with process compliance or focus on clinical areas with high rates of adverse outcomes. For example, the NSQIP reports risk-adjusted morbidity and mortality rates to every hospital. Surgeon champions and quality improvement personnel will target improvement efforts to areas where performance is statistically worse than expected.

Improving Quality Measurement

Although the science of surgical quality measurement has come a long way in the past decade, it is still in its infancy. We will review several improvements to quality measurement currently on the horizon. These improvements focus on addressing the problems with the process of care and outcome measures discussed above.

We ultimately need to develop a better understanding of the processes of care that explain differences in outcome across hospitals. Once these "high leverage" processes of care are known, they can be promoted as best practices to improve care at all hospitals. Such research should use the tools of clinical epidemiology to isolate the root causes of variation in outcomes. For example, a recent study by Ghaferi and colleagues shed light on the mechanisms underlying variations in surgical mortality rates. Ghaferi et al., using detailed, clinically rich data from the NSQIP, ranked hospitals according to risk-adjusted mortality [17]. When comparing the "best" to "worst" hospitals, they found no significant differences in overall (24.6% vs. 26.9%) or major (18.2% vs. 16.2%) complication rates. However, the so-called "failure to rescue" (death following major complications) was almost twice as high in hospitals with very high mortality as in those with very low mortality (21.4% vs. 12.5%, $p < 0.001$). This study highlights the need to focus on processes of care related to the timely recognition and management of complications – aimed at eliminating "failure to rescue" – to reduce variations in surgical mortality.

Recent emphasis has been placed on improving the efficiency of risk-adjustment techniques [18]. At present, most clinical registries collect a large number of clinical data elements from the medical record for risk adjustment. This "kitchen sink" approach to risk adjustment is largely based on the assumption that each additional variable improves our ability to make fair hospital comparisons. However, recent empiric data suggests that only the most important variables contribute meaningfully to risk-adjustment models. For example, Tu and colleagues demonstrated that a five-variable model provides nearly identical results to a 12-variable model for comparing hospital outcomes with cardiac surgery [19]. Using data from the NSQIP, we have demonstrated similar results for both general surgical procedures [18]. These results should be used to streamline the collection of data for risk adjustment, which will decrease the costs of data collection and lower the bar for participation in these important clinical registries.

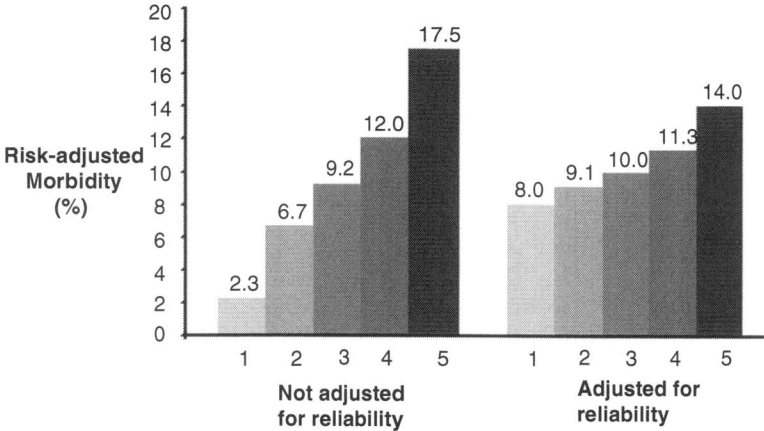

Fig. 1.2. Comparison of ventral hernia repair morbidity rates across hospital quintiles (1 = "best hospitals" and 5 = "worst hospitals") before and after adjusting for statistical reliability. After adjusting for reliability, the apparent variation across hospitals is greatly diminished.

There is also increasing emphasis on using advanced statistical techniques for addressing the problem with "noisy" outcome measures [20]. As discussed above, imprecision from small sample size is the Achilles heel of outcomes measurement. These new techniques rely on empirical Bayes theory to adjust hospital outcomes for reliability. In this approach, the statistical "noise" is explicitly measured and removed by shrinking the observed outcome rate back toward the average rate. For example, Fig. 1.2 shows risk-adjusted hospital morbidity rates across quintiles for ventral hernia repair, before and after adjusting for reliability. Before adjusting for reliability, rates of morbidity varied eightfold (2.3–17.5%) from the "best" to "worst" quintile. However, after removing chance variation (i.e., "noise") by adjusting for reliability, rates of morbidity varied less than twofold (8.0–14.0%) from the "best" to "worst" quintile.

While this approach has many advantages, reliability adjustment makes the assumption that small hospitals have average performance. Although this approach gives small hospitals, the benefit of the doubt (i.e., they are innocent until proven guilty), under certain circumstances it could bias hospital rankings. For instance, given the well-known relationship between volume and outcome in surgery, these small hospitals may actually have performance below average. Incorporating information about hospital volume could address this bias. We have developed a novel technique for performing reliability adjustment by shrinking to a conditional average (i.e., the outcome expected given hospital volume) to address this problem [6]. This approach is considered a composite measure as it includes two inputs (mortality and volume).

This general approach can also be used to create more sophisticated composite measures of quality. As discussed above, most current approaches for combining measures are flawed. To address this problem, we have developed a method for empirically weighting input measures [21]. Briefly, we first identify a gold standard quality measure, such as mortality or serious morbidity. We then determine the relationship between each candidate measure and this gold standard measure. Finally, each input measure is given a weight based on (1) the reliability with which it is measured and (2) how correlated it is with the gold standard measure. These empirically weighted composite measures been shown to be better predictors of future performance than individual measures alone [21].

Conclusions

Each type of quality measure – structure, process, and outcome – has its unique strengths and limitations. Structural measures are strongly related to important outcomes and are readily available. Unfortunately, however, structural measures are proxies for quality and do not discriminate among individual providers. Process measures are extremely useful because they are actionable for quality improvement. But the most high leverage processes in surgery are not yet known. Outcomes are the bottom line in surgery and everyone agrees that they are important. Because of small sample size at most hospitals, however, they are often too "noisy" to reliably reflect hospital quality. Ultimately, when choosing among these different approaches, surgeons need to be flexible and consider the specific procedure and policy application prior to choosing a measure.

Selected Readings

1. Osborne NH, Nicholas LH, Ghaferi AA, et al. Do popular media and internet-based hospital quality ratings identify hospitals with better cardiovascular surgery outcomes? J Am Coll Surg. 2010;210:87–92.

2. Rosenthal MB, Dudley RA. Pay-for-performance: will the latest payment trend improve care? JAMA. 2007;297:740–4.

3. Birkmeyer JD, Shahian DM, Dimick JB, et al. Blueprint for a new American College of Surgeons: National Surgical Quality Improvement Program. J Am Coll Surg. 2008;207:777–82.

4. Dimick JB, Osborne NH, Nicholas L, et al. Identifying high-quality bariatric surgery centers: hospital volume or risk-adjusted outcomes? J Am Coll Surg. 2009;209:702–6.

5. Birkmeyer JD, Dimick JB, Birkmeyer NJ. Measuring the quality of surgical care: structure, process, or outcomes? J Am Coll Surg. 2004;198:626–32.

6. Dimick JB, Staiger DO, Baser O, et al. Composite measures for predicting surgical mortality in the hospital. Health Aff (Millwood). 2009;28:1189–98.

7. Birkmeyer JD, Siewers AE, Finlayson EV, et al. Hospital volume and surgical mortality in the United States. N Engl J Med. 2002;346:1128–37.

8. Hawn MT. Surgical care improvement: should performance measures have performance measures. JAMA. 2010;303:2527–8.

9. Stulberg JJ, Delaney CP, Neuhauser DV, et al. Adherence to surgical care improvement project measures and the association with postoperative infections. JAMA. 2010;303:2479–85.

10. Neuman HB, Michelassi F, Turner JW, et al. Surrounded by quality metrics: what do surgeons think of ACS-NSQIP? Surgery. 2009;145:27–33.

11. Khuri SF, Daley J, Henderson WG. The comparative assessment and improvement of quality of surgical care in the Department of Veterans Affairs. Arch Surg. 2002;137:20–7.

12. Dimick JB, Welch HG. The zero mortality paradox in surgery. J Am Coll Surg. 2008;206:13–6.

13. Dimick JB, Welch HG, Birkmeyer JD. Surgical mortality as an indicator of hospital quality: the problem with small sample size. JAMA. 2004;292:847–51.

14. Iezzoni LI. The risks of risk adjustment. JAMA. 1997;278:1600–7.

15. O'Brien SM, DeLong ER, Dokholyan RS, et al. Exploring the behavior of hospital composite performance measures: an example from coronary artery bypass surgery. Circulation. 2007;116:2969–75.

16. Birkmeyer JD, Dimick JB, Staiger DO. Operative mortality and procedure volume as predictors of subsequent hospital performance. Ann Surg. 2006;243:411–7.

17. Ghaferi AA, Birkmeyer JD, Dimick JB. Variation in hospital mortality associated with inpatient surgery. N Engl J Med. 2009;361:1368–75.

18. Dimick JB, Osborne NH, Hall BL, et al. Risk adjustment for comparing hospital quality with surgery: how many variables are needed? J Am Coll Surg. 2010;210:503–8.

19. Tu JV, Sykora K, Naylor CD. Assessing the outcomes of coronary artery bypass graft surgery: how many risk factors are enough? Steering Committee of the Cardiac Care Network of Ontario. J Am Coll Cardiol. 1997;30:1317–23.

20. Dimick JB, Staiger DO, Birkmeyer JD. Ranking hospitals on surgical mortality: the importance of reliability adjustment. Health Serv Res. 2010;45:1614–29.

21. Staiger DO, Dimick JB, Baser O, et al. Empirically derived composite measures of surgical performance. Med Care. 2009;47:226–33.

2. Never Events

Josef E. Fischer

"Never Events"

The term "Never Events" was first introduced in 2001 by Dr. Ken Kizer, M.D. in response to a series of medical errors which he felt were completely avoidable, such as "wrong side surgery." This was against a background of the 1999 Institute of Medicine report which proclaimed that between 44,000 and 98,000 patients died each year as a result of medical errors in US hospitals. That the report probably considerably exaggerated the number of patients injured is immaterial. No patient should die from medical errors. The fiscal impact amounted to an estimated $9.3 billion dollars annually and 2.4 million extra hospital days. The report has been widely criticized because of extrapolation which is inappropriate, but it does not matter – it is part of our national culture.

Dr. Kizer and the National Quality Forum (NQF) proposed a series of serious reportable events to increase public accountability and consumer access to critical information and healthcare performance. The NQF approved 28 events in 6 categories: surgical, products or device, patient protection, care management, environmental, and criminal.

Dr. Kizer and the NQF claimed that these categories shown in Table 2.1 are the result of "widespread discussion among representatives of all parts of the health care system." While I am not certain this is entirely the case, and I will take issue with several of the "Never Events," compared with what followed from CMS, these seem highly reasonable with some caveats. My concern, however, is that, however well intentioned these efforts are, they do not seem to bear in mind that there is a downside to all of these "improvements" in medical practice. This is the issue of whether physicians are professionals or employees. I would argue that any "improvement" which increases the feeling that physicians are employees, rather than professionals, ultimately damages patient care to a much greater extent than anyone realizes. I will return to this theme later.

D.S. Tichansky, J. Morton, and D.B. Jones (eds.), *The SAGES Manual of Quality, Outcomes and Patient Safety*, DOI 10.1007/978-1-4419-7901-8_2,
© Springer Science+Business Media, LLC 2012

Table 2.1. The National Quality Forum's Health Care "Never Events" (2006).

Surgical events

Surgery performed on the wrong body part

Surgery performed on the wrong patient

Wrong surgical procedure performed on a patient

Unintended retention of a foreign object in a patient after surgery or other
    procedure

Intraoperative or immediately postoperative death in an American Society of
    Anesthesiologists Class I patient

Artificial insemination with the wrong sperm or donor egg

Product or device events

Patient death or serious disability associated with the use of contaminated
    drugs, devices, or biologics provided by the health care facility

Patient death or serious disability associated with the use or function of a device
    in patient care, in which the device is used for functions other than as intended

Patient death or serious disability associated with intravascular air embolism
    that occurs while being cared for in a health care facility

Patient protection events

Infant discharged to the wrong person

Patient death or serious disability associated with patient elopement
    (disappearance)

Patient suicide, or attempted suicide resulting in serious disability, while being
    cared for in a health care facility

Care management events

Patient death or serious disability associated with a medication error (e.g.,
    errors involving the wrong drug, wrong dose, wrong patient, wrong time,
    wrong rate, wrong preparation, or wrong route of administration)

Patient death or serious disability associated with a hemolytic reaction due to
    the administration of ABO/HLA-incompatible blood or blood products

Maternal death or serious disability associated with labor or delivery in a
    low-risk pregnancy while being cared for in a health care facility

Patient death or serious disability associated with hypoglycemia, the onset of
    which occurs while the patient is being cared for in a health care facility

Death or serious disability (kernicterus) associated with failure to identify and
    treat hyperbilirubinemia in neonates

Stage 3 or 4 pressure ulcers acquired after admission to a health care facility

Patient death or serious disability due to spinal manipulative therapy

Environmental events

Patient death or serious disability associated with an electric shock or electrical
    cardioversion while being cared for in a health care facility

Any incident in which a line designated for oxygen or other gas to be delivered
    to a patient contains the wrong gas or is contaminated by toxic substances

Patient death or serious disability associated with a burn incurred from any
    source while being cared for in a health care facility

Patient death or serious disability associated with a fall while being cared for in
    a health care facility

(continued)

Table 2.1. (continued)

Patient death or serious disability associated with the use of restraints or bedrails while being cared for in a health care facility

Criminal events

Any instance of care ordered by or provided by someone impersonating a physician, nurse, pharmacist, or other licensed health care provider

Abduction of a patient of any age

Sexual assault on a patient within or on the grounds of the health care facility

Death or significant injury of a patient or staff member resulting from a physical assault (i.e., battery) that occurs within or on the grounds of the health care facility

---

Comments on "Never Events"

One cannot argue that surgery performed on the wrong side, on the wrong patient, or the wrong surgical procedure performed on a patient are not egregious. However, some comments on the NQF "Never Events" are warranted:

1. "Unintended retention of a foreign object in a patient after surgery or other procedure."

   While I agree that this should never happen, the surgeon does not control the situation in which this does happen. Complicated operative procedures that go on for 7 or 8 hours are not unusual in academic medical centers. Operations of such long duration rarely have just one scrub tech or nurse or one circulating nurse. Instead, the surgeon usually has three different technical or nursing teams, not including breaks for lunch and other mandated breaks. The setting in which sponges are retained or, more likely, laparotomy pads (since surgeons such as myself do not use sponges anymore because they are too likely to get lost) is that there are counts when the team is switching over and these are put in plastic bags. These counts are done quickly so as not to delay the operative procedure. At the end of the procedure, there is a count in which there is confusion as to how many lap pads were actually used and sometimes the count is wrong. By this time, the surgeon has started closing the abdomen and then asked whether there is anything in the abdomen. With the abdomen partially closed, one does not have a clear look at the abdomen because the incision is partially closed and, rather than open the incision again, one does the best they can. Some institutions such as the Mayo Clinic have dispensed with counts.

They completely close the patient and do an X-ray on the way to the recovery room. Most operating rooms do not have the setup or the space to do this. Of course any "witch hunt," as to the responsible person, usually ends up on the back of the surgeon, rather than the system, thanks mostly to our "friends" from the plaintiff's bar.

2. "Intraoperative or immediately postoperative death in a Class I patient."

    I agree that this should never happen, but I can think of one situation in which it may. Malignant hyperthermia usually affects a young, very highly muscled male who is a "very good candidate for general anesthesia." Whether one thinks of this possibility and the response of the anesthesiologist or nurse anesthetist determines whether the patient dies.

3. "Product or device events."

    I have no quarrel with product or device events. In addition, some of the patient protection events are clerical errors, such as the infant discharged to the wrong person, and undoubtedly reflect on the quality of the staff performing the duty. This may appear to be simple, but it can result in disastrous consequence. Patients' elopement and/or suicide relate to the ability to keep track of every single patient, 60 min an hour and 24 h a day. The current economics of hospitals are such that they have too much "administration," some of which is occasioned by the joint commission and some of which is simple inefficiency. Whatever the reason, there are too few people on the line and too many people who are staff. This has nothing to do with physicians and surgeons and more to do with the administrative structure, of which physicians have lost control.

I have difficulty with several other areas, as follows.

4. Maternal death or serious disability in a relatively normal delivery should be very rare. However, amniotic fluid embolism, even if promptly recognized, may be fatal. It may be a reportable event, but is not culpable.

5. I do not believe that it is possible to absolutely prevent elderly patients from falling in a healthcare facility, nor do I believe that it is possible to prevent elderly patients, including those who are disoriented and infirm, from falling while trying to get out of bed when the bed rails are up. Similarly, with respect to criminal events, I doubt that it is possible, to prevent all of these

without an army of security people, which will detract from the nursing ratio. Determined criminals can evade any security net with enough skill.

The CMS List of "Never Events" and the "No Pay" Initiative

The CMS Initiative

The reason for the CMS initiative is not entirely clear. For the most part, the CMS initiatives follow the NQF list. The CMS initiative was put forth in the recent Federal Register [1]. In this publication, the CMS lists a series of HAC (hospital-acquired conditions) for which payment to hospitals will be withheld. The amount of money is trivial, $20 million, but the purpose, according to Kerry Weems, Acting Administrator, was to make the hospital safer for patients. Unfortunately, the CMS lists of events, and especially those for which payment will be withheld, are not totally preventable. I will now go through some of the events and HAC for which Medicare will withhold, or least proposes to withhold, hospital funds, discussing several of the hospital-acquired conditions (HAC) which I will show are not only not "Never Events" but also cannot be defended as "No Pay" events. The reader is referred to an interesting editorial by Lembitz and Clarke entitled: "Clarifying 'never events' and introducing 'always events'" in which they provided evidence that the "No Pay" category is not only inappropriate but also dead wrong [2].

Specific Events

1. *Prevention of falls.* In a recent editorial, Inouye et al. in the *New England Journal of Medicine* pointed out that "falls are often the result not of medical errors but of disease impairments and appropriate use of medications and other treatments. Falls and injuries can occur even when hospitals provide the best possible care" [3]. As I have pointed out previously in this article, even with bed rails, dementia may lead patients to try and get out of bed, thus falling and injuring themselves.

2. *Catheter-associated urinary tract infection.* Even with the best care, patients with indwelling urinary catheters will develop infections. There is no possible way that the infection rate will be zero. Patients also pick at the catheter and the meatus, thus leading to urinary tract infections.

3. *Vascular catheter-associated infections.* I know a little about this, having organized several programs in hospitals for the administration of TPN. Even at the University of Cincinnati Hospital, in which we had three excellent TPN nurses in a hospital of 600 beds and in which we reduced the infection rate from 27%, when the residents were mixing TPN on the floor, to 0.77%, the rate was not zero. In addition, in the ICU, when patients have a tracheostomy, a subclavian catheter site will inevitably become contaminated, making the catheter prone to infection. Including vascular catheter-associated infection may be well-intentioned, but it is just plain wrong. It bespeaks a group of individuals who clearly do not have any clinical experience in this and no idea of what actually transpires (Dr. Peter Provonost through the Michigan Colloborative has been able to accomplish a zero rate).

4. *Surgical site infection following coronary artery bypass graft-mediastinitis.* It is certainly possible to decrease the incidence of mediastinitis by careful attention to detail, control of blood sugar, preoperative showering with chlorhexidine, and the appropriate use of antibiotics. However, the rate will never be zero, though it may approach 1% as de La Torre and his colleagues have shown [4]. In that paper, a maximum blood sugar of 120 mg/dl was the target. At this time, the consensus is that 120 is too low because of the frequency of hypoglycemia, but a target of below 150 mg/dl accomplishes the same result without the hypoglycemia.

5. *Surgical site infection following bariatric surgery.* This category shows how out of touch the individuals who put together the list really are. While the incidence of surgical site infection is less in laparoscopic bariatric surgery, it probably is about 4–6%. This does not belong on the "No Pay" list.

6. *Surgical site infection following orthopedic procedures.* The orthopedic surgical community has made great strides in decreasing the surgical site infection, but it will never be zero.

7. *Deep vein thrombosis and pulmonary embolism in total knee and hip replacement.* The orthopedic literature in the prevention of deep vein thrombosis led by Harris, among others, was a

great scientific accomplishment. The rate has been greatly reduced and further attempts at reduction will lead to hematomas and infection and loss of the prosthesis. The American Academy of Orthopedic Surgeon has recently recommended different prophylaxis regimens from those proposed by the American College of Chest Physicians.

Surgeons: Professionals or Employees

While I believe the attempts by CMS are well-intentioned, I think they miss the point. A critical issue for me is a gradual transformation of physicians and surgeons from professionals to employees. This has profound implications for the care that patients will receive in this country. Professional obligations are without limit of time and surgeons are always responsible for the patient. Professionals take emergency calls. Employees do not, unless they are paid to do so. Professionals care for the indigent. Employees do not unless they are paid to. Each time another rule is passed by a governmental agency, however well-intentioned, it drives a further nail into the coffin of professionalism. The patient is the loser.

As I have said earlier, "the beatings will continue until morale improves" and it seems the beatings go on. When you finally reduce a once proud profession to employees, you will have shift workers and finally there will be a physicians union. I know that physicians unions are illegal, but there will be strikes. Over a decade ago, when I served as a Governor of the American College of Surgeons, I called attention to the newsreels of Walter Reuther leading the strikes in Detroit for the AFL-CIO and the strikers being beaten by police. I certainly hope that it does not come to that but, at the rate we are going, I believe that a union is inevitable. Not a professional organization but a union. Already the medical students have unions and some of the resident organizations have unions, so as these physicians grow into practice, they will have unions. There will be new work rules.

The Quality of Individuals Who Become Physicians and Surgeons

Many of us who had been involved in surgical education and the education of medical students believe that the quality of the people going into medicine has diminished over the past decade. A congressman from

Table 2.2.

---

1. "Never" and "No pay"

Events which overlap between the NQF and CMS definitions of "never events"

- Surgery on the wrong body part
- Surgery on the wrong patient
- Wrong surgery on a patient
- Foreign object left in patient after surgery
- Death/disability associated with intravascular air embolism
- Death/disability associated with incompatible blood
- Death/disability associated with hypoglycemia (HAC's include diabetic ketoacidosis, nonketotic hyperosmolar coma, hypoglycemic coma, secondary diabetes with ketoacidosis, secondary diabetes with hyperosmolarity)
- Stage 3 or 4 pressure ulcers after admission
- Death/disability associated with electric shock
- Death/disability associated with a burn incurred within facility
- Death/disability associated with a fall within facility

2. "Never"

Events which should never happen according to the NQF, but are not listed on the CMS "never events"

- Postoperative death in a healthy patient
- Implantation of wrong egg
- Death/disability associated with the use of contaminated drugs, devices, or biologics
- Death/disability associated with the use of device other than as intended
- Infant discharged to wrong person
- Death/disability due to patient elopement
- Patient suicide or attempted suicide resulting in disability
- Death/disability associated with medication error
- Maternal death/disability with low risk delivery
- Death/disability associated with hyperbilirubinemia in neonates
- Death/disability due to spinal manipulative therapy
- Incident due to wrong oxygen or other gas
- Death/disability associated with the use of restraints within facility
- Impersonating a health care provider (i.e., physician and nurse)
- Abduction of a patient
- Sexual assault of a patient within or on facility grounds
- Death/disability resulting from physical assault within/on facility grounds

3. "No pay"

The list of controversy: Adverse events which are classified by the CMS as non-reimbursable "never events", but lack the according definition by the NQF

- Catheter-associated urinary tract infection
- Vascular catheter-associated infection
- Surgical site infection following coronary artery bypass graft (CABG) – mediastinitis
- Surgical site infection following bariatric surgery (laparoscopic gastric bypass, gastroenterostomy, laproscopic gastric restrictive surgery)

(continued)

Table 2.2. (continued)

- Surgical site infection following orthopedic procedures (spine, neck, shoulder, and elbow)
- Deep vein thrombosis (DVT)/pulmonary embolism (PE) in total knee replacement and hip replacement
---

Comparison of "never events", as defined by the NQF ("serious reportable events") versus CMS ("non-reimbursable serious hospital-acquired conditions").
Lembitz and Clarke *Patient Safety in Surgery* 2009 3:26 doi:10.1186/1754-9493-3-26

a southern state recently told me that he had always attended an annual meeting of 400 of the best college students in southern universities. He told me of a recent meeting he attended in which he asked his usual question of how many in the audience were pre-med, only one hand went up in that room of 400 students. He then said that, 10 years ago, half the students in the room would have raised their hands. I will close with another well-known quote: "So shall ye reap the whirlwind" (Table 2.2).

Selected Readings

1. "Preventable Hospital-Acquired Conditions (HACs), Including Infections," Federal Register 75, no. 157 (Aug 2010):50080.
2. Lembitz A, Clarke TJ. Clarifying "never events" and introducing "always events". Patient Saf Surg. 2009;3:26–31.
3. Inouye SK, Brown CJ, Tinetti ME. Medicare nonpayment hospital falls and unintended consequences. N Engl J Med. 2009;360:2390–3.
4. Carr JM, de la Torre R. Implementing tight glucose control after coronary artery bypass surgery. Ann Thorac Surg. 2005;80(3):902–9.

3. Creating a Surgical Dashboard for Quality

Tim Plerhoples and John Morton

Introduction

It has been estimated that 234 million operations are performed worldwide every year, a rate higher than childbirth. Since the Institute of Medicine's report "To Err is Human", there has been a sharp increase in interest in programs to decrease medical errors, especially in surgical care. Complications from operative care result in 11% of total disease burden, of which nearly half is estimated to be preventable. Despite numerous efforts to improve patient safety, rates of errors, and complications continue to rise nationwide.

Health care has begun to look outside to other fields of high-risk endeavor for solutions, such as in the utilization of crew resource management (CRM) that exists for airlines to improve team communication in the operating room. As hospitals, practitioners, and professional organizations begin to do a better job tracking and quantifying quality of care, the explosion of available data makes real interpretation difficult, often resulting in little practical change.

A *dashboard* – a tool for overcoming this hurdle – has a history of demonstrated use in other fields (including finance, the airline industry, and nuclear power plants). It is an information system user interface that allows the visual display of an array of data in a manner easy to read. Similar to the one found in a car or airplane, a dashboard provides a decision maker with the relevant input to make the system work – that is to "drive" it. The concept has been around since the 1970s, but the advent of the internet and widespread computing increased their use in business and technology in the late 1990s. The graphical nature allows for ready identification of trends, and the automated aspect encourages real-time information synthesis. In recent years, hospitals and professional organizations have become more interested in such medical "quality

D.S. Tichansky, J. Morton, and D.B. Jones (eds.), *The SAGES Manual of Quality, Outcomes and Patient Safety*, DOI 10.1007/978-1-4419-7901-8_3, © Springer Science+Business Media, LLC 2012

dashboards" for helping diagnose areas of needed improvement, for tracking the effects of interventions, and in aiding comparison among colleagues.

Surgical quality dashboards[1] are beginning to appear throughout the country to give a near-continuous progress report to physicians and administrators. As more and more data – patient medical records, care characteristics, and other variables – becomes computerized, physicians are provided with a wealth of information to aid in clinical decision making. However, not all pieces of data are created the same, leaving many clinicians in want of a means to quickly digest such streams of information. This is true not only for making clinical decisions for individual patients but also for improving systems of care to impact many patients. The inclusion of processed and adjusted patient safety and quality data allows for recognition of performance gaps.

Characteristics of a Surgical Quality Dashboard

A quality dashboard should possess several characteristics to ensure optimal functionality (Fig. 3.1). There should be some understanding of overall performance at a quick glance; that is, it must have an ease of review. Some dashboards use simple emoticons (happy or sad faces), traffic lights (green for excellent, yellow for good, and red for needs improvement), or a star system (one through five stars) which correlate with performance measures. Data may be conveyed on any level of detail, from the national, regional, or hospital-wide level down to the individual practitioner level (if enough data is collected to be deemed representative). Since many aspects of health care delivery are team-oriented, most dashboards tend to focus on departments or divisions.

One of the most valuable aspects of the dashboard is the ability to benchmark one's own performance against that of similar groups. Even individual practitioners can be compared. Comparisons may be made using data adjusted for severity of patient illness and complexity of the operation. Recently, however, there has been a move away from risk adjustment toward tracking absolute reduction in risk. Some groups have

---

[1] It should be noted that the term *dashboard* has also been used in health care to denote the computer interface used to monitor operating room progress. Among the data on such dashboards may be some quality data, but the purpose is primarily for moving surgical cases through the operating room in an efficient manner.

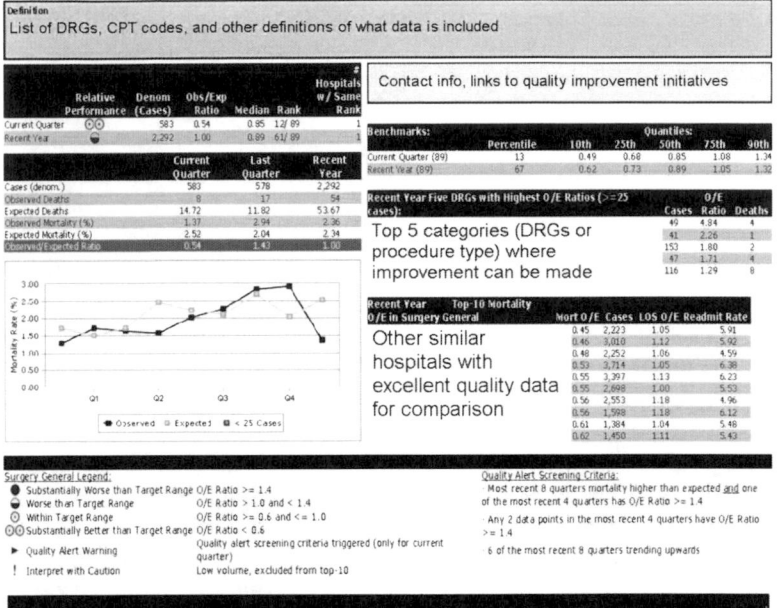

Fig. 3.1. Quality dashboard.

demonstrated that a goal of zero complications may be possible and that a complication such as a surgical site infectious is as unacceptable for a high-risk patient as it is for a low risk one. Also important is the dynamic nature of the dashboard. Tracking changes over time can help document success of interventions and quality improvement programs, as well as act as an impetus for change (the graphical format tends to be convincing even for the most entrenched surgeon). Typically, the dashboard shows measures during the present quarter and year and gives values for the last quarter and year for comparison.

The dashboard's greatest strength – its graphical nature – allows for clear prioritization. The area given to a particular aspect should convey to the user its relative importance. Similar to the front page of a newspaper, the location on the dashboard is also important. Organizations may prioritize one diagnosis-related group (DRG) or current procedural terminology (CPT) code by changing its location or relative size. Graphs and charts can be used rather than tables for additional emphasis.

Taxonomy of Complications and Quality Measures

Data included on a quality dashboard will typically stem from two sources: administrative (or billing) data and clinical data. Administrative data is required by insurance companies, Medicare, and other groups for billing. It is typically automated in a near real-time manner. While easy to collect and consistent, such data does not always lend itself to simple conversion to patient safety and quality parameters. Clinical data – that is, data gleaned prospectively from patient charts or through close follow up – is much better for discerning quality, but can be extremely onerous and expensive to gather. Often additional staff is required to maintain such a program. Administrative data is best used as an early warning or to help prioritize issues to examine more closely by linking to clinical data. An area of academic interest presently is to develop a way to connect administrative data to prospectively collected clinical data to yield an automated integrated method to tracking progress on institutional performance and to compare with both internal and regional benchmarks.

Mortality

Patient mortality is the most basic (and simplest to collect and least controversial) variable that should be displayed on a dashboard. It is typically readily available from administrative data sources and is very accurate. There are well-defined national standards of mortality for specific procedures; this readily allows for adjustment by comparing the "observed to expected" (O/E) ratio. In addition, this allows for easy ranking and understanding where one falls in the gradient of performance. The time period typically ranges from inpatient to 30-day postoperatively.

Hospital Admissions Data

Another easy source of data for the dashboard comes from admissions data. Length of stay and readmission rates do not give the entire picture, but can be helpful benchmarks. Both of these measures are under more regulatory scrutiny with payors threatening not to pay for readmissions. Length of stay (LOS) may not give an entirely comprehensive view of complications given other factors such as patient preference, availability of care facilities, and course of disease may affect it. However, LOS may be a useful surrogate marker for complications given that patients with complications tend to have longer LOS. These can also be adjusted against expected results for more appropriate comparison. Although not specifically applicable to quality, many hospitals gather patient satisfaction data that clinicians may be interested in tracking.

PSI

Patient safety indicators (PSI) are hospital-level administrative data designated by the Agency for health care research and quality (AHRQ) to reflect the quality of care inside hospitals by focusing on complications (Table 3.1). This data is viewed as surrogate measures for a broad level of quality, and a poor result typically triggers closer investigation. PSIS are widely used in surgical quality dashboards, since they are broadly applicable, easily attainable, and regularly updated in a timely manner.

Table 3.1. Patient safety indicators.

Complications of anesthesia (PSI 1)
Death in low-mortality DRGs (PSI 2)
Decubitus ulcer (PSI 3)
Failure to rescue (PSI 4)
Foreign body left in during procedure (PSI 5)
Iatrogenic pneumothorax (PSI 6)
Selected infections due to medical care (PSI 7)
Postoperative hip fracture (PSI 8)
Postoperative hemorrhage or hematoma (PSI 9)
Postoperative physiologic and metabolic derangements (PSI 10)
Postoperative respiratory failure (PSI 11)
Postoperative pulmonary embolism or deep vein thrombosis (PSI 12)
Postoperative sepsis (PSI 13)
Postoperative wound dehiscence in abdominopelvic surgical patients (PSI 14)
Accidental puncture and laceration (PSI 15)
Transfusion reaction (PSI 16)
Birth trauma – injury to neonate (PSI 17)
Obstetric trauma – vaginal delivery with instrument (PSI 18)
Obstetric trauma – vaginal delivery without instrument (PSI 19)
Obstetric trauma – cesarean delivery (PSI 20)

Table 3.2. SCIP targets.

Inf	Prophylactic antibiotic received within 1 h prior to surgical incision
	Prophylactic antibiotic selection for surgical patients
	Prophylactic antibiotics discontinued within 24 h after surgery end time
	Cardiac surgery patients with controlled 6 AM postoperative blood glucose
	Surgery patients with appropriate hair removal
	Urinary catheter removed on postoperative day 1 (POD 1) or postoperative day 2 (POD 2) with day of surgery being day zero
	Surgery patients with perioperative temperature management
Card	Surgery patients on beta-blocker therapy prior to arrival who received a beta-blocker during the perioperative period
VTE	Surgery patients with recommended venous thromboembolism prophylaxis ordered
	Surgery patients who received appropriate venous thromboembolism prophylaxis within 24 h prior to surgery to 24 h after surgery

Administering organizations must provide a consistent baseline for describing complications and for the priority each PSI is given. This can be "personalized" for individual physicians for their particular areas of focus.

SCIP

The surgical care improvement project (SCIP) is a national partnership of several organizations that aims to reduce surgical morbidity and mortality. The program's goal is to reduce complications by focusing on specific target areas (Table 3.2): infection (Inf), cardiac (Card), and venous thromboembolism (VTE). These areas have the strongest scientific evidence showing that specific interventions can reduce the incidence of such complications. SCIP is viewed as the *process* to improve surgical care. These measures are appropriate for both individual- and hospital-level performance.

NSQIP

The national surgical quality improvement program (NSQIP) is a venture by the American College of Surgeons (ACS) to improve surgical care. It is a data-driven, risk-adjusted, outcomes-based surgical quality improvement program that uses sampling of clinical data. It uses a prospective, peer controlled, validated database to quantify 30-day risk-adjusted surgical outcomes. Notably, the program focuses mainly on systems and not individuals, although physician-specific data is available. Membership in the program requires a dedicated reviewer to collect the data, which is accomplished via sampling over an 8-day cycle by including the first 40 cases that meet inclusion criteria. A total of 135 data points are gathered for each case: 74 preoperatively, 19 intraoperatively, and 42 postoperatively. At present, there are over 250 participating sites and growing. The program aims for quality over quantity and can be very valuable in a surgical quality dashboard as central focus points.

Connecting to Quality Improvement

The real benefit of a quality dashboard lies in the easy way to connect to improvement programs and to monitor their success. Surgical dashboards in the future will need to move away from simple trends and instead employ a "Six Sigma" approach of process management specifically around measurement. As the ACS NSQIP has now adapted, "run" charts are ideal to determine whether change has truly occurred. By establishing clinical borders 1 or 2 standard deviations from the norm, current progress can have quantifiable goals.

Once an area of concern is identified, predetermined "suggestions" for specific quality improvement actions for remediation can be set. For example, if there is poor performance on DVT/PE reduction (either rising rates or failure to meet reduction goals), immediate information can be given on hospital policy for prevention (i.e., how to set up and comply with order sets for sequential compression devices or pharmaceutical prophylaxis). Using the plan-act-review-improve model for implementing change, the dashboard can be used in the planning stage by identifying areas of weakness as well as in the review stage to see, if the action had any consequences. This forces a "closing of the loop" to identify a problem, act on it, and review the results of the intervention. Low end performance can be flagged for review by a Professional Practice Evaluation Committee (PPEC), whose responsibility it is to oversee the data that makes up the dashboard. Such peer review committees are tasked with investigating substandard performance through close inspection of the medical record. In deciding what triggers such an investigation, it is important for committees to clearly define standards of performance beforehand. This avoids any aspect of ex post facto effect and encourages a real sense of fairness. To encourage to most improvement, committees should take care to make feedback as objective, equitable, defensible, and timely as possible.

Accountability and transparency are important aspects of the quality dashboard. An individual's performance should be made available not only to themselves but also to their department, the entire organization, and even the public. Some organizations customize dashboards in different ways for different groups (general quality information for patients, more specific data for practitioners and supervisors). While there is some concern for a "chilling effect", where physicians shy away from difficult cases due to the worry of worse outcomes, it has been our experience that transparency's benefits far outweigh the challenges. The highest performing surgeons have always and will continue to be referred the most challenging cases. The dashboard can play an important part in the training of residents and other staff, emphasizing a culture of safety.

Integrating a surgical quality dashboard into an organization has many challenges. This includes technical issues, such as getting different data collection systems to communicate with each other to form a unified output. Having a review committee for investigating poor performance and collecting clinical data is labor intensive and not without cost. Politically, it may be difficult to get convince all parties of its importance. Many clinicians find easy excuses to their quality problems, suggesting that the dashboard fails to fairly showcase the entire picture of clinical care. While there are some challenges, the value of investing in a system shown to decrease errors, improve patient care, and ultimately lead to better outcomes is clear. In the end, to the surgeon, the dashboard is a way to think (and compare) globally but act locally in changing one's own practice.

Selected Readings

1. Baskett L, LeRouge C, Tremblay MC. Using the dashboard technology properly. Health Prog. 2008;89(5):16–23.
2. Beaulieu PA, Higgins JH, Dacey LJ, Nugent WC, Defoe GR. Likosky DS. Qual Saf Health Care: Transforming administrative data into real-time information in the Department of Surgery; 2010.
3. Behal R, Finn J. Understanding and improving inpatient mortality in academic medical centers. Acad Med. 2009;84(12):1657–62.

4. Frith KH, Anderson F, Sewell JP. Assessing and selecting data for a nursing services dashboard. J Nurs Adm. 2010;40(1):10–6.

5. Gates PE. Think globally, act locally: an approach to implementation of clinical practice guidelines. Jt Comm J Qual Improv. 1995;21(2):71–84.

6. Loeb BB. A dashboard for medical staff goals. Trustee. 2010;63(3):35–6. 1.

7. Nelson EC, Batalden PB, Homa K, Godfrey MM, Campbell C, Headrick LA, et al. Microsystems in health care: Part 2. Creating a rich information environment. Jt Comm J Qual Saf. 2003;29(1):5–15.

8. Pronovost P, Needham D, Berenholtz S, Sinopoli D, Chu H, Cosgrove S, et al. An intervention to decrease catheter-related bloodstream infections in the ICU. N Engl J Med. 2006;355(26):2725–32.

9. Roberts DH, Gilmartin GS, Neeman N, Schulze JE, Cannistraro S, Ngo LH, et al. Design and measurement of quality improvement indicators in ambulatory pulmonary care: creating a "culture of quality" in an academic pulmonary division. Chest. 2009;136(4):1134–40.

10. Wolpin S. An exploratory study of an intranet dashboard in a multi-state healthcare system. Stud Health Technol Inform. 2006;122:75–9.

4. Patient-Centered Outcomes: Patient Satisfaction and Quality of Life Assessment

Vic Velanovich

Traditionally, to assess the value of an intervention, physicians have used objective, "physician-centered" outcome measures. These measures would include such endpoints as survival of cancer patients, recurrences after hernia repair, increased blood flow after vascular bypass, incidence of stroke after carotid artery surgery, and the like. Although such measures are valuable, they do not tell the whole story in the patient's experience. In some respects, they are surrogates for the true endpoint – is the patient feeling better and can he or she function and enjoy life? It is this aspect of measuring patient-perceived functional improvements that the field of quality of life research developed [1]. The addition of quality of life to other objective measures of outcomes leads to an "algebra" of sorts to determine the "net benefit" of an intervention for the patient [1]. Many patients understand intuitively and value this algebra – "I don't want to exchange my quality of life for quantity of life." The purpose of this chapter is to provide the foundation for understanding the patient-centered outcomes of satisfaction and quality of life.

A *patient-reported outcome* is defined as "any endpoint derived from patient reports, whether collected in the clinic, in a diary, or by other means, including single-item outcome measures, event logs, symptom reports, formal instruments to measure health-related quality of life, health status, adherence, and satisfaction with treatment" [2]. This concept has lead to an explosion of research in quality of life. In fact, a Medline literature search from 1996 to 2010 using "quality of life" as the keyword identified over 50,000 articles. Quality of life can be used both

D.S. Tichansky, J. Morton, and D.B. Jones (eds.), *The SAGES Manual of Quality, Outcomes and Patient Safety*, DOI 10.1007/978-1-4419-7901-8_4, © Springer Science+Business Media, LLC 2012

for research purposes [3] and in clinical practice [4]. Clearly, the ability to assimilate and use this information is becoming increasingly important to surgeons.

How is one to use quality of life measurement in surgical research or practice? Donaldson [5] enumerates the potential benefits of quality of life measurement in clinical practice:

1. *Assessment*: Description of the patient's status upon entering treatment, and the detection of treatable problems that may have been overlooked. An example of documenting a patient's status would be assessing the level of symptom severity of a patient with gastroesophageal reflux disease prior to treatment using a disease-specific questionnaire. An example of detecting an overlooked problem would be identifying depression in a pancreatic cancer patient by reviewing the mental health component of a generic questionnaire.

2. *Monitoring*: Evaluation of disease progression and treatment response. An example of this would be to assess pain severity periodically in a patient treated for chronic pancreatitis.

3. *Diagnosis*: Detection, measurement, and identification of the causes of decreased functioning. Differentiation of physical, emotional, and other problems. Detection of treatment side effects or toxicity. Prediction of the course of the disease.

4. *Treatment*: Application of the results of clinical studies to treatment choices. This concept is probably the most important use of quality of life research. Particularly for those interventions designed primarily to improve symptoms or function, having standardized measurable changes will help the clinician decide on the value of competing treatments.

5. *Facilitate communication*: Foster shared decision-making to improve treatment planning and guide changes in therapeutic plans that are consistent with patient preferences. Provide feedback to patients about their progress and explore goals and expectations. Foster patient adherence to medical advice. Improve satisfaction with care. By seeing the changes in quality of life scores, many patients feel that this validates their subjective feelings. In addition, the physician may become aware of other health issues that were not communicated during the routine clinical encounter.

Therefore, the next step is to understand quality of life instruments.

Primer on Quality of Life Instruments

Quality of life is measured by questionnaires completed by the patient. These questionnaires are called *instruments*. The questions in each instrument are called *items*. If an instrument measures more than one aspect of quality of life, such as physical functioning, pain, or social activities, each of these aspects is called a *domain*. The instrument is scored, and these scores "quantitate" quality of life.

This approach can beg the question of "why is having a quality of life score valuable?" Why cannot we just ask the patient how are they feeling? Wright [6] perhaps gives the most cogent answer: Patients come to doctors with unique, individual concerns, and this communication is the fundamental interchange between the physician and patient. Patient-centered measures are a particular type of measurement that allow patients to state their individual concerns and weigh their relative importance; therefore, these questionnaires provide the physician a standardized method of assessing patient status. These quantitated responses can then be analyzed statistically to obtain scientifically sound results.

There are three basic types of instruments: *generic, disease-specific, and symptom severity* [1, 3]. Generic instruments are designed to be applicable broadly across a wide range of types and severity of diseases, across different medical treatments or health interventions, and across demographic and cultural subgroups. Disease-specific instruments are designed to assess specific diagnostic groups or patient populations, especially with the goal of measuring "clinically important changes." Symptom severity instruments focus only on the symptoms produced by a given disease process without addressing other quality of life issues, such as social interactions or psychological stresses.

The instrument can take on one or more of three broad functions [7]. It can be *discriminative*. The instrument can separate groups of patients based on its results. It can be *predictive*. That is, the pretreatment scores can predict posttreatment outcomes. Or, it can be *evaluative*. The instrument can be used to assess change in status over time.

Each instrument has essentials properties that have to be assessed prior to use by either the surgical research or practitioner.

1. *Validity.* Does the instrument measure what it intended to measure? In fact, there is no one type of validity. An instrument's validity can be assessed in several ways [8]. *Content validity* relates to the adequacy of the content of the instrument to the quality of life characteristics it intends to measure. An aspect of

content validity is *face validity*; that is, whether the instrument appears to cover the issues of the disease as determined by those familiar with the disease. *Criterion validity* involves measuring the instrument against a "gold standard." This gold standard can be another quality of life instruments, the "standard" clinical assessments of a disease, or physiological tests of the disease. A subtype of criterion validity is *concurrent validity*; that is, the scores of the instrument change with the change in quality of life or functional status as measured by the gold standard. Another subtype is *predictive validity*; that is, the instrument is able to predict change in status. Lastly, *construct validity* is an assessment of the degree to which an instrument measures the theoretical construct that it was designed to measure. A subtype of construct validity is *known-groups* validity; that is, it would be expected that similar groups would have similar scores and differing groups would have different scores. Another subtype of construct validity is *discriminant validity*, in which instruments which do not measure the same aspects of quality of life would have scores which poorly correlate.

2. *Reliability.* The instrument must produce the same results on repeated administrations when the patient has the same level of quality of life [3, 4]. That is to say, it is free from random error [8]. This is usually measured by the test–retest methodology, in which patients whose reported status has not changed should have the same (or close to the same) scores.

3. *Responsiveness (sensitivity to change).* The instrument must be able to detect and measure change over time or after an intervention. From the standpoint of the clinical surgeon, this is one of the most important characteristics. If clinically important changes in quality of life or functional status occur as a result of an operation, but the instrument does not measure this change, it is not an appropriate instrument for the study.

4. *Appropriateness.* The instrument must be appropriate for health issues affected by the disease and the likely range of effects, both positive and adverse, of the treatment.

5. *Practicality.* This refers to the ease of use of the instrument. For example, simple and easy to understand instruments may be self-administered; while instruments that are long or complex may require trained personnel to administer.

In addition, consumers of these instruments need to assess if clinically meaningful changes have occurred. This may be a simple matter of appropriate statistical analysis and understanding the behavior of quality of life data [9]. However, it may also relate to understanding *minimally important* difference; that is, the smallest change in score that reflects a patient-perceived change in status. Lastly, comparisons of an individual patient's score to population norms can be valuable to gauges "where a patient is at."

Patient Satisfaction

Surgeons want their patients to be satisfied with their episode of care. Measuring this satisfaction can be more difficult that is apparent.

As with quality of life, patient satisfaction research leads to understanding the components of satisfaction [10]. This can include satisfaction with the clinical encounter independent of surgical outcome, satisfaction with the surgical outcome, satisfaction with the interaction of the surgeon with the patient and family, and satisfaction with the administrative processes independent of clinical care, among others. Therefore, as with quality of life measurement, it is important to understand what is being measured. This also requires attention to the same details as with the assessment of quality of life as described above [10].

Conclusions

Quality of life and patient satisfaction are two measures of patient-centered outcomes that have become critical in understanding the patient experience. Understanding how these endpoints are measured and interpreted will insure that surgical researchers will choose the best instruments for their purposes and consumers of this research will understand the information being presented.

Selected Readings

1. Testa MA, Simonson DC. Assessment of quality-of-life outcomes. N Engl J Med. 1996;334:835–40.
2. Willke RJ, Burke LB, Erickson P. Measuring treatment impact: A review of patient-reported outcomes and other efficacy endpoints in approved product labels. Controlled Clin Trials. 2004;25:535–52.

3. Velanovich V. Using quality of life instruments to assess surgical outcomes. Surgery. 1999;126:1–4.

4. Velanovich V. Using quality of life measurements in clinical practice. Surgery. 2007;141:127–33.

5. Donaldson MS. Taking stock of health-related quality-of-life measurement in oncology practice in the United States. J Natl Cancer Inst Monogr. 2004;33:155–67.

6. Wright JG. Evaluating the outcome of treatment: Shouldn't we be asking patients if they are better? J Clin Epidemiol. 2000;53:549–53.

7. Kirshner B, Guyatt G. A methological framework for assessing health indices. J Chron Dis. 1985;38:27–36.

8. Fayers PM, Machin D. Quality of life: Assessment, analysis, and interpretation. Chichester: Wiley; 2000.

9. Velanovich V. Behavior and analysis of 36-item short-form health survey data for surgical quality of life research. Arch Surg. 2007;142:473–8.

10. Chow A, Mayer EK, Darzi AW, Athanasiou T. Patient-reported outcome measures: The importance of patient satisfaction in surgery. Surgery. 2009;146:435–43.

5. Quality, Safety, and the Electronic Medical Record

Carter Smith and Gretchen Purcell Jackson

Introduction

Electronic medical records (EMRs) are becoming increasingly prevalent across clinical settings, and as any other new technology, they have the potential both to enhance and to compromise the quality of medical care and patient safety. This chapter provides an introduction to the basic quality and safety issues pertinent to the adoption and use of EMRs by practicing surgeons.

Security and Privacy

EMRs provide a large amount of confidential information in a single, often easily searchable place. Concerns of healthcare providers, administrators, and patients regarding the use of EMRs commonly involve issues of privacy and security. This section describes the procedures and policies necessary for protecting electronically stored health information.

Authentication

Authentication is the process of verifying the identity of a person who accesses the medical record. Login procedures requiring individual usernames and passwords are the most common form of authentication. To provide robust security, the passwords must be increasingly complex to prevent unauthorized access. The best way to enhance the strength of a password is to increase the total number of possible character combinations, usually by requiring a greater number of characters and the use of upper

D.S. Tichansky, J. Morton, and D.B. Jones (eds.), *The SAGES Manual of Quality, Outcomes and Patient Safety*, DOI 10.1007/978-1-4419-7901-8_5, © Springer Science+Business Media, LLC 2012

case, lower case, numerical, and special characters. Remembering these long and complex passwords is difficult, but may be simplified by system integration so that one password is recognized across all systems. Ultimately passwords are a relatively vulnerable security measure. A computer program can systematically generate thousands or even millions of passwords per second until it guesses correctly or make more intelligent attempts using dictionary words or user information such as family names and birth dates. Malicious software can record username and password combinations as they are entered. System-level protections against such threats include login delays after the entry of incorrect passwords or lockouts after multiple failed attempts. Virus protection and regular system re-imaging, a process that reinstalls clean copies of software on shared workstations periodically, can reduce the risk of exposure to malicious software.

To enhance the security, many systems utilize some form of *multifactor authentication*, which necessitates more than one independent method to identify a user. Identify verification may occur through something a user knows, such as a password or personal identification number (PIN); something a user has, such as a digital token or smart card; or biometrics, such as fingerprints or retinal scans. These systems can be costly and are not without failures, but they are much more secure than password-only systems.

Authorization

Authorization is the permission for a user to access specific data or to perform certain actions (cm, such as writing orders). In an ideal world, only providers who need a patient's record should be able to access to it, but many EMRs provide broad authorization to all healthcare providers. Some systems allow individuals or groups of users to be assigned varied privileges so that they can only see or use the parts of the chart that are relevant to them. These safeguards can protect patients from malicious breaches in confidentiality and prevent a well-intended clinician from inadvertently reading the wrong chart or writing an order on an incorrect patient.

Encryption

The personal health information contained in an EMR is vulnerable to security breaches not only during active clinical use, but also during storage and transmission. Most EMRs employ some form of encryption.

Encryption is the process of transforming information to make it unreadable to anyone or anything without specific key or algorithm used to convert the data to a readable form.

Network-Level Security

Most EMRs reside on computer networks that not only interact within a healthcare system but also allow broad access to the Internet. Network-level security protects confidential health information from threats that can occur through such network connections. Firewalls are employed in many networks to monitor and restrict data communications. A *firewall* is a hardware and/or software barrier between networks that inspects the communications between them and stops unauthorized transmissions.

Clinicians often need access to EMRs from locations remote from their primary hospital or clinic, and they may need to use public networks that are far less secure than those provided by their institution. A *virtual private network* (VPN) allows users from outside of a firewall to share secure access to a network as if they were within it. There are various types and implementations of VPNs, but most use a combination of authentication and data encryption methods to protect the communications between the remote user and the network. These technologies offer safe access of patient information to healthcare providers while at home, traveling, or practicing at off-site locations.

User-Level Security

Clinicians who adopt EMRs are important components of security process, and they often must learn new behaviors to fulfill their responsibilities to protect confidential patient health information. Passwords should never be written down, shared with other users, or sent over email, text messages, or telephone. Healthcare providers should adopt strong security practices for password selection and maintenance. Using upper and lower case letters, as well as numbers, and creating longer passwords make the possible combinations larger and protect against brute force attacks. Changing passwords often prevents old password breaches from turning into new ones. It is extremely bad practice to use identical passwords for multiple accounts, and providers who use the same or similar passwords for accessing EMRs and personal electronic accounts (e.g., banks, email, or social networks) threaten their personal information in addition to that of their patients.

Secondary devices for authentication such as secure identification tokens or smart cards must be secured and reported if missing, just as one might report a lost license or credit card. Laptops and now even cellular telephones can be portals into the personal health information of patients. Users must remember to log out, and any device used to access the medical record should never be left unattended. Stolen or missing communication tools should also be reported promptly, especially if logins to secure systems are done automatically [1, 2].

Quality and Safety Issues

The implementation and adoption of an EMR is a complex social, organizational, and technological process that often requires not only a substantial investment in hardware, software, and technical support, but also significant workflow redesign, employee education, and ongoing process evaluation. The EMR can potentially impact every aspect of quality and safety in hospital and ambulatory care, and the informatics literature provides evidence for both considerable benefits and alarming adverse events resulting from the introduction of EMRs. This section focuses on strategies for maximizing benefits and minimizing harm to improve quality of care and patient safety through use of EMRs, based on the recommendations of several leading experts [3, 4].

Questions to Address When Selecting and Implementing an EMR

The goals of minimizing harm and maximizing benefit are accomplished by both the selection of EMR software, its implementation, and monitoring of the system. The answers to the questions below can guide the EMR committee through this process.

1. *Are we selecting appropriate software and hardware?* The EMR software must be able to accomplish the required clinical activities and not disrupt clinician workflow. Emergency departments and operating rooms function very differently than inpatient or outpatient environments. The proposed software must also seamlessly interface with or replace existing hospital infrastructure such as the laboratory and radiology systems.

In addition, the software must be supported by proper hardware. Potential hardware additions and upgrades should be included in the selection process and budget. For example, additional computer workstations may be needed to facilitate clinician access.

2. *Is the system content up to date?* With the EMR, there is great potential for benefit through use of clinical decision support. The content used to drive such features must be evidence based, up to date, and error free. Logic controlling medication allergies and interactions, clinical alerting and reminders, order-entry safety checks, and specialty-specific features (e.g., postoperative order sets) must be properly implemented and maintained. It is important to identify how errors will be corrected and how new information will be incorporated in a timely manner. Additionally, adherence to communication and vocabulary standards like the Systematized Nomenclature of Medicine – Clinical Terms (SNOMED CT) and Health Level Seven electronic interchange standard encourage the application of advanced clinical decision support and information exchange through uniform and defined languages.

3. *How does the user interface affect groups of users?* It is important to consider how the system delivers information to each group of users. The specific needs of the surgeon are discussed in the next section. Pertinent information may vary across provider types, clinical environments, and specialty groups, and each may have separate needs for data entry and display. A system should be flexible enough to address diverse needs without creating confusion and communication breakdown with excessive customization. The modern clinician may want to use advanced technologies such as voice recognition and mobile devices to enter and access clinical data, and careful consideration must be given to the associated advantages and costs (e.g., interface adaptation and user training).

4. *What support personnel will we have?* It is crucial that ample support personnel be identified whether from within the institution or through outside agreements. Training staff is vital to implementation as well as integration of new users. Software engineers and other technical staff are needed to provide continued software updates and address issues as they arise, especially after hours. Inpatient facilities and other practices that care for patients overnight may need a special system to

solve problems that arise outside of typical business hours. Personnel needs in all of these areas may be significantly higher during the initial implementation of a new system.

5. *How will workflow be affected by this new system?* The implementation of an EMR usually requires changes to existing workflows. A thorough review of existing and proposed communication processes and information exchanges can potentially improve safety and optimize workflow; a failure to understand such changes can introduce errors and frustrate users. This process may require a multidisciplinary team of software designers, developers, trainers, policy makers, clinicians, and maintenance staff. Analysis of clinical workflows should be initiated early and continue through implementation to address risks that are foreseen as well as those that arise during use.

6. *What methods for testing the system are in place both before and after implementation?* System testing may be able to identify problems and workflow issues so that they can be addressed before there is potential for patient harm. Testing may be undertaken by the software manufacturer, by the local institution, or both. It is important to develop a plan for robust usability and performance testing both before implementation and during ongoing use. Testing may require time commitment of clinical staff as well as support personnel, and the associated costs must be anticipated.

7. *How will we report and study bugs, safety flaws, and incidents?* To address user concerns and to enhance EMR safety, it is important to have well-established internal and external processes for reporting and addressing flaws and incidents as they are identified. Each institution and its supporting vendors must specify a system for reporting of events and developing solutions to them. It is critical to recognize the limitations of local and institutional support personnel and to know when problems or errors require higher level intervention. Several authors have proposed federal oversight of this process as well as federal reporting to produce aggregate data [3, 4]. Partnering with other groups with common patients, software systems, or infrastructure may allow for creation of a knowledge base of risks, adverse events, and solutions. Collaborative groups can be invaluable in identifying common patterns of errors and deficiencies.

8. *What are the most recent state and federal regulations for EHRs and does our system address them?* Both the Health Insurance Portability and Accountability Act (HIPAA) of 1996 and the American Recovery and Reinvestment Act (ARRA) of 2009 have placed specific requirements on EMRs, and many details of the latter regulations are still in evolution [5, 6]. Both federal and state legislation have the potential to change and vary as more institutions implement electronic systems and federal oversight increases. Individuals and institutions with systems that meet the most current requirements may be eligible for financial incentives, and those that do not may be subject to a variety of penalties or punishments.

EMR Functions for the Surgeon

Surgeons as a group have unique needs from the EMR, and each surgical specialty may require particular functions or customizations for their practices. Surgeons are encouraged to participate in EMR advisory committees and test groups to insure their requirements are being met. This section discusses essential and desirable EMR features for surgeons.

Some general requirements for EMRs are shared across specialties. The surgeon practices from many locations including the emergency room, outpatient clinics, the operating room, and the intensive care unit, or even from home or while traveling. The EMR must be *accessible* from a variety of locations and ideally *portable* with access through the Internet and smart phones. *Installation services* and *training* are essential pieces of the overall package from the EMR vendor, and as are superior *service* and *support*. Ongoing support both during the installation period and after are important considerations. These services can be undertaken by the vendor or by the institution, but adequate support is absolutely essential. The *customizability* of the system for the needs of individual specialties or practice groups is a desirable feature. System-wide or specialty-wide customization is more practical than tailoring at the user level due to the difficulty of providing support when each user setup is unique. Because the implementation of a complete system or specialty-specific features may be prohibitive due to cost, training, or workflow limitations, a system's *modularity* and *extensibility* can allow for integration of additional components or customization as resources become available. In addition, *interoperability* between the new system and existing information systems is vital. It may be necessary to consider upgrades or replacements to existing laboratory, radiology, billing, dictation, and pathology systems to support compatibility. Finally, there must be plan for maintaining or integrating old records, either paper or electronic formats.

Surgery is an anatomically oriented specialty, and thus, it is particularly important that EMRs be able to incorporate *clinical and radiographic images*. Images may be acquired using the Diagnostic Image Communication Of Medicine (DICOM) transmission standard, or in non-DICOM formats (e.g., wound photographs and intraoperative photos), so inclusion of both DICOM and non-DICOM images is desirable, as is the ability to include and display and annotate a variety of multimedia from anatomic drawings to operative videos. If the institution uses an external picture archiving and communication system (PACS), it is useful for this system to be integrated with the EMR.

Many EMR vendors now support *electronic informed consent*, which can be particularly useful for procedurally oriented specialties. Such modules may also incorporate *educational materials, preoperative and postoperative instructions*, and relevant anatomic drawings, which can expedite clinical workflow and reduce liability risks. Surgeons should ask about the availability of such information in various *languages* and for *multiple reading levels* [7, 8].

User-Level Quality and Safety Guidelines

Provider behaviors can contribute significantly to both the benefits and harms that result from use of EMRs. EMR systems vary substantially, but most require new approaches to clinical documentation. This section provides some practical guidelines for safe EMR use to provide high quality care.

Each document in the EMR should serve as a succinct, effective communication tool to facilitate care of the patient. As with paper records, providers should take the time to carefully and thoroughly record an assessment and plan. This synthesis of applicable data is arguably the most important part of a provider's documentation and what marks a good clinician. Depending on individual skills and system support, this process may take longer than jotting a note in a paper chart, but users should not cut corners on any critical documentation (e.g., consent and procedure notes).

Similarly, important recommendations should not be buried in pages of erroneous data simply because it is easy to incorporate information from previous documents. EMR users should avoid excessive "reuse" or "copy and paste" functions because these tools inevitably introduce errors without careful editing. Although the duplication of information is often motivated by documentation requirements for maximal reimbursement, payers may deny compensation if the information is clearly copied, especially when incorrect data are introduced (e.g., a postoperative day or incorrect preoperative diagnosis is not updated). The same principles apply to using templates that automatically fill documents with data from other sources or standard text. These tools should be used with caution, and all text should be reviewed carefully for accuracy before saving.

Clinical decision support in the form of warnings and recommendations provide great potential for improvement of patient care and prevention of medical mistakes as well as common sources of EMR user frustration. It is important not to blindly click through such notifications. Likewise, it is critical that clinicians insist that the rules that drive the clinical alerts are driven by solid evidence and practice guidelines. Warnings must be clinically important and consistently relevant to the situation to be heeded and to avoid establishing a reflex reaction to ignore such alerts. It is essential that practicing clinicians participate actively in creating useful and pertinent decision support modules, and their contributions to quality and safety be evaluated in an ongoing manner [4].

Regulatory Issues

The Legal Electronic Medical Record

The EMR must meet regulatory requirements for a legal medical record. While the complete specifications for a legal medical record are beyond the scope of this chapter, this section highlights some of the most important considerations.

A unique record must exist and be maintained for each patient, and some key components of documentation must be included. The author, time, and date must be recorded accurately for each element added to the record. It is important to determine how successive versions of documentation are treated both before and after a signature is applied. The signature procedure must meet qualifications both legally and professionally. All corrections, amendments, or clarifications must be clearly noted.

The safe guards that are in place to prevent access without authorization must also prevent unauthorized alterations in both the individual record and system databases. Access audits and document version histories should be available to reproduce event timelines if needed. Additionally, policies and procedures should be defined for alterations and amendments to system components including templates and clinical decision support as well as for record retention, archiving, data reporting, and other forms of data abstraction [9].

Health Insurance Portability and Accountability Act

The Health Insurance Portability and Accountability Act (HIPAA) of 1996 specified two rules – the privacy and security rules – as they apply to patient identifiable information and those who transmit and receive this information. The privacy rule established a standard for the protection of personal health information. The security rule defined a national set of security standards for protecting certain health information that is held or transferred in electronic form. It specified how this information may be disclosed and what protections must be in place to prevent unauthorized access or disclosure. It also required that covered entities must create privacy policies and train workforce members as well as safeguard their data and mitigate harmful effects caused by disclosure of this type of information. Most clinicians are familiar with the concept that protected health information may only be transmitted and disclosed under certain guidelines according to this legislation. For the implementation of an EMR system, four types of security are needed: (1) physical security – the data storage must be in a location that prevents theft of data; (2) user security – efforts to prevent unauthorized access need to be in place; (3) system security – procedures and policies must protect the information from damage or destruction, and backup files in remote locations may be needed to safeguarded from fire, flood, or system crashes; and (4) network security – protection of the data while in transit and storage, and prevention of access to data from outside of the system [6].

The American Recovery and Reinvestment Act

The American Recovery and Reinvestment Act of 2009 (ARRA) is an economic stimulus package that was signed into law in February of 2009 and includes the Health Information Technology for Economic and

Clinical Health (HITECH) Act, which allocated $19.2 billion in funding to increase the use of EMRs. In the HITECH Act, Congress provides Medicare and Medicaid payment incentives to individual providers and hospitals that adopt certified EMR technologies and achieve "meaningful use." Short-term incentives that begin in 2011 are replaced by penalties in 2015 for failure to accomplish meaningful use of a certified EMR.

One of the most controversial aspects of this legislation is the definition of "meaningful use." Stage I criteria for meaningful use were issued in July of 2010 with planned biennial updates to these criteria to achieve "health care that is patient-centered, evidence-based, prevention-oriented, efficient, and equitable." To qualify for incentive payments, individual providers must complete 15 core and 5 additional of 25 meaningful use objectives; hospitals must achieve 14 core and 5 additional of 24 meaningful use objectives. Core objectives include the use of computerized order entry, maintenance of up-to-date problem, medication, and allergy lists, implementation of clinical decision support rules, and providing patients with electronic copies of health information and discharge summaries. Optional objectives include recording advanced directives for patients 65 years old or older and sending reminders for preventative care to patients according to their preferences. In addition to meeting these objectives, individuals must report 6 and hospitals must report 15 clinical quality measures to achieve meaningful use criteria. Examples of clinical quality measures are blood pressure measurements and tobacco use assessments for individual providers and measures of emergency department throughput for hospitals.

Realistically, the financial incentives are small compared to the costs of adopting and maintaining high quality EMRs, and thus, they are not the best reason to strive for meaningful use of EMR technologies. The proper application of healthcare information technology can lead to improvements in the quality and safety of care provided, and this legislation represents an emerging trend toward government requirements and oversight for EMR use [5, 10].

Selected Readings

1. Shortliffe EH, Cimino JJ. Biomedical informatics: computer applications in health care and biomedicine. New York: Springer; 2006.
2. Security aspects in electronic personal health record: data access and preservation. http://www.digitalpreservationeurope.eu/publications/briefs/security_aspects.pdf.

3. Sittig DF, Classen DC. Safe electronic health record use requires a comprehensive monitoring and evaluation framework. JAMA. 2010;303:450–1.

4. Walker JM, Carayon P, Leveson N, Paulus RA, Tooker J, Chin H, et al. Stewart WF: *EHR safety: the way forward to safe and effective systems.* J Am Med Inform Assoc. 2008;15:272–7.

5. 42 CFR Parts 412, 413, 422 et al. Medicare and Medicaid Programs.

6. Electronic Health Record Incentive Program. Final Rule. *Federal Register.* 2010;75:44314–588.

7. Health Information Privacy [http://www.hhs.gov/ocr/privacy/hipaa/understanding/coveredentities/index.html].

8. Mukherjee K, Jackson GP. Optimal EMR system criteria offered. Surgery News. 2009;5:3–4.

9. Schwaitzberg SD. Successful implementation of EMR in your practice: I work in a large hospital. If they ask me what I need, what should I tell them? Presentation at the American College of Surgeons 94th Annual Clinical Congress, San Francisco, CA.

10. The legal electronic medical record [http://www.himss.org/content/files/LegalEMR_Flyer3.pdf].

11. Baron RJ. Meaningful use of health information technology is managing information. JAMA. 2010;304:89–90.

6. Leading and Managing Change: Systems Improvement

Nestor F. Esnaola and Kate Atchley

Change management is a structured, proactive, coordinated approach to transition individuals and organizations from a current state to a desired future state to achieve lasting change. As such, change is viewed not as an event, but rather, as a planned process that occurs within a specified period of time. A successful change management initiative is usually guided by a strong model or framework that anticipates and mitigates resistance along the way and outlines a stepwise, gradual process of transition.

Most current models of change management represent variations of Kurt Lewin's "Unfreeze-Change-Refreeze" model. Lewin, one of the founders of social psychology, presented a simple model in the 1940s for changing how people think and act consisting of three phases or stages:

1. The "unfreezing" stage, in which individuals and organizations are made ready for change, and if necessary, shocked out of the status quo.
2. The change (or transition) stage, in which the previously "unfrozen" individuals (or organizational units) are gradually led to make the changes needed to achieve the desired end state.
3. The "refreezing" stage, in which the adjustments made during the transition are embedded or hardwired into the system to ensure lasting change.

Irrespective of which change management model is used, a positive attitude toward change, effective communication, persistence, and active listening are needed to successfully lead change in any organization. This chapter outlines the steps involved in the change management process and explains how to plan and enact lasting change within one's organization (Table 6.1).

D.S. Tichansky, J. Morton, and D.B. Jones (eds.), *The SAGES Manual of Quality, Outcomes and Patient Safety*, DOI 10.1007/978-1-4419-7901-8_6, © Springer Science+Business Media, LLC 2012

Table 6.1. Steps involved in leading and managing organizational change.

Planning for change
Step 1: Understand the Need for Change

DO: Continually scan the external environment and perform internal diagnostics

DON'T: Become complacent

Step 2: Build the Guiding Change Team

DO: Enlist other individuals with expertise, credibility, leadership/management skills, and "position power"

DON'T: Act alone

Step 3: Create a Vision/Strategy for Change

DO: Make it simple, tangible/attainable, and desirable; engage key stakeholders (ensure "shared ownership")

DON'T: Ignore silos/power centers that pose potential barriers to change

Implementing change
Step 4: Create a Sense of Urgency

DO: Use tangible/dramatic evidence from both within/outside the organization to make a case for change

DON'T: Rely on a dry business case (rather, create a burning platform); create a sense of urgency without proposing solutions (which breeds anxiety/uncertainty)

Step 5: Communicate the Vision/Strategy for Change

DO: Make the change vision simple and compelling; present the right message, in the right format(s), at the right time

DON'T: Under-communicate; fail to "walk the talk"

Step 6: Empower Broad-Based Action

DO: Recognize/reward individuals who have "bought into" and promote the change vision/strategy

DON'T: Try to remove all barriers at once; ignore intractable resisters

Step 7: Generate Short-Term Wins

DO: Ensure and celebrate quick/visible/meaningful wins early on

DON'T: Launch too many projects at once (which leads to burnout); declare absolute victories

(continued)

Table 6.1. (continued)

Planning for change
Step 8: Exploit Gains to Produce More Change

DO: Promote "change champions"; continually reinvigorate the change process with new people/projects

DON'T: Let up; tie yourself to a rigid plan (rather, allow for flexibility/take advantage of unforeseen opportunities)

Step 9: Hardwire Change

DO: Ensure the change "roots" itself into the organizational culture; use the orientation/promotion process to create new advocates

DON'T: Rely on individuals/structures/processes *alone* to hold major changes in place

Planning for Change

Planning for change and engaging an effective, core change team is central to any change initiative *and must take place before any action is taken*. In fact, the planning stage could comprise 50–60% of the time allotted for the change, depending on the scope of the change being initiated.

Step 1: Understand the Need for Change. All successful organizations recognize that change is unavoidable, shun complacency, and take a proactive, rather than reactive, approach to change. It is important to continually scan the external environment for signs of change and perform internal diagnostics using varied data sources and individuals to uncover "threats to the system" and identify strategic opportunities for change and innovation. When problems are identified, it is important to look for root causes hidden beneath symptoms before attempting to generate effective solutions, and that key stakeholders be involved in this process if they are to understand and agree on the need for change.

Step 2: Build the Guiding Change Team. At the center of any change initiative is a change agent or leader. This individual must be enthusiastic, instill confidence in others, and be able to motivate the eventual target audience. Successful change leaders never act alone, but rather, stand at the helm of a guiding change coalition with whom they work closely to plan and execute the transformation process.

Before creating the core change team, the change leader should map potential support and resistant to the initiative taking into account the typical distribution of champions (10%), helpers (10%), bystanders (60%), and resisters (20%) to change in most organizations. Although bystanders can often be the most difficult to identify, their inclusion on the guiding change team (along with champions and helpers) can be extremely helpful in ensuring more rapid, widespread support for the initiative.

When selecting members for the guiding change team (Fig. 6.1), it is critically important to select individuals with:

- Expertise (to ensure better, more credible decisions)
- Credibility and/or a proven track record in the organization
- Leadership and management skills
- "Position power" (e.g., ability to secure resources, strategic reporting relationships, etc.)

Tools for mapping support/resistance to organizational change, such as a power/influence map (Fig. 6.1a) and stakeholder diagnostic grid (Fig. 6.1b), can be of significant value when selecting members for the guiding change team. Change efforts that rely on a single person (or no one) or a weak task force without the required skills or power to get the job done are doomed to failure.

Step 3: Create a Vision/Strategy for Change. Once the core change team has been enlisted, a compelling vision and sets of strategies for change must be drafted. The change vision is a description of the desired end state (i.e., to become a low outlier for SSI among participating hospitals in ACS NSQIP). The vision must be simple, tangible, and attainable. The vision must "speak" to all the members of the guiding team and should ideally be perceived as desirable by the relevant target audience (i.e., must pass the "what's-in-it-for-me" test).

Once the vision has been created, a change strategy should be drafted to determine "how you will get there." The strategy will help guide day-to-day operational decisions for the change initiative, and like any good strategy, should be based on the experience/knowledge of key individuals and be the result of an open debate of alternative options.

Before moving forward, it is imperative that the change vision and strategy is supported by as many of the relevant, key stakeholders in the organization to ensure "shared ownership" of the change initiative and increase its chances of success, (see Fig. 6.2).

a

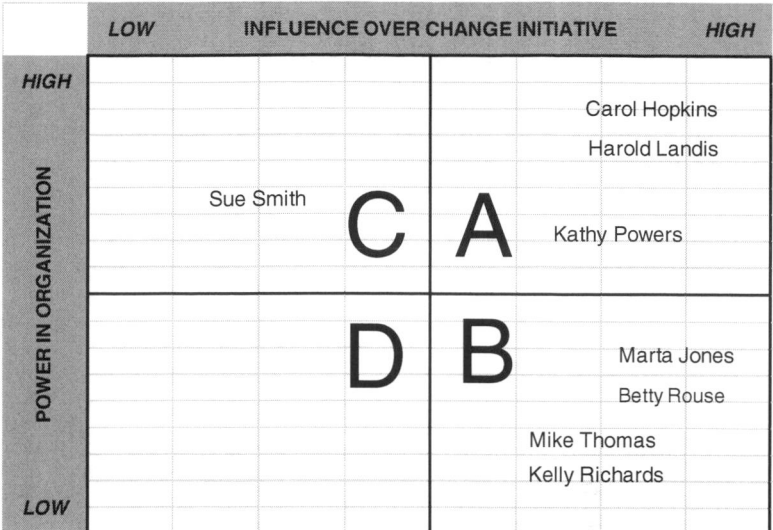

b

	Stakeholder	Role	Power/ Influence	Impact of Change on Stakeholder	Current/Desired Support					Reasons for Support/ Resistance
					Strongly Opposed	Opposed	Neutral	Supportive	Champion	
1	Sue Smith	Infection Prevention & Control, Head	C	Low				●		Reduce SSI rates
2	Harold Landis	Department of Anesthesia, Quality Officer	A	Medium			○———→			Optimize perioperative outcomes
3	Carol Hopkins	Department of Surgery, Quality Officer	A	High					●	Optimize perioperative outcomes
4	Betty Rouse	County Hospital OR, Charge Nurse	B	High		●————→				"More work"/"bad cop"
5	Marta Jones	University Hospital OR, Charge Nurse	B	High	○—————→					"More work"
6	Mike Thomas	Administrative Chief Resident, Anesthesia	B	Medium	○—●——→					Erodes resident autonomy?
7	Kelly Richards	Administrative Chief Resident, Surgery	B	Medium	●———→					Erodes resident autonomy?
8	Kathy Powers	OR Pharmacy, Director	A	Low	●—→					Optimize work flow

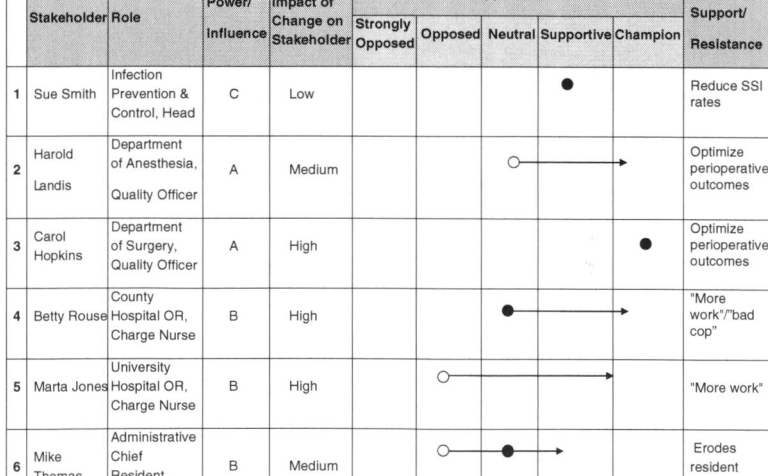

○ *Assumed* position　　● *Confirmed* position　　——→ Where they *need* to be

Fig. 6.1. (**a** and **b**) Tools for mapping support/resistance to organizational change and selecting members for the guiding change team. (**a**) Power/influence map, (**b**) Stakeholder diagnostic grid.

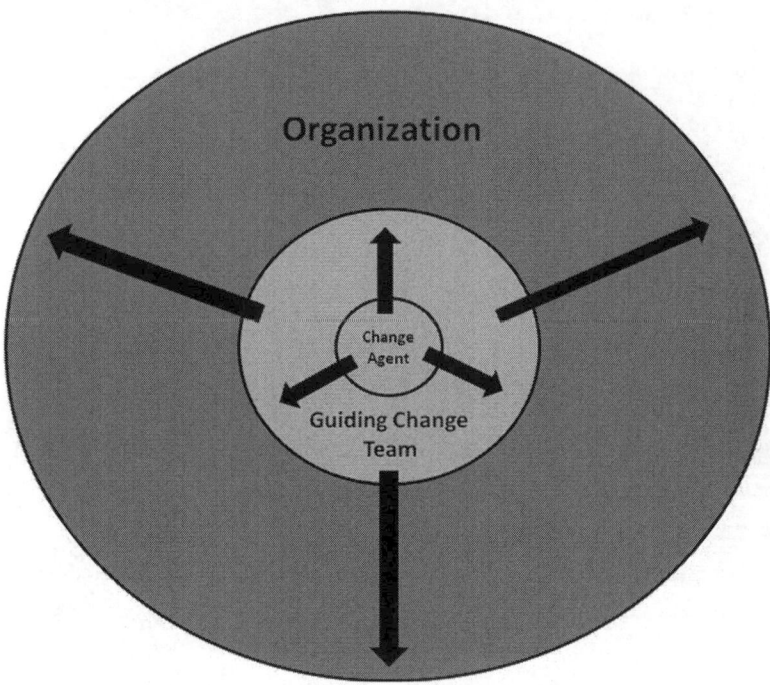

Fig. 6.2. Role of change agent, core team, and stakeholders in planning (*light gray area*) and implementing (*dark gray area*) organizational change. The change agent initiates the call for change (the "why"), the core/guiding change team helps build the case for change and create the vision/strategy for change (the "what"), and the key stakeholders (*black arrows*) help implement change outwards throughout the organization (the "how"). [Adapted from figure created by leadership simulation experts at ExperiencePoint, Inc.].

Implementing Change

Leaders must have a coherent, effective persuasion strategy to motivate change before any actions can be taken. Once the need for change has been communicated and accepted, the transformation is launched via sequential, purposeful adjustments to align systems, structures, and processes with the change vision and strategy.

Step 4: Create a Sense of Urgency. In any organization, the status quo often breeds a false sense of security. As such, a focused persuasion campaign is often necessary to overcome "business as usual," and in some instances, shock the system out of complacency. Change leaders must identify and discuss external threats to the system and explain the organizational *and personal* consequences of clinging on to status quo. Rather than creating a dry business case, it is better to use dramatic evidence from within/outside the organization to create a "burning platform" for change. For example, sharing financial data or other metrics that show that the current state is not sustainable can be a powerful tool for helping people understand the need for change. Ideally, at least 75% of the relevant people must be persuaded that the status quo is no longer acceptable, else complacency, fear, and anger will eventually undermine and sink the change initiative.

Step 5: Communicate the Vision/Strategy for Change. An effective persuasion campaign must increase urgency by tempering external threats with viable solutions; otherwise, it may result in widespread anxiety and uncertainty. It is important to make the change vision simple and compelling. Repetition using symbols and slogans across multiple channels (e.g., buttons, posters, and flyers) and forums (e.g., Morbidity and Mortality Conference, staff meetings, town hall meetings, etc.) is needed to avoid under-communicating the change vision/strategy. The change leader and other member of the guiding team must also visibly "walk the talk"; else, the change initiative may soon lose credibility and momentum.

It is not uncommon for major change to breed uncertainty and resistance. Time and support is needed to help affected individuals understand, process, and accept the need for change. As such, it is imperative that change leaders continually present the right message, in the right format, at the right time to remind people where they are heading (and why).

Step 6: Empower Broad-Based Action. If the change initiative is to take hold, obstacles preventing individuals from acting on the vision must be identified and removed (so they would not grow discouraged) and creativity should be solicited, encouraged, and rewarded in carrying out the vision/strategy. Supervisors (i.e., resisters), systems, and/or structures that undermine the change should be aligned with the change vision by updating training programs, realigning reward/incentive systems, reassigning of roles or tasks, and creating cross-working teams across "functional silos." If the obstacle is an individual who is actively resisting and even damaging progress, transfer or termination of that employee may be necessary.

Step 7: Generate Short-Term Wins. Careful selection of small, manageable projects that are more likely to result in highly visible, quick wins is imperative to ensure early success of the change and to encourage growing acceptance across the organization. These quick wins provide ready credibility for the change and facilitate recruitment of additional manpower and resources. In contrast, slower, less visible wins are less compelling to bystanders and may not be perceived as clearly related to the change, sapping its momentum.

Step 8: Exploit Gains to Produce More Change. Although it is important to stop and celebrate the attainment of short-term objectives, it is important not to claim absolute victories. Rather, these opportunities should be used to set tougher goals and further change systems, structures, and processes not congruent with the change strategy. Successful change leaders ensure momentum by strategically choosing what project to tackle next and promoting/developing people who implement the change vision. In addition, they avoid "burnout" and continually reinvigorate the process by bringing on new people and projects that will perpetuate the change vision/strategy.

Step 9: Hardwire Change. Despite successful implementation of the "unfreezing" and "change" phases cited above, major change is often short-lived and individuals/organizations soon revert back to the previous state. As such, it is imperative that explicit steps are taken to "re-freeze" new beliefs and behaviors, encourage acceptance and stability, and ensure lasting change. It is important to continually highlight connections between new beliefs and actions and organizational success to help "root" change within the organizational culture (i.e., explain to providers how recent hospital-wide, surgical site infection prevention protocols reduced wound infections rates, improved the hospital's reputation within the community, and reduced costs). Means to ensure leadership development and succession congruent with the new transformation (e.g. revamped reward/promotion criteria) should be also developed.

An Example of Leading and Managing Organizational Change

The Department of Surgery's Quality Officer for Hospital A notes that her hospital remains a high outlier for surgical site infection (SSI) in the most recent American College of Surgeons National Surgical Quality

Improvement Program semiannual report despite monthly reporting of detailed SSI data at Morbidity and Mortality Conference. SSIs are still viewed by some providers (including nurses, residents, and staff) as trivial postoperative occurrences. Previous, hospital-wide initiatives to optimize use of perioperative antibiotic prophylaxis and reduce SSI rates have met with limited, short-lived success. How can the Quality Officer change providers' attitudes about SSIs and more effectively roll out best practices to prevent SSIs across her organization?

Step 1: Understanding the Need for Change. Further investigation into the semiannual report reveals that Hospital A's SSI rate is unacceptable high (almost 15%) among gastrointestinal (GI) surgery patients. Among patients who underwent GI surgery, less than 80% of patients received any antibiotic prophylaxis within 1 h prior to incision time and less than 60% received the appropriate antibiotic(s). An informal survey of surgical residents/staff uncovers poor understanding of the need for timely antibiotic prophylaxis prior to GI surgery (as well as which agents are most appropriate according to the type of procedure being performed). This information is shared with the Chairs of Surgery and Anesthesia, the hospital's Quality Officer, and the Director of Pharmacy Services. Shortly thereafter, a hospital-wide, quality improvement initiative to optimize use of perioperative antibiotic prophylaxis and reduce SSI rates in surgical patients is approved and launched.

Step 2: Building the Guiding Change Team. With the Department of Surgery's Quality Officer at the helm, a core change team is enlisted including the Head of Infection Prevention and Control (who reports directly to the hospital's Quality Officer), the Department of Anesthesia's Quality Officer, the Director of the Operating Room Pharmacy, and charge nurses from the Operating Room. Potential support/resistance to the initiative is mapped, as a result of which Administrative Chief Residents from Surgery and Anesthesia are added to the team.

Step 3: Creating a Vision/Strategy for Change. The core change team sets "low outlier status for SSI on the ACS NSQIP semiannual report within 12 months" as a goal. It plans to achieve this goal by (a) educating residents/nurses/pharmacists/staff about the association between antibiotic prophylaxis and postoperative SSI rates and (b) ensuring that all surgical patients receive timely/appropriate antibiotic prophylaxis. Potential improvement strategies include perioperative standing orders for antibiotic prophylaxis (depending on the type of surgery being performed), daily stocking of anesthesia case carts with antibiotics commonly used for perioperative prophylaxis, and modification of the intraoperative "time out" protocol to include a team discussion around antibiotic prophylaxis.

Step 4: Creating a Sense of Urgency. The change team prepares a PowerPoint presentation outlining the clinical/economic impact of SSIs, risk factors for SSIs (in particular, failure to provide optimal antibiotic prophylaxis prior to surgery), the hospital's high outlier status for SSI, rates of postoperative SSIs across surgical services, potential expansion of the Center of Medicare and Medicaid's non-payment policy for hospital acquired conditions to include all SSIs (and its potential impact on the hospital's "bottom line"), and growing interest/public reporting of hospital process and outcome data (and in particular, SSIs). Members of the guiding team are assigned to give the presentation across multiple forums (e.g., Morbidity and Mortality Conferences, resident teaching conferences, nursing staff meetings) to create a "burning platform" for the change.

Step 5: Communicating the Vision/Strategy for Change. Ways to reduce the risk of postoperative SSIs (timely/appropriate use of prophylactic antibiotics) are discussed at the end of these presentations/at each of these forums. Key slides from the PowerPoint presentation are posted at strategic sites (e.g., Operating Room lounge, resident work rooms, nursing staff break rooms, etc.), buttons with the slogan "NO BUGS" are distributed to surgical staff/residents/nurses, and screen savers with the message "Help stomp out SSIs" are rolled out across the hospital.

Step 6: Empowering Broad-Based Action. Anesthesia case carts are stocked with antibiotics on a daily basis (and restocked throughout the day in "high turnover" operating rooms), operating room staff are instructed and empowered to delay incision times until the surgery/anesthesia team has discussed antibiotic prophylaxis and the appropriate agent has been administered, and data fields for "time of antibiotic prophylaxis" and "type of antibiotic prophylaxis" are created in the nursing/anesthesia computerized perioperative records. Patients/families are provided with education sheets outlining ways to prevent SSIs (to help reinforce appropriate provider adherence and encourage self-protective behaviors).

Step 7: Generating Short-Term Wins. Standing order templates for antibiotic prophylaxis are agreed upon by the various surgical/anesthesia teams and made readily available on the hospital's Intranet. Laminated protocols outlining which patients require perioperative antibiotic prophylaxis are posted in all the operating rooms. "Wins" resulting from these improvements (e.g. rate of patients who received antibiotic prophylaxis within 1 h of incision time, rate of GI surgery patients who received appropriate antibiotic prophylaxis, etc.) and the names of their respective physician/nurse/pharmacy champions are posted in the Operating Room lounge each month.

Step 8: Exploiting Gains to Produce More Change. As the initiative gains momentum, staff/nurses from all surgical services are tapped/ encouraged to identify other patient populations who require perioperative antibiotic prophylaxis and develop similar improvement plans. A "SSI Prevention Module" is created and incorporated into the orientation program for all new nursing staff. Nurse-driven, perioperative antibiotic prophylaxis orders (that do not require surgeon/physician cosignature) are agreed upon by the various surgery/anesthesia teams and incorporated into the hospital's computerized physician order entry system.

Step 9: Hardwiring Change. Connections between the change initiative, increased rates of appropriate antibiotic prophylaxis, reduced rates of SSIs (and potential morbidity/mortality/costs avoided) are highlighted and disseminated periodically across various private/public forums. Physician/nurse/pharmacy champions of the change initiative are openly recognized and rewarded. Soon, the new standard-of-care becomes "just the way we do things around here" and becomes rooted within the hospital's culture of quality and safety.

Selected Readings

1. Kotter JP. Leading change. Boston, MA: Harvard Business School; 1996.
2. Kotter JP, Cohen D. The heart of change. Massachusetts: Harvard Business School; 2002.
3. Bridges W, Susan M. Leading Transition: a New Model for Change. Leader to Leader. 2000;16 (Spring):30–6.
4. Kanter RM. The Enduring Skills of Change Leaders. Leader to Leader. 1999;13(Summer): 15–22.
5. Garvin DA, Roberto MA. Change through persuasion. Harv Bus Rev. 2005;83(2): 104–12.

Helpful Websites for More Information

ExperiencePoint: http://www.experiencepoint.com/

7. Surgical Timeout and Retained Foreign Bodies – Patient Safety in the Operating Room

Eric Weiss and Cybil Corning

There has been much debate about patient safety after the release of the landmark report *To Err is Human: Building a Safer Health System* in 1999 by the Institute of Medicine (IOM) [1]. The authors report 44,000–98,000 deaths per year due to medical errors in the United States. The IOM called for more than 50% decrease in the number of deaths within the 5 years following that publication establishing goals and strategies to achieve this result. These goals include: (1) Establishing a national focus to create leadership, research, tools, and protocols to enhance knowledge. (2) Identifying and learning from errors by developing a nationwide, public, mandatory reporting system, and by encouraging healthcare organizations and practitioners to develop and participate in voluntary reporting systems. (3) Raising performance standards and expectations for improvements in safety through the actions of oversight organizations, professional groups, and group purchasers of healthcare. (4) Implementing safety systems in healthcare organizations to ensure safe practices at the delivery level.

As surgeons, we are potentially intimately involved in some of the errors that are among the most costly to individual morbidity and mortality. More globally, there are institutional and healthcare costs, societal losses of productivity, and other factors due to medical errors. Patient care in any setting from outpatient clinic encounters to ambulatory care centers to intensive care units can be subject to medical errors. The hospital units where errors are *most* likely to occur, and to cause an adverse event, are the intensive care units, the emergency room, and the operating room [1]. In the operating room, these errors include wrong site surgery and retained surgical foreign bodies. Although there are other possible errors such as lack of equipment availability, equipment failure, poor knowledge of patient history, lack of surgeon preparation, fire, medication administration errors, and others, they are beyond the focus of this chapter [2].

D.S. Tichansky, J. Morton, and D.B. Jones (eds.), *The SAGES Manual of Quality, Outcomes and Patient Safety*, DOI 10.1007/978-1-4419-7901-8_7, © Springer Science+Business Media, LLC 2012

Wrong Site Surgery and the Universal Protocol

What is wrong site surgery? In the literature, the term *wrong site surgery* usually encompasses the breadth of wrong patient, wrong site, and wrong side surgery. A procedure is considered wrong site surgery if the operation begins at the wrong site, even if the error is identified and corrected by the end of the operation without apparent injury. For example making an incision on the opposite side, even if only through the skin and recognizing this and then performing the correct surgery is still considered wrong site surgery. Wrong site surgery has been included in the list of "Serious Reportable Events"(SRE) (Table 7.1) by the

Table 7.1. Serious Reportable Events, National Healthcare Quality Report, Agency for Healthcare Research and Quality, 2007.

Surgical Events

Surgery performed on the wrong body part

Surgery performed on the wrong patient

Wrong surgical procedure performed on a patient

Unintended retention of a foreign object in a patient after surgery or other procedure

Intraoperative or immediately postoperative death in an ASA Class I patient

Product or Device Events

Patient death or serious disability associated with the use of contaminated drugs, devices or biologics provided by the healthcare facility

Patient death or serious disability associated with the use or function of a device in patient care in which the device is used or functions other than is intended

Patient death or serious disability associated with the intravascular air embolism that occurs while being cared for in a healthcare facility

Patient Protection Events

Infant discharged to the wrong person

Patient death or serious disability associated with patient elopement (disappearance)

Patient suicide, or attempted suicide, resulting in serious disability while being cared for in a healthcare facility

Care Management Events

Patient death or serious disability associated with a medication error

Patient death or serious disability associated with a hemolytic reaction due to the administration of ABO/HLA incompatible blood or blood products

Maternal death or serious disability associated with labor or delivery in a low-risk pregnancy while being cared for in a healthcare facility

Patient death or serious disability associated with hypoglycemia, the onset of which occurs while the patient is being cared for in a healthcare facility

(continued)

Table 7.1. (continued)

Death or serious disability (kernicterus) associated with failure to identify and treat hyperbilirubinemia in neonates

Stage 3 or 4 pressure ulcers acquired after admission to a healthcare facility

Patient death or serious disability due to spinal manipulative therapy

Artificial insemination with the wrong donor sperm or wrong egg

Criminal Events

Any instance of care ordered by or provided by someone impersonating a physician, nurse, pharmacist, or other licensed healthcare provider

Abduction of a patient of any age

Sexual assault on a patient within or on the grounds of a healthcare facility

Death or significant injury of a patient or staff member resulting from a physical assault (i.e., Battery) that occurs within or on the grounds of a healthcare facility

Environmental Events

Patient death or serious disability associated with an electric shock while being cared for in a healthcare facility

Any incident in which a line designated for oxygen or other gas to be delivered to a patient contains the wrong gas or is contaminated by toxic substances

Patient death or serious disability associated with a burn incurred from any source while being cared for in a healthcare facility

Patient death or serious disability associated with a fall while being cared for in a healthcare facility

Patient death or serious disability associated with the use of restraints or bedrails while being cared for in a healthcare facility

National Quality Forum, a nonprofit organization composed of public and private healthcare consumers, hospitals, physicians, nurses, healthcare technology companies and other quality research groups with the goal of improving healthcare [3, 4]. Beginning in 2003, The Joint Commission on Accreditation of Healthcare Organizations (JCAHO) has required reporting of SRE or sentinel events for root cause analysis. Root cause analysis is a method of thoroughly investigating all of the thoughts and actions which preceded the adverse event to identify the true underlying cause, which if corrected may prevent the event in the future. Although there are several methods to complete an analysis or investigation, the analysis is typically conducted *after* an adverse event. When used appropriately by a team experienced in these methods, it can also be an important *preventive* tool that a healthcare system must utilize to mitigate hazards and prevent recurrence.

The Universal Protocol was initiated by the Joint Commission Board of Commissioners to prevent wrong site, wrong procedure, and wrong patient procedures. This was in response to continuing and increasing occurrences of wrong site, wrong procedure, wrong patient surgery as well as several high visibility cases [5]. The protocol was created in 2003 and implemented in 2004. It was further revised in 2009 after obtaining endorsement and consensus from groups including the American Medical Association, American Hospital Association, American College of Physicians, American College of Surgeons, American Dental Association, and the American Academy of Orthopaedic Surgeons and other leading professional associations [6]. The three principle components of the Universal Protocol are conducting a pre-procedure verification process, marking the procedure site, and performing a time out before the procedure [6].

The incidence of wrong site surgery is unknown. Due to the concerns for litigation and inconsistent reporting, current national estimates probably underestimate the true occurrence of wrong site surgery. Near misses and wrong site surgeries without drastic consequences are also unlikely to be included in these estimates. Yet extrapolated data from malpractice claims during a 20-year period estimate that one wrong site procedure occurs in 112,994 total procedures performed, while other studies estimate one in every 15,000–30,000 procedures performed [3], or in busy hospitals one case in every 5–10 years [7]. The most described wrong site surgery is actually wrong side surgery. Reports demonstrate 50% or more of wrong site surgeries are performed on the incorrect side, only 11–15% of procedures are the wrong procedure, and only 3–13% of procedures are performed on the wrong patient [3, 7]. It is estimated that a surgeon who operates on bilateral structures has an almost 25% lifetime risk of wrong site surgery in their career [3, 8].

Numerous factors have been identified that may increase the risk of wrong site surgery. These frequently include multiple surgeons participating in the same operation. Also, multiple procedures during one operation, or other factors such as time pressures, emergency surgery, abnormal anatomy, and morbid obesity increase the risk of wrong site surgery [9]. An inordinately large number of insurance claims have been identified with orthopedic cases, but this percentage must be weighed with the volume of cases and frequent laterality of procedures. Additionally, wrong site surgery occurs with some frequency in spine cases where the wrong vertebral level is operated on. This has prompted specific protocols to properly identify the proposed vertebral level in spine surgery [10]. This is particularly germane to minimally invasive surgeons who provided laparoscopic access to the chest or retroperitoneum for spine surgery. Other cited factors identified in individual root cause analyses include poor communication, competing tasks assigned to OR personnel, unusual equipment or setup, staffing problems, and changes in nursing staff during the case, all of which underscore the importance of the accurate flow of information [4, 5, 11].

In the ensuing years after implementation of the Universal Protocol, and particularly the surgical timeout, evidence of decreased medical errors and decreased patient deaths has not been realized to the extent the authors of the IOM report required [2, 3, 9, 10]. There have been various degrees and inconsistent implementation of the IOM recommended strategies to achieve their stated goals and there has been little evidence that the goals have been achieved. Much speculation is published about the reasons for failure; inaccurate reporting systems, infrequent occurrence of such events and others. Gawande et al. [2] believe that we are not using the appropriate tools to evaluate success. In an effort to interpret currently published data the authors explain that if one looks only at the absolute decrease in number of individual deaths or decrease in preventable injuries, implementation of the Universal Protocol has not been effective. The success, however, of the Universal Protocol, may be better appreciated if you evaluate additional important outcomes, such as evidence-based improvement in quality and performance of the healthcare system as a whole or improvements in statistical lives saved, a method of looking at improved outcomes in a broad population. This may be more difficult to measure in a quantitative way, and the outcomes will not necessarily be observed immediately, but there is some evidence already that these outcomes are improving.

In 2008, in an effort to further improve patient safety and postoperative outcomes the World Health Organization (WHO) expanded upon the Universal Protocol. A 19-point checklist was suggested in their Safe Surgery Saves Lives Campaign/Global Patient Safety Challenge. Briefly, the checklist includes three portions: (1) a surgical *sign in* prior to the induction of anesthesia where the patient's identity is confirmed and the patient risk is assessed and the perioperative plan is discussed, (2) a *time-out* prior to incision confirming patient identity, team member identification, antibiotic administration, critical events, and (3) a *sign-out* before the patient leaves the operating room which discusses handling of the specimen, correct documentation of the procedure performed and key findings. In an effort to validate the WHO recommendations, the Safe Surgery Saves Lives Study Group designed a study to evaluate the effectiveness of the checklist. This was a multi-institutional, multinational study set in eight cities with prospectively collected data on processes and outcomes. The primary endpoints included the rate of complications and death during hospitalization and over the following 30 days. The study found an average of 36% decrease in postoperative complications and deaths over all of the sites [12, 13]. This expanded checklist is not yet a JCAHO requirement, but many institutions such as the Cleveland Clinic Florida have begun using the checklist in the operating rooms.

As the name implies, Universal Protocol is applicable to all surgical procedures. How the protocol is implemented depends on the nature of the surgery and the institution's regulations. For laparoscopic and endoscopic surgeons, there are many opportunities to observe the surgical timeout and implement changes which may improve patient safety and eliminate wrong site surgery. These may range from reviewing operative strategy with OR staff preoperatively reviewing pertinent radiography and running through the operative procedure with the other operating staff and assistants. Additionally, discussing equipment needs preoperatively is particularly important in laparoscopic procedures which require very specialized equipment, e.g., energy devices, staplers, assistant requirements, etc. Confirming tumor location and preoperative endoscopic marking in patients with colon cancers or polyps, and requiring the primary surgeon to be present for and to assist with patient positioning may be other strategies to consider. The post-procedure time-out or debriefing is another important opportunity in laparoscopy. During this time, the team has the assignment to review equipment malfunctions, inspect the instruments that were used and discuss any events or near misses which delayed, complicated or improved the case. It is important to foster an environment in the operating room of patient safety above all else. This process levels the traditional hierarchies to create an environment where any team member is encouraged and expected to speak up and appropriately discuss any concerns he or she may have about patient safety and specifically wrong site surgery. This must be a top-down process in order for it to be effective and requires the surgeons to champion this process.

Retained Foreign Bodies

Another important patient safety issue that involves surgical patients is postoperatively retained foreign bodies. Retained foreign bodies have long been described in medical literature, including instruments, retractors, needles, and laparotomy pads in any and all cavities. The first case reported was a lost "sea sponge" in 1859 [14]. Since then this topic has been the subject of much debate, literature, and litigation. The most commonly reported retained foreign body is either a 4×4 gauze sponge or a laparotomy pad. No surgical specialty and no operative field are without risk for retained foreign bodies. There have been reports of sponges found years after spine surgery, as well as retained foreign bodies in the eye, the mandible, the chest, and most commonly the abdomen and pelvis, including the vagina.

Retained foreign bodies can manifest in many different ways depending on the object left behind and the cavity or site in which it is retained. Given that more than half of foreign bodies are left in the abdomen, abdominal pain and or mass is the most common presentation. About 50% of abdominal retained foreign bodies become symptomatic, with symptoms including the aforementioned abdominal pain, erosion into the bowel or vessels, abscess formation, fistula formation, obstruction, or bleeding. [15]. Needles and sharps may also be retained in the patient, but there are fewer reported cases. Needles smaller than 13 mm are difficult to identify on plain radiographs; however, it has been suggested that needles of this size are rarely symptomatic and clinically relevant. [14]. Although foreign bodies have been found up to 30 years after being left in the patient, or even at autopsy, the median time to discovery is less than 1 month after surgery [16].

Since 2005, JCAHO mandates reporting of retained foreign bodies. It requires hospitals to perform a root cause analysis after each sentinel event. The incidence of retained foreign bodies is reported at approximately one case per 8,000–18,000 operations, or about one case per year in a busy institution [7, 10, 14]. As with wrong site surgery, the actual incidence is likely much higher in reality for the following reasons. Despite the JCAHO reporting mandate, many retained foreign bodies are either not discovered, discovered much later or are not reported due to fear of litigation or loss of public confidence and lost revenue. That is why it is important to maintain a certain level of suspicion if a patient has unexplained complaints after an operation, even after many years. Currently, computerized tomography (CT) is the best imaging method to detect items inadvertently left behind [14, 15]. It is not, however, without its limitations. Sponges or needles can be mistaken for calcifications, wires, or surgical clips. Surgical instruments are retained less frequently, but can be more easily identified on plain radiographs or other imaging.

After the 1999 IOM report *To Err is Human* and the increased awareness about patient safety, there has been a lot of effort placed on determining the factors that increase the risk of leaving a surgical foreign body in a patient. Many factors have been suggested to contribute to the risk. Those factors identified most consistently in the literature include emergency operations, unplanned changes in the operative plan, and increased body mass index of the patient or poor communication. Other studies identify multiple procedures at one time, multiple surgical teams, and an incorrect sponge count [11, 14–17]. Other factors considered important but not identified as statistically significant include changes in nursing staff, increased blood loss, and fatigue of the surgical team [13]. It should be noted, however, that a falsely correct count is identified in 88% of cases. The surgical count, therefore, is unfortunately not enough to prevent these occurrences and relies heavily on human performance and is, as such, subject to error.

Strategies to prevent retained foreign bodies will need to be applicable across a wide variety of situations. As one review points out, there is no mandatory method of performing surgical counts or any other method to prevent retaining surgical items. The only standard is that no item be left unintentionally in the patient [16]. Performing needle, instrument and sponge counts as mentioned earlier may be subject to many errors of miscounts which include counting items more than once, not at all, or just errors in addition. Other factors that distract the count process include frequent interruptions and time constraints. In addition, the failure of the surgeon to appropriately address incorrect counts can lead to retained foreign bodies. In many institutions, not all operations even require counts, despite published data showing retained foreign bodies in nearly all procedures large or small.

Although imperfect, the surgical count is an important process in the frontline of preventing retained objects. Improvements can be made by standardizing the way the count is performed, and specifically requiring it be performed for every procedure performed, including gynecologic procedures and vaginal deliveries. A hospital should be obligated to provide the appropriate personnel, funds, and policy enforcement needed to carry out surgical counts in a responsible manner. In addition to improving the performance of counts, the surgeon should make a focused effort to methodically evaluate the cavity prior to closing. One proposed strategy to prevent retained objects, Gibbs et al. suggest a technique which emphasizes using both sight and touch to thoroughly investigate major cavities in a standardized fashion [13]. The surgeon should also require the use of only those sponges and products which are appropriate for use in the designated cavity. For example, by limiting or altogether avoiding the use of small 4×4 gauzes in an open abdomen, or choosing only towels with radio-opaque markers instead of draping towels if such an item must be used. Additionally, the surgeon should be aware of when the count is being performed, accept the time commitment required to complete this thoroughly and accurately, minimize interruptions or requests for instruments and make every effort to have completed at least one correct count prior to closure of the cavity. Another proposed strategy which should be strongly considered by each institution is developing an institutional policy to address incorrect counts. We have created a sample algorithm to address this (see Fig. 7.1). This will decrease the potential for variability or conflict when an incorrect count is identified.

To overcome human error, other strategies for preventing retained foreign bodies prior to closing or leaving the OR have been suggested. One good strategy that has been implemented by some institutions is selectively requiring plain radiographs prior to leaving the OR (closing films), while others mandate radiographs with every surgical procedure. These techniques are not fail-proof either. It is important to recognize that the interpretation of radiographs can be faulty as well. Films should be reviewed by the operating surgeon along and a radiologist, as it has been shown to be statistically less likely to retain a surgical foreign body when films are read by the radiologist rather than relying only on the surgeon. Film quality varies, objects can be misinterpreted, and thus radiographic imaging cannot be the sole method relied upon for detecting or preventing retained foreign bodies. When used in conjunction with a well-performed count, radiography should prove cost-effective and the benefits provided will outweigh the negligible radiation exposure to the patient and OR personnel. This is particularly true in high risk situations, such as those patients with a high body mass index, emergency operations, those with intra-operative changes in procedure, or procedures with an incorrect count.

The need for patient safety has spurred the adaptation of existing technologies and invention of new technologies with remarkably good results. Some that deserve mentioning are the electronic article surveillance, use of two-dimensional bar codes on sponges, and radiofrequency identification tags [14]. Electronic Article Surveillance adapts current technology used in video stores and other places. The target, specifically the sponge is specifically tagged with a magnetic marker, and a portable detecting device is swept over the cavity. A sound is emitted when a retained marker is identified. Similarly, a radiofrequency identification tag may be incorporated into sponges and detected with a handheld wand. These chips are smaller and act as transponders, receiving and sending signals from the scanner. Both systems were found to have

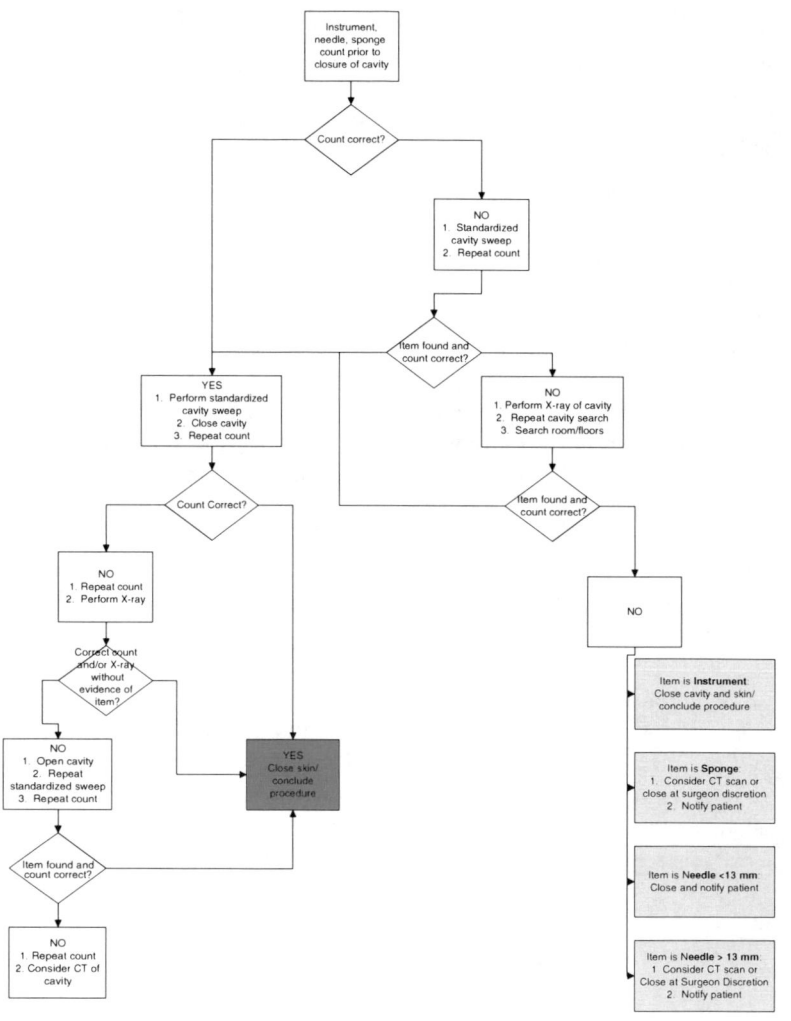

Fig. 7.1. Incorrect Count Algorithm.

nearly 100% sensitivity and specificity in cadaver studies. The bar code system also involves labeling sponges. The item with a bar code is scanned using an electronic scanner similar to that in a department store. Sponges are scanned prior to being placed on the instrument table and after coming off the back table. The device records which items are scanned in and out, identifies if one is left behind at the end of the case, and can print out a "receipt" at the end of the case. Some of these technologies are already in use at various hospitals across the country. It is important to remember that these tools can be used in conjunction with the previously mentioned efforts at preventing retained foreign bodies. Accuracy should be dramatically improved when responsible counts are performed, appropriate techniques and items are used during the operation, and new technologies are applied appropriately.

Minimally invasive surgeries present a unique set of circumstances for inadvertently leaving behind a foreign body. Although used less frequently, surgical sponges can be introduced into the operative cavity and must be accurately accounted for prior to and after the case. The field of vision is limited and the possibilities of retaining a surgical instrument or part of an instrument, sponge, or needle are potentially increased. The use of trocars and other instruments with multiple parts provides the opportunity to retain an item which might be difficult to detect radiographically. There are multiple reports of fragments of trocars, instrument tips, and surgical needles breaking off and being left within the abdomen after laparoscopic surgeries. Specimens intended for removal are frequently set aside, either in a collection bag or unmarked and can easily be forgotten. In addition to performing the surgical counts, it would be wise to inspect laparoscopic instruments and trocars as part of the count or include this inspection as part of the sign-out as described earlier in the chapter. The sign-out should also include instructions to the nursing team on how to handle the specimen. If the specimen remains in the patient, it should be identified at this time, prior to end of anesthesia and leaving the operating room. Despite the unique risk they present for leaving behind a foreign body, minimally invasive techniques have been just as widely described in the literature for retrieving retained foreign bodies. Typically this is better accomplished early in the postoperative course and is not accomplished as easily with retained sponges, however, laparoscopy and thoracoscopy have been used as late as 14 years after the original procedure with good success.

The best detection method is prevention. Communication with OR staff, anesthesiologist and radiologists is important and cannot be overemphasized. If an object is left behind, the surgeon should avoid delay in diagnosis to the best of his or her ability. Be upfront and honest about the event and accept responsibility for remedying the problem. With heightened awareness and rapidly emerging techniques and technologies, the goal of completely eliminating these "never events" becomes more achievable.

Selected Readings

1. To Err is Human: Building a Safer Health System. http://www.iom.edu/~/media/Files/ Report%20Files/1999/To-Err-is-Human/To%20Err%20is%20Human%201999%20 %20report%20brief.ashx.

2. Brennan T, Gawande A, Thomas E, Studdert D. Accidental deaths, saved lives, and improved quality. N Engl J Med. 2005;353:1405–9.

3. Clark J, Johnston J, Blanco M, Martindell D. Wrong-site surgery: can we prevent it? Adv Surg. 2008;42:13–31.

4. Christian CK, Gustafson ML, Roth EM, et al. A prospective study of patient safety in the operating room. Surgery. 2006;139(2):159–73.

5. Gibbs VC, Coakley FD, Reines HD. Preventable errors in the operating room – part 2: retained foreign objects, sharps injuries, and wrong site surgery. Curr Prbl Surg. 2007;44:352–81.

6. Facts about the Universal Protocol – Joint Commission. 2010. http://www. jointcommission.org/PatientSafety/UniversalProtocol/up_facts.htm. Accessed 19 May 2010.

7. Kwaan M, Studdert D, Zinner M, Gawande A. Incidence, patterns, and prevention of wrong-site surgery. Arch Surg. 2006;141:353–8.

8. Canale ST. Wrong-site surgery, a preventable complication. Clin Orthop Relat Res. 2005;433:26–9.

9. Michaels R, Makary M, Dahab Y, et al. Achieving the national quality forum's "never events" prevention of wrong site, wrong procedure, wrong patient operations. Ann Surg. 2007;245:526–32.

10. DeVine J, Chutkan N, Norvell DC, Dettori JR. Avoiding wrong site surgery, a systematic review. Spine. 2010;35:S25–36.

11. Gibbs VC. Patient safety practices in the operating room: correct-site surgery and nothing left behind. Surg Clin N Am. 2005;85:1307–19.

12. Weiser TG, Hanes AB, Dziekan G, Berry WR, Lipsitz SR, Gawande AA. Effect of a 19-item surgical safety checklist during urgent operations in a global patient population. Ann Surg. 2010;251:976–80.

13. Haynes A, Weiser T, Berry W, et al. A surgical safety checklist to reduce morbidity and mortality in a global population. N Engl J Med. 2009;360:491–9.

14. Gibbs VC, Coakley FD, Reines HD. Preventable errors in the operating room: retained foreign bodies after surgery – Part I. Curr Probl Surg. 2007;44:281–337.

15. Wan W, Le T, Riskin L, Macario A. Improving safety in the operating room: a systematic literature review of retained surgical sponges. Curr Opin Anaesthesiol. 2009;22:207–14.

16. Gawande A, Studdert D, Orav EJ, Brennan T, Zinner M. Risk factors for retained instruments and sponges after surgery. N Engl J Med. 2003;348:229–35.

17. Lincourt AE, Harrell A, Cristiano J, Sechrist C, Kercher K, Henifor BT. Retained foreign bodies after surgery. J Surg Res. 2007;138:170–4.

8. SAGES Laparoscopic Surgery Safety Checklist

Esteban Varela and L. Michael Brunt

Introduction

Laparoscopic surgery has become the preferred approach for a wide variety of intra-abdominal pathology. As a result, hundreds of thousands of laparoscopic procedures are undertaken in the USA every year. For example, approximately 500,000 laparoscopic cholecystectomies and 200,000 laparoscopic gastric bypasses alone are being performed yearly. Surgical complications such as wound infections and postoperative bleeding account for nearly half of all surgical adverse events and many of these are thought to be potentially preventable [1].

Laparoscopic surgery has increased the complexity of commonly performed abdominal procedures which require not only additional surgical expertise, but also involve the use of sophisticated laparoscopic and energy equipment as well as increased demands on the operating room staff for set-up and troubleshooting of equipment. It has been shown that structured surgical team behaviors and preoperative checklists and briefings improve perioperative outcomes [2, 3]. Furthermore, a surgical safety checklist has demonstrated to significantly decrease morbidity and mortality in global populations [4]. Therefore, a safety checklist specific to laparoscopic surgery appears to be a reasonable strategy given the additional complexity that laparoscopy brings to the operating environment and may prove in the future to provide similar beneficial outcome effects.

In this chapter, we present the evidence for preoperative surgical safety checklists and propose the use of the SAGES Laparoscopic Surgery Safety Checklist during laparoscopic surgery.

D.S. Tichansky, J. Morton, and D.B. Jones (eds.), *The SAGES Manual of Quality, Outcomes and Patient Safety*, DOI 10.1007/978-1-4419-7901-8_8, © Springer Science+Business Media, LLC 2012

Surgical Safety Checklists

In 2008, the World Health Organization (WHO) and the Safe Surgery Saves Lives Program published safety guidelines for surgical patients with the goal to strengthen the commitment of clinical staff to address safety issues within the operative environment [5]. These guidelines included improving anesthetic safety practices, ensuring correct site surgery, minimizing the risk of surgical site infections, and improving communication within the surgical team. A 19-item checklist was then designed and intended to reduce overall perioperative surgical complications (Appendix 1). However, it has been suggested that these checklists need to be customized by specialty, since items that are not relevant to the surgical specialty may actually adversely impact patient's safety [6].

The elements of the WHO Guideline for Safe Surgery checklist include a sign in before the induction of anesthesia; a time out before skin incision is made; and a sign out before the patient leaves the operating room. Using the 19-item WHO checklist, Haynes et al. showed in a prospective pre- and postintervention study that after the implementation of a surgical safety checklist, the rate of postoperative deaths and complications decreased significantly in a diverse group of hospitals [4]. Remarkably, postoperative complications and death rates fell by 36% each, the majority of which was due to a reduction in the incidence of surgical site infections. The mechanism of improvement was thought to be multifactorial which involved both system and behavioral team changes. A prospectively collected multicenter outcomes study in 1,750 patients undergoing urgent noncardiac surgery was also associated with an approximately one-third reduction in morbidity due primarily to fewer surgical infections and a lower incidence of major blood loss [7].

Similarly, during a commonly performed laparoscopic procedure, Buzink and colleagues demonstrated that the combined use of an integrated operating room system with the *Pro/cheQ* tool, a digital procedure-specific checklist, the number of risk-sensitive events was reduced by 65% during laparoscopic cholecystectomy when compared to an operating room integrated system alone [8]. Integrated operating room systems may also help prevent technical problems, improve ergonomics, reduce operating room clutter, and enhance efficiency by decreasing turnover time and improving the flow of information [9, 10].

The use of equipment checklists during laparoscopic surgery has shown to prevent problems with laparoscopic equipment by over 50% [11]. Verdaasdonk and colleagues developed a 28-item checklist based on problems that arose frequently with laparoscopic equipment.

They then piloted this checklist in 60 laparoscopic cholecystectomy cases in which half utilized the checklist and half did not. Fewer episodes of wrong patient positioning and wrong settings and connections of the equipment were noted in the checklist group and overall the checklist resulted in a 53% lower incident rate per procedure compared with controls. Another group found that a 10-step checklist during laparoscopic cholecystectomy was associated with a reduction in conversion rates to open cholecystectomy [12]. These observations suggest that a laparoscopic-specific checklist is feasible and would help reduce equipment problems and potentially improve outcomes for these commonly performed procedures. It has also been suggested that surgeons' skills coupled with basic team performance and basic surgical equipment may enable a surgeon to achieve a 90% success rate in high-risk operations [13]. In other words, poor team performance and poor equipment may lead to frustration on the part of the surgeon and, thereby, have detrimental effects on his/her performance.

The utilization of checklists in the operating room must have a full commitment from the entire surgical team and should be carried out with conscious effort and not in a superficial or perfunctory manner [14]. Checklist misuse can also have potentially detrimental effects on safety and teamwork in the operating room. In aviation, a badly performed checklist has shown to provide a false sense of security [15]. Therefore, a careful and rigorous implementation plan is required to ensure that the checklist is used routinely and correctly [16].

SAGES Laparoscopic Surgery Safety Checklist

Laparoscopic surgery, because of its inherent reliance on high technology equipment and potential for equipment failure or other technologic problems that may interfere with the conduct of the operation, requires that staff be able to solve the myriad of equipment problems that may arise. In response to this perceived need, in the 1990s the SAGES Continuing Education Committee developed the SAGES Troubleshooting Guide which was revised and updated in 2005. The guide addresses strategies to deal with problems in eight broad categories: (1) poor insufflation/loss of pneumoperitoneum; (2) excessive insufflation pressure; (3) inadequate lighting; (4) lighting too bright; (5) problems with monitor picture; (6) image quality problems; (7) inadequate suction/irrigation; and (8) problems with electrocautery. The Troubleshooting Guide is available in laminated copies or as a pdf download from the SAGES website [17].

As a part of the process to update the Troubleshooting Guide, the SAGES Laparoscopic Surgery Safety Checklist was developed to guide surgical teams in ensuring that equipment, patient position, and safety checkpoints were carried out. Much like an aviation preflight check, this document divides checklist responsibilities into three general categories: circulator nurse pre-patient entry checks, scrub nurse/technician pre-patient entry checks, and a series of checklist items that should occur after patient entry. The checklist is not intended to add to the burden of documentation that is already required by the circulating RN in the operating room, but instead should be viewed as a mechanism to eliminate reliance on human memory and to ensure that the necessary equipment is available, operational, and connected and that the OR table, patient and monitors are all properly positioned and should be used as an adjunct to the general safety parameters that are in the WHO checklist. These measures are intended to enhance efficiency, performance, and safety in the complex environment of a laparoscopic surgery suite.

The original checklist has recently been updated and modified by the SAGES Quality, Outcomes, and Safety Committee and is shown in Appendix 2. This laparoscopic checklist may be used either as the sole checklist employed on operative cases or it may be used in conjunction with the WHO or institution-specific checklists that deal with issues of patient and procedure verification, antibiotics and DVT prophylaxis, imaging availability, and others. SAGES is in the process of partnering with the Association of Operating Room Nurses (AORN) to trial the Laparoscopic Safety Checklist in multiple centers across the USA to evaluate its utility and impact on safety and efficiency in laparoscopic surgery.

Summary

The proper use of a Surgical Safety Checklist improves surgical team communication and efficiency that translates into a significant reduction in morbidity and mortality. The SAGES Laparoscopic Surgery Safety Checklist is yet another tool aimed to decrease adverse events during laparoscopic surgery. Surgical teams should work together to ensure that checklists become a routine part of every operating room culture.

Appendix 1

Surgical Safety Checklist

World Health Organization | Patient Safety
A World Alliance for Safer Health Care

Before induction of anaesthesia

(with at least nurse and anaesthetist)

Has the patient confirmed his/her identity, site, procedure, and consent?
☐ Yes

Is the site marked?
☐ Yes
☐ Not applicable

Is the anaesthesia machine and medication check complete?
☐ Yes

Is the pulse oximeter on the patient and functioning?
☐ Yes

Does the patient have a:

Known allergy?
☐ No
☐ Yes

Difficult airway or aspiration risk?
☐ No
☐ Yes, and equipment/assistance available

Risk of >500ml blood loss (7ml/kg in children)?
☐ No
☐ Yes, and two IVs/central access and fluids planned

Before skin incision

(with nurse, anaesthetist and surgeon)

Confirm all team members have introduced themselves by name and role.

Confirm the patient's name, procedure, and where the incision will be made.

Has antibiotic prophylaxis been given within the last 60 minutes?
☐ Yes
☐ Not applicable

Anticipated Critical Events

To Surgeon:
☐ What are the critical or non-routine steps?
☐ How long will the case take?
☐ What is the anticipated blood loss?

To Anaesthetist:
☐ Are there any patient-specific concerns?

To Nursing Team:
☐ Has sterility (including indicator results) been confirmed?
☐ Are there equipment issues or any concerns?

Is essential imaging displayed?
☐ Yes
☐ Not applicable

Before patient leaves operating room

(with nurse, anaesthetist and surgeon)

Nurse Verbally Confirms:
☐ The name of the procedure
☐ Completion of instrument, sponge and needle counts
☐ Specimen labelling (read specimen labels aloud, including patient name)
☐ Whether there are any equipment problems to be addressed

To Surgeon, Anaesthetist and Nurse:
☐ What are the key concerns for recovery and management of this patient?

This checklist is not intended to be comprehensive. Additions and modifications to fit local practice are encouraged   Revised 1 / 2009   © WHO, 2009

Appendix 2: SAGES/AORN Laparoscopic/MIS Surgery Safety Checklist

1. Pre-patient entry

A. Circulating nurse duties

Parameter	Actions
Surgeon Preference Card	☐ Reviewed
OR Table Position	☐ Correct orientation and weight capacity
	☐ Bean bag mattress (if indicated)
	☐ Table accessories (e.g., spreader bars/leg supports/foot board (as indicated)
	☐ Positioned for fluoroscopy if indicated
Power sources	☐ Connected and linked to all devices
CO_2 insufflator	☐ Check CO_2 volume, pressure, and flow
	☐ Backup cylinder and accessories (wrench and key) in place
	☐ Filter for CO_2 unit or tubing
Video monitors	☐ Position per procedure
	☐ Test pattern present
Suction/irrigation	☐ Cannister set
	☐ Irrigation and pressure bag available
Alarms	☐ Turned on and audible
Video documentation	☐ Recording media available and operational (DVD, print, etc.)

B. Scrub Person Duties

Parameter	Actions
Reusable instruments	☐ Check movement handles and jaws, all screws present
	☐ Check sealing caps
	☐ Instrument vents closed
	☐ Check cautery insulation
Veress needle	☐ Check plunger/spring action
	☐ Flush needle and stopcock
	☐ Saline solution available
Hasson cannula	☐ Check valves, plunger, and seals
Trocars/Ports	☐ Check appropriate size/type
	☐ Close stopcocks
Laparoscope	☐ Appropriate size and type (0° or 30°, 5 or 10 mm) for case
	☐ Check lens clarity
	☐ Anti-fog solution or warmed saline for lens cleaning

2. After Patient Entry

Parameter	Actions
Patient position	☐ Secured to OR table, safety strap on
	☐ Pressure sites padded
	☐ Arms out or tucked per procedure
Sequential compression device	☐ On and connected to device
Electrosurgical unit	☐ Ground pad applied
Foot controls	☐ Positioned for surgeon access
Power sources (camera, insufflator, light source, monitors, cautery, ultrasonics, and bipolar)	☐ Turned on
Miscellaneous	☐ Foley catheter (if indicated)
	☐ Naso- or orogastric tube (bougies if indicated)
Antibiotics	☐ Given as indicated

3. After Prep and Drape

Parameter	Actions
Electrosurgical unit	☐ Cautery cords connected to unit
Monopolar cautery	☐ Tip protected
Ultrasonic or bipolar device	☐ Connected to unit
	☐ Activation test performed
Line connections	☐ Camera cord
	☐ Light source (on standby)
	☐ CO_2 tubing (connected and flushed)
	☐ Suction/irrigation (Suction turned on)
	☐ Smoke evacuation filter connected
Local anesthetic	☐ Syringe labeled and filled with anesthetic of choice, needle connected
Fluoroscopy case	☐ Mix and dilute contrast appropriately and label
	☐ Clear tubing, syringe, catheter of air bubbles, label syringes

This checklist has been developed by SAGES and AORN to aid operating room personnel in the preparation of equipment and other duties unique to laparoscopic surgery cases. It should not supplant the surgical time out or other hospital-specific patient safety protocols. For equipment problems during laparoscopic cases, refer to the SAGES Troubleshooting Guide (www.sages.org/publications/troubleshooting/).

Selected Readings

1. Gawande AA, Thomas EJ, Zinner MJ, Brennan TA. The incidence and nature of surgical adverse events in Colorado and Utah in 1992. Surgery. 1999;126:66–75.
2. Mazzocco K, Petitti DB, Fong KT, et al. Surgical team behaviors and patient outcomes. Am J Surg. 2009;197:678–85.
3. Lingard L, Regehr G, Orser B, et al. Evaluation of a preoperative checklist and team briefing among surgeons, nurses, and anesthesiologists to reduce failures in communication. Arch Surg. 2008;143:12–7. discussion 8.
4. Haynes AB, Weiser TG, Berry WR, et al. A surgical safety checklist to reduce morbidity and mortality in a global population. N Engl J Med. 2009;360:491–9.
5. WHO. Patient Safety: Safe Surgery Saves Lives. 2009. http://wwwwhoint/patientsafety/safesurgery/en/indexhtml Acccession date 7/15/2011.
6. Clark S, Hamilton L. WHO surgical checklist. Needs to be customised by specialty. BMJ. 2010;340:c589.
7. Weiser TG, Haynes AB, Dziekan G, Berry WR, Lipsitz SR, Gawande AA. Effect of a 19-item surgical safety checklist during urgent operations in a global patient population. Ann Surg. 2010;251:976–80.
8. Buzink SN, van Lier L, de Hingh IH, Jakimowicz JJ. Risk-sensitive events during laparoscopic cholecystectomy: the influence of the integrated operating room and a preoperative checklist tool. Surg Endosc. 2010;24(8):1990–5.
9. Kenyon TA, Urbach DR, Speer JB, et al. Dedicated minimally invasive surgery suites increase operating room efficiency. Surg Endosc. 2001;15:1140–3.
10. Herron DM, Gagner M, Kenyon TL, Swanstrom LL. The minimally invasive surgical suite enters the 21st century. A discussion of critical design elements. Surg Endosc. 2001;15:415–22.
11. Verdaasdonk EG, Stassen LP, Hoffmann WF, van der Elst M, Dankelman J. Can a structured checklist prevent problems with laparoscopic equipment? Surg Endosc. 2008;22:2238–43.
12. Robb WLJ, Falk G, Waldron R, Khan W. A ten-step intra-operative checklist for laparoscopic cholecystectomy reduces conversion rates to an open procedure. Br J Surg. 2009;96:50.
13. Vincent C, Moorthy K, Sarker SK, Chang A, Darzi AW. Systems approaches to surgical quality and safety: from concept to measurement. Ann Surg. 2004;239:475–82.
14. Keane MJ, Marshall SD. Implementation of the World Health Organisation Surgical Safety Checklist: implications for anaesthetists. Anaesth Intensive Care. 2010;38:397–8.
15. Degani A, Wiener EL. Procedures in complex systems: the airline cockpit. IEEE Trans Syst Man Cybern A Syst Hum. 1997;27:302–12.
16. Vats A, Vincent CA, Nagpal K, Davies RW, Darzi A, Moorthy K. Practical challenges of introducing WHO surgical checklist: UK pilot experience. BMJ. 2010;340:b5433.
17. SAGES. The Society of American Gastrointestinal Endoscopic Surgeons Laparoscopy Troubleshooting Guide & Operative Checklist. 2010. http://wwwsagesorg/publications/troubleshooting/ Acccession date 7/15/2011.

9. Faculty Hour: A Model for Interdisciplinary Quality Improvement in the Perioperative Setting

Sharon Muret-Wagstaff and Brett A. Simon

Background

Clinicians who are committed to quality and patient safety frequently lack the means and infrastructure to implement and sustain the interdisciplinary collaboration needed to actualize system improvement. Insufficient time and opportunities exist to build communication, consensus, respect, collaboration, and teamwork. Clinical schedules prevent operating room-based faculty and staff from participating in both service meetings and career development training, and it is increasingly difficult to engage faculty in activities that could lead to clinical improvements because of production demands. Additionally, many clinicians feel that current performance benchmarks are created top-down and do not fully reflect the thoughtful, skillful, insightful, experienced care that they provide.

To address these barriers, we created Faculty Hour, an interdepartmental partnership initiative uniting departments of surgery, anesthesia, nursing, orthopedics, obstetrics and gynecology, and others in a 621-bed, two-campus New England academic medical center. We were encouraged by historical successes of local discrete projects, such as the interdisciplinary development of cardiac surgery guidelines for clinicians and patients, outstanding performance on Surgical Care Improvement Project (SCIP) measures, and implementation of interdisciplinary briefings and checklists. However, we recognized the need to support and spread these kinds of efforts systematically as well as create an outlet for provider-initiated care improvement projects.

D.S. Tichansky, J. Morton, and D.B. Jones (eds.), *The SAGES Manual of Quality, Outcomes and Patient Safety*, DOI 10.1007/978-1-4419-7901-8_9, © Springer Science+Business Media, LLC 2012

Overview

Faculty Hour affords surgeons, anesthesiologists, nurses, and others the opportunity to meet together at the start of the day once each week to advance quality and outcomes for patients, to accelerate learning and innovation, and to foster mutual joy in work. Each Tuesday, start time for all operating rooms is moved forward by 30 min (8:00 a.m.) to accommodate 6:45 a.m. Faculty Hour sessions. This allows unopposed 45-min meetings for multiple groups as well as travel and clinical preparation time to be carved out.

Getting Started

We began by soliciting input and securing support from hospital leaders and department chairs, and by reviewing hospital and department missions. We also were cognizant of the hospital's two bold goals: (1) eliminate all preventable harm and (2) rank in the top 2% of US hospitals for creating a consistently excellent patient experience by January 1, 2012. We used a Baldrige-based assessment of organizational performance [2], clinical data review, results from a Hospital Survey on Patient Safety Culture [1] elucidating staff attitudes, and a faculty development survey to determine faculty and perioperative needs and priorities. A steering committee composed of department chairs, senior faculty, and nursing leaders then created a balanced scorecard of metrics [8] to guide formation of initial chartered teams, infrastructure, support, communication mechanisms, and scheduling and logistics.

Components

Each 90-day cycle of Faculty Hour is composed of multiple, simultaneous weekly offerings (Table 9.1), including:

- Two chartered interdisciplinary project teams (10–12 members) that meet weekly
- Sustain the Gains meetings monthly or quarterly for prior chartered teams
- Quarterly meetings for 13 traditional anesthesiology department divisions (e.g., cardiac and thoracic) and cross-cutting groups (quality and education)

Table 9.1. Faculty Hour model – 90-day cycle by week (Tuesdays, 6:45–7:30 a.m.).

Group	Month 1				Month 2				Month 3			
Chartered teams	X	X	X	X	X	X	X	X	X	X	X	X
Sustain the gains		X					X				X	
Departmental division meetings	X				X				X	X		
Interdisciplinary division meetings		X				X						
Departmental faculty development theme			X	X			X	X			X	
Quarterly review												X
Combined patient safety grand rounds (Wednesday)	X											

- Quarterly interdisciplinary division meetings for 11 groups of surgeons, anesthesiologists, and nurses
- Several faculty development theme sessions in departments
- Quarterly review of departmental highlights, metrics, and upcoming plans
- Quarterly review of Faculty Hour results during multidisciplinary Patient Safety Grand Rounds and plans for the next 90-day cycle.

Each 90-day chartered team has an aim and scope statement endorsed by the steering committee, a steering committee sponsor, and, in some cases, a management engineering facilitator. Triad leadership of each team consists of a surgeon, an anesthesiologist, and a nurse chosen for both their content expertise and their strong relationship and communication skills. They meet in advance with steering committee members to refine the scope statement and recruit a balanced team from all relevant disciplines, from frontline staff to division directors. The team has great flexibility in how it addresses its aim. For example, a Reducing Hazards in the OR Team fashioned its splash injury reduction plans based in part on a successful community health intervention focused on use of eyewear by Latino farm workers [6]. A discovery subgroup from each chartered team also makes one trip outside the usual environment to stimulate learning and innovation. Examples of chartered teams include the following:

- A "Joint Replacement" Team worked to optimize multiple aspects of perioperative care of patients undergoing arthroplasty, including reorganizing the operating room layout to minimize traffic near the sterile field to reduce surgical site infection risk.

- A "Communicating for Safety in the OR" Team elicited more than 200 responses from perioperative staff to determine local priorities for better communication and organized an interactive grand rounds for multidisciplinary education.
- An "OR Team Training with Simulation" Team developed and launched a 5-h, high fidelity simulation-based training curriculum focused on the use of checklists, speaking up, and closed loop communication – issues determined through analysis of local claim data. The training is now offered monthly to interdisciplinary OR groups in the simulation center at our hospital. CRICO/RMF, a patient safety and medical malpractice company, provides a 10% insurance discount for surgeons who complete the training.
- A "Bridge Flow Diagnostics" Team analyzed pre- to postoperative patient flow patterns that had frustrated patients and staff alike for 13 years, resulting in a follow-up implementation project "Optimizing Patient Arrival in the OR" Team.
- A "Reducing Hazards in the OR" Team worked on splash injury protection, and spawned evidence-based projects to promote blunt needle use and to establish safe passing zones for sharps to reduce injuries.

Our ultimate portfolio of projects is intended to be a mix of big bets, promising midrange ideas to be tested, and a broad base of early-stage ideas or incremental innovations [7].

We learned early that team accomplishments can easily be lost without a plan for sustainability, and thus we established "Sustain the Gains" follow-up sessions during Faculty Hour for teams to reunite periodically to monitor new processes and make changes as needed. The leaders and team members also must continue to build coalitions and advocate for the team's efforts with others in order for their solutions to be well-received, supported, and diffused in the mainstream institution.

Separate from the chartered team projects, subspecialty divisions form a basis for quarterly intra- and inter-departmental faculty development, academic, and care improvement activities. Within the Department of Anesthesiology, each division sets its own goals, metrics, and proposed projects aligned with the Faculty Hour balanced scorecard. One division, for example, set the goal of training all division faculty in the performance of transversus abdominis plane (TAP) blocks while another designed a protocol to improve readiness for early extubation in cardiac surgery patients. To ensure productive interdisciplinary division meetings, the division chiefs create formal meeting agendas that are agreed upon in advance by the respective team leaders and that are appropriate and of interest to each constituency. Interdisciplinary specialty-specific approaches have included case conferences addressing complex or controversial management issues, design of perioperative clinical research projects to address areas where evidence for best practices is lacking, and joint efforts to find solutions to mutual challenges, such as the multidisciplinary structuring of hand-offs for neurosurgical cases in the operating room.

On alternate weeks from the division meetings, department members who are not part of chartered teams participate in sessions planned by each department. In Anesthesia, for example, faculty have participated in clinical innovation workshops to refresh clinical skills and introduce new techniques and technologies, and carried out a 90-day initiative in which faculty explored and adapted educational methods that demonstrably improved the frequency and usefulness of clinical performance feedback given to residents.

Preliminary Results

In the first year of operation, each chartered team has achieved at least one planned, tangible result to improve clinical care, operations, or staff safety and satisfaction. A newly formed hospital Patient and Family Advisory Council has agreed to provide input to teams and review Faculty Hour progress, which we anticipate will increase the effectiveness and patient-centeredness of our work. Clinicians take pride in team accomplishments and comment on new levels of respect and the pleasure of joint problem-solving. No one has refused an invitation to lead or be part of a team. The steering committee has received a growing number of new ideas generated by staff for ways to use Faculty Hour to improve patient care quality and outcomes, and conflicts are arising as clinicians must sometimes choose between work on two or more different projects. Ironically, on-time starts in the operating room are more frequent on Faculty Hour Tuesdays than on any other day of the week.

Discussion

The Faculty Hour model affords clinicians new opportunities to collaborate and communicate among disciplines to improve not only care delivery, but organizational performance on multiple levels in ways that matter to patients and clinicians. While collaboration, communication, and teamwork are central to good outcomes for surgical patients as well as staff recruitment and retention [4, 9, 10], infrastructure and mechanisms to learn and improve together in the fast-paced, high-intensity operative environment often are lacking. Leape and colleagues assert that "safety does not depend just on measurement, practices and rules, nor does it depend on any specific improvement methods; it depends on achieving a culture of trust, reporting, transparency and discipline." Furthermore, they point to evidence that "caregivers cannot meet the challenge of making healthcare safe unless they feel valued and find joy and meaning in their work" (2009, pp. 424–5).

Achieving such a culture is not easy. In particular, simply making time for interdisciplinary relationship-building and improvement is challenging. For example, in a recent 32-site study to improve perioperative communication and teamwork, researchers resorted to shutting down operating rooms for a day to carry out the core intervention. Participants noted "how rare and valuable it was to have all OR staff in one room at the same time and discuss how to improve communication" [11].

Finally, ineffective faculty development approaches such as didactic presentations persist despite new understandings of better ways to advance interprofessional efforts and learning, such as through series of interactive sessions [3, 5, 12].

We sought an approach that would overcome these obstacles and foster innovation [7] without disrupting the organization [8]. The Faculty Hour model is broad in scope yet tightly focused through chartered team initiatives and a set of overall goals that are clarified and communicated through a balanced scorecard; regular and ongoing overall while segmented in well-defined, 90-day participatory cycles; and sustainable due to its simplicity. It is designed to be responsive and molded to meet emerging faculty and clinical needs and interests. Ninety-day projects, in addition to targeting specific clinical needs, have created numerous new opportunities for the development of leadership skills and professional ties that may spill over into enhanced system operations. We anticipate that Faculty Hour will continue to evolve in both structure and function as these needs change and new opportunities to improve quality and safety arise.

Conclusions

We have demonstrated the feasibility of a simple but promising approach to removing common barriers that surgeons, anesthesiologists, nurses, and others face in attempts to work synergistically to improve healthcare systems and outcomes in the demanding perioperative setting. The Faculty Hour model, built on evidence gleaned from studies in improvement science, interprofessional collaboration, faculty development, and innovation, can be adapted and implemented in a systematic and sustainable way without restructuring, closing the OR, or suffering adverse impact on daily operating room efficiency.

Selected Readings

1. Agency for Healthcare Research and Quality. Hospital Survey on Patient Safety Culture. Gaithersburg, MD: AHRQ, 2010. http://www.ahrq.gov/qual/patientsafetyculture/. Accessed 19 Oct 2010.
2. Baldrige Performance Excellence Program. Are We Making Progress? Gaithersburg, MD: National Institute of Standards and Technology, 2008. http://www.nist.gov/baldrige/publications/progress.cfm. Accessed 19 Oct 2010.
3. Bloom BS. Effects of continuing medical education on improving physician clinical care and patient health: A review of systematic reviews. Int J Technol Assess Health Care. 2005;21(3):380–5.
4. Committee on Quality of Health Care in America, Institute of Medicine. Crossing the Quality Chasm: A New Health System for the 21st Century. Washington, DC: National Academy Press; 2001.
5. Davis D, O'Brien MAT, Freemantle N, Wolf FM, Mazmanian P, Taylor-Vaisey A. Impact of formal continuing medical education. Do conferences, workshops, rounds, and other traditional continuing education activities change physician behavior or health care outcomes? JAMA. 1999;282(9):867–74.
6. Forst L, Lacey S, Chen HY, Jimenez R, Bauer S, Skinner S, et al. Effectiveness of community health workers for promoting use of safety eyewear by Latino farm workers. Am J Ind Med. 2004;46:607–13.
7. Kanter RM. Innovation: the classic traps. Harv Bus Rev. 2006;84(11):72–83. 154.
8. Kaplan RS, Norton DP. How to implement a new strategy without disrupting your organization. Harvard Bus Rev. 2006;84(3):100–9. 150.
9. Leape L, Berwick D, Clancy C, Conway J, Bluck P, Guest J, et al. Transforming healthcare: a safety imperative. Qual Saf Health Care. 2009;18:424–8.
10. Neily J, Mills PD, Young-Xu Y, Carney BT, West P, Berger DH, et al. Association between implementation of a medical team training program and surgical mortality. JAMA. 2010;304(15):1693–700(a).

11. Neily J, Mills PD, Lee P, Carney B, West P, Percarpio K, et al. Medical team training and coaching in the veterans health administration; assessment and impact on the first 32 facilities in the programme. Qual Saf Health Care. 2010;19:360–64 (b).
12. Zwarenstein M, Goldman J, Reeves S. Interprofessional collaboration: effects of practice-based interventions on professional practice and healthcare outcomes. Cochrane Database Syst Rev. 2009;8(3):CD000072.

10. Creating Effective Communication and Teamwork for Patient Safety

Pascal Fuchshuber and William Greif

Effective Communication within a Culture for Patient Safety

> "Healthcare culture does not support high performing teamwork (…and culture eats strategy for lunch)" (IHI)

Patient Safety cannot exist outside a conducive set of behavioral norms defined as safety culture. Teamwork, effective communication, and safety culture are part of a multidimensional framework that determines quality of care (Figs. 10.1 and 10.2). Good teamwork relies on effective communication, mutual respect, problem solving, and sharing of ideas. Without that care cannot be delivered in a safe and reliable way. This is far from being the norm in today's health care environment. Many health care providers, particularly physicians, do not have a good understanding of the importance of good communication skills and where they fall short. Many nurses, when surveyed, will admit that their ability to communicate is hindered and that they would be hesitant to point out mistakes made by physicians, even though they judge good teamwork by their ability to speak up. Physicians see good teamwork and communication as the ability and effectiveness to tell others what to do and get it done.

This chapter describes who to overcome these barriers and use the tools of effective communication as the basis for delivery of safe patient care. Failed communication is the most common reason for harm to the recipient of health care. In the context of a clinical setting, effective communication is the accurate handoff and transfer of information between two or more providers. Communication fails when it is incomplete, ineffective, or inappropriate. The result is patient harm, i.e., substandard care because of missing and inadequate information. The importance of

D.S. Tichansky, J. Morton, and D.B. Jones (eds.), *The SAGES Manual of Quality, Outcomes and Patient Safety*, DOI 10.1007/978-1-4419-7901-8_10, © Springer Science+Business Media, LLC 2012

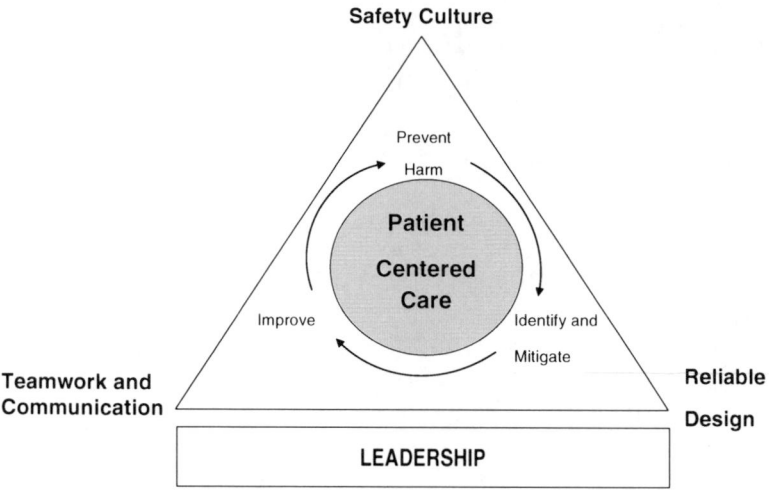

Fig. 10.1. Delivering Safe care – Institute of Health Care Improvement Model (IHI Boston Patient Safety Officers Curriculum, 2010).

The top 5 most commonly identified contributing factors of preventable adverse outcomes

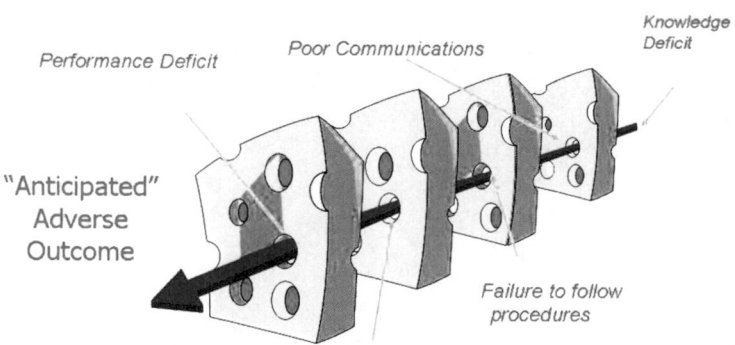

Fig. 10.2. Effective Communication is one of the five basic tools to prevent patient harm. (IHI Boston Patient Safety Officers Curriculum, 2010).

understanding why this happens and what is the context of communication within health care organizations cannot be overemphasized.

The primary root causes of failed communications are poor handoffs, the failure to read back and confirm the information given, the inability to share information due to fear of authority and retaliation, and the assumption that outcome and safety of care is as expected and does not need to be checked.

The foundation of effective communication is an environment that promotes consistent high-quality care, is free of retaliation and blame, encourages learning from mistakes, supports interactions between patients, families, and providers within a safe, satisfying and rewarding work place.

There are many reasons why it is difficult to achieve effective communication within a health care organization. Briefly, some of the fundamental and pervasive issues are:

(a) *Teamwork* – Clinical medicine is a very complex environment with quickly changing parameters, unpredictability, incomplete data, and frequent task interruptions. Building on teamwork does largely mitigate the negative impact of these circumstances, thus the strong impetus to build a team approach to patient safety and care delivery.

(b) *Leadership* – Failure of leadership to recognize the importance and prioritize the implementation of effective communication and teamwork.

(c) *Training* – Failure to create and train providers to form teams that can effectively interact and are accountable for maintaining effective communication skills.

(d) *Culture* – Creating "buy-in" and the organizational value for team approaches over individual expert-thinking, particularly among health care providers steeped in autonomy and lacking effective leadership training.

(e) *Hierarchy/Psychological Safety* – Psychological safety is a belief that one will not be punished or humiliated for speaking up with ideas, questions, concerns, or mistakes. Hierarchical barriers are inherent to health care systems based on vertical authority and prevent people from "speaking-up" when a decision is questionable or a problem arises. Effective leadership by a surgeon should emphasize "flat hierarchy" by using people's name, sharing the plan of action, inviting other team members to participate in the communication and ask people directly to share questions or concerns. Psychological safety matters most in systems with a rapidly changing knowledge base, a high need for collaboration and a short decision time – classic attributes of a health care organization.

(f)   *Lack of structure* – Absence of processes that include a structured "handoff" template to ensure completeness of information, respect for all participants, and engagement in effective communication.

(g)   *Abusive and disrespectful behavior* – Failure to create a culture of universal mutual respect leading to increased risk as recognized in the Joint Commission "Sentinel Event Alert" [1]: "Intimidating and disruptive behavior can foster medical errors, contribute to poor patient satisfaction and to preventable adverse outcomes, increase the cost of care, and cause qualified clinicians, administrators, and managers to seek new positions in more professional environments." For example, if a surgeon loses temper in the OR and treats its team with disrespect, leadership has to intervene and ensure psychological safety for the members of the team. This is best done by timely intervention and demonstrating that disrespectful behavior is not tolerated within the organization. CEO, Chief Medical Officer or Patient Safety Officer are responsible to reinforce desired behavior with disregard to the vertical hierarchy of the team. For example, a surgeon behaving rudely and disrespectful in the OR is made to apologize to the team and nursing staff as soon as possible.

(h)   *Setting the tone* – Negative Example: *A surgeon runs into the OR loudly announcing that he has a meeting he cannot miss in 3 hours and a whole lot of cases to do. Get going !* Setting the stage and tone occurs within a few seconds from the beginning of a verbal communication and has a profound effect on the effectiveness of communication in the clinical setting. It is an important, trainable leadership skill for the surgeon [2]. Ideally, the surgeon as a leader tries to create a positive tone immediately by greeting each person of the team by name and setting the stage by communicating that the common value is the care of the patient, the team effort, and respectful, open collaboration. Non-negotiable mutual respect in every interaction, every day as well as accessibility, humility, and determination to get things done right are key elements of a successful surgeon team leader.

Structured Communication, Handoffs and SBAR: The Tools of the Trade

To assure effective communication in situations where specific and complex information must be exchanged and acted upon in a timely manner, structured communication techniques become essential tools. Below is a brief list of such structured communication tools with a description of their definition and use. Some of these tools are described in more detail in other chapters of this manual:

(a) *Briefings* – concise exchange of information essential to operational effectiveness involving others by (1) asking for their input, (2) using first names to encourage familiarity and lower barriers to speak up, and (3) making eye contact as well as facing the other person to reinforce their contribution and value. Briefings are most effective in procedural areas (OR, ICU, ambulatory care, etc.). It may be difficult to gain "buy-in" for briefings in the OR, particularly from surgeons inherently adverse to interference with what they perceive as their "realm." Getting physician support for briefings may be facilitated by team-training exercises in the OR, by showing the particular provider how briefings will increase the likelihood for an effective day in the OR (correct equipment, more engagement by other team members, faster turn-around) and greater patient safety by ensuring correct side surgery and therefore lower malpractice risk.

(b) *Debriefings* – should occur at the end of procedures to allow learning from what happened during the process and set the stage for the next procedure. Briefings and debriefings depend on each other and both should be as specific and detailed as possible. Typical debriefing questions:

- What was the procedure?
- Are specimens correct?
- What went well?
- What could have gone better?
- What are the next steps for this patient?
- What did we learn?
- How did we document (specimen, wound class, etc.)?
- What do we need for the next case?

(c) *Assertive Language* – It describes a communication that "speaks up" and states the information with appropriate persistence until there is resolution. The lack of assertive language skills often leads to patient harm, particularly when it is pared with the pervasive vertical authority encountered in health care organizations which inhibits the ability to speak up and to brake down hierarchical barriers. It is known that up to 40% of nurses report hesitance to speak up about mistakes in Safety Attitude Questionnaires. Because of these barriers information is typically communicated in an unclear, oblique, and indirect manner with a "hint of hope that what I said must have been heard" and "something didn't seem right but a proposed action did not occur." Effective assertion does not mean aggressive and confrontational communication but rather a polite and pleasant form of making sure one is heard in a timely and clear manner. Training and practice among team members in assertive language can be very helpful. A typical checklist to help understand the meaning and technique of assertive language is shown here:

- get the attention of the other(s)
- use names
- use eye contact
- face the other person
- state the problem concisely
- state your concern
- propose an action
- recheck if concern and action were understood
- reassert if necessary
- expect a decision that is understood by all members of the team
- escalate if no result

Assertive communication skills can be trained and are very helpful in creating a culture of safety and effective communication.

(d) *Critical Language* – briefly this is the ability to use language during a stressful and dangerous situation to avert patient harm. Again, this will work best if a flattened hierarchy has already been established. Typical sentences to illustrate this type of language are: "I am concerned/scared," "may I have a little clarity" or "let's hold for a minute and make sure we are all on the same page" or "excuse me, doctor, but I need some clarity about which breast you are going to do the mastectomy."

After the fourth or fifth breast case of the day I can easily imagine the effect of such a comment by the nurse when the tired surgeon is about to cut on the wrong side.

(e) *Common Language* – this communication tool describes a specific language around a specific event in a clinical setting that is adopted and understood by all team members. It creates a "benchmark" of how to communicate around certain event. A good example is the standardized terminology and language describing fetal heart rates by the National Institute of Child Health and Human Development (NICHD). This assures good understanding by all providers in the clinical setting of the fetal heart tracing [3]. An agreed upon language around checklists and timeout procedures is another example of the use of common language to assure reliable and effective communication.

(f) *Closed Communication Loops* – it consists of the use of read-back, whereby the recipient repeats back the concisely stated information by the sender and the sender in turn acknowledges the read-back. Corrections are made as necessary to the communicated content. This type of communication is necessary when critical content cannot be lost, for example when communicating in a dangerous environment such as a nuclear submarine, but also in the clinical setting, when confirming sponge count in the operating room or when giving telephone orders for medications. This is recognized by the Joint Commission who requires a read-back process for verbal or telephone orders as defined in the National Patient Safety Goal 2.

(g) *Callouts* – as surgeons we commonly use this communication technique in the OR to clearly indicate the timeline of the procedure in progress. Callouts should be communicated in clearly and loudly spoken simple phrases so that all team members can understand and hear. Good examples are "we are closing," "we are having difficulty and will convert to open procedure in 5 min," "we will be closing in 15 min," "start the sponge count," "I will need the ultrasound machine in 30 min."

(h) *Handoffs – "Gentlemen, it is better to have died as a small boy than to fumble this football" – John Heisman (1869 – 1936)* Handoffs are an essential part of effective communication when information is transferred from one team to another or between providers. This occurs innumerable times each day in hospitals, offices, and laboratories. These transition points of care are prone to error and can be dangerous as each handoff carries the potential for information loss or misinterpretation. Errors at the time of transition of care are among the most common errors in health care. Handoffs occur between different providers (change of shift in the ER, change of call provider on the floor) or can involve the physical location change of a patient (transfer from floor to ICU, from hospital to skilled nursing facility, discharge home). The key for a successful handoff is accurate transfer of information, preferably through standard protocols. Common aspects of a good handoff are interaction, timeliness, appropriate information content, review of relevant data, and lack of interruptions. To achieve that goal it is helpful to designate specific times and locations for handoffs to minimize distraction, cover all possible scenarios and use structured language and checklists for communication. Within the National Patient Safety Goals, The Joint Commission requires a structured process for patient handoffs (see Chap. x). Table 10.1 depicts a simple mnemonic for a safe and effective handoff [4].

(i) *SBAR (Situation, Background, Assessment, Recommendation)* – SBAR is a communication technique using a standardized template similar to the SOAP model (subjective/objective/assessment/plan) as shown in Table 10.2. It can be used in verbal and written communications to set the expectations within a dialogue. Its structure assures that relevant and critical informational content is communicated every time a patient or an issue is discussed. It forces the communicators to acknowledge the goals of all involved parties – as they may diverge. For example, physicians tend to focus on problem solving ("what do I need to do" – "in a nutshell this is the problem") while nurses are trained to be narrative and descriptive. They may need to understand the background and more specific aspects of the problem. Similarly, when used in a performance improvement project, written communication by SBAR will concisely communicate the fundamental framework and context of a project, describe its goal and how to achieve it (Table 10.2). To be effective and enhance predictability of the communication, SBARs need to be crisp to the point and promote critical thinking.

In addition to the above list of communication tools, organizations may want to use additional communication structures such as *multidisciplinary rounds* and *red rules*.

Table 10.1. Mnemonic for safe and effective Handoffs: "ANTICipate" (modified from 4).

Administrative	Name and location of patient
New Information	Update of clinical situation, brief H + P, problem list, meds, current status, significant events
Tasks	To Do list (use "if/then" statements)
Illness	Assessment of the severity of current illness
Contingency Plan(s)	Prepare cross-coverage for best way to manage based on what did and did not work in the past

Table 10.2. SBAR: Situation, Background, Assessment, Recommendation. A situational briefing tool. Three examples in clinical practice.

Clinical Examples for SBAR

S – State patient name and call out problem: "*Doctor, I am worried about Ms Flagherty's wound. I think it is infected*"

B – State the pertinent medical history and treatment to date: "*She is diabetic and had a colon resection two days ago*"

A – What is your assessment and what is the clinical picture: "*I am concerned because her wound is red and she had a high temperature and chills last night*"

R – State what you would like to see done: "*I think she needs her wound to be opened. I need you to come and see her*"

S – "*Jim, I know you are getting ready to wake up the patient, but the instrument count is wrong*"

B – "*We looked and counted 2 times, but it is still incorrect. We need to find the missing instrument*"

A – "*The count is incorrect, we need an X-ray*"

R – "*Don't wake the patient up until we have done the X-ray and the radiologist has seen it. Lets get the film now*"

Performance Improvement Example for SBAR

S – Finding the standard for surgical prep solution to reduce surgical site infections

B – We do not have a standard for adult surgical skin prep solutions. Evidence suggests the solutions A and B to be superior than Y and Z

A – The most common prep solution we use is Y and Z. Infection rate is measurably less when using prep solution A and B

R – Use of prep solution A and B for all adult skin prep. Eliminate solutions Y and Z from OR and procedure rooms. Exceptions listed

S – Situation: What is this about? Establish the topic of the communication (Punch Line).

B – Background: What information is needed, Why are we talking about this? (Context).

A – Assessment: Describe and state the problem/situation (Patient Status, Problem).

R – Recommendation: What should we do? When are we doing it? (Clarify action)

Multidisciplinary rounds assemble all members of the care team for walk rounds on each patient. Teams are encouraged to use structured communication tools such as SBAR and briefings to enhance their ability to effectively speak to each other about the current care issues. The success of such multidisciplinary rounds depends largely on the ability of the leadership to create a culture of safety and flattened hierarchy that gives every team member the confidence to speak up.

Red rules are adopted from the nuclear power industry to provide non-negotiable rules when necessary. In a health care environment these might be "always do a time out," "always check sponge count before closing," "always wash hands before and after entering a patient's room." These hard rules need to have the "buy-in" of everybody on the team, should be completely nonambiguous and carry immediate consequences for violating them. Because of this stringent normative setting, the number of red rules within an organization should be limited.

Structured communications, handoffs, and SBARs are part of effective teamwork and communication skills that are not inherent to the nature of health care providers. They require specific training and practice that should be provided by any health care organizations striving for best outcomes in patient safety and care. Specific teamwork training sessions should include all members of a care team and be led by a trained professional (Institute of Health Improvement trained Patient Safety Officer, for example). Key elements of these training sessions are realistic scenarios to provide education on team behavior, communication strategies, and safe culture. Essential attributes of a team include non-negotiable mutual respect, inclusiveness of all concerns and acknowledgment of failure, thrive for excellence, conflict resolution, and use of structured communication tools. Observations of team climate, behavior, and work are essential to continued improvement and should include assessment of effective communication (see Chap. x on Safety Attitude Questionnaire)

Rapid Response Team

The purpose of a rapid response team (RRT) is to assemble a team of experts around the bedside of a patient within a short time frame (minutes) anytime there is a concern because:

-   a staff member is worried
-   there is an acute change in vital signs such as change in systolic blood pressure (<90), heart rate (<40 >130), and respiratory rate (<8 >30)

- there is an acute change in oxygen saturation <90%
- there is a change in mental status
- there is drop in UO to < 50 ml in 4 h

The team consists typically of a hospitalist or intensivist, an ICU nurse and a respiratory therapist. The team can be called upon by anyone involved in the patient's care including clinicians, nurses, patients, and family members, whenever the patient meets certain criteria posted throughout the hospital. The role of the RRT is to:

- assess the health status of the patient
- stabilize the patient
- communicate with all involved health care providers and nurses to make sure the primary attending is notified
- provide support and expertise for the staff caring for the patient
- assist with transfer to a higher level of care when necessary

Good RRTs are allotted time by their organization to make rounds on all patients assigned to them, so potential problems and harm can be anticipated and acted upon. It helps foster a good relationship between floor staff and the RRT which encourages the use of RRTs. In essence, there is no "bad" reason to call on the RRT and the willingness of the team to help in any situation should never be called into question. The characteristic of a good RRT is a positive attitude: always ask "how can I help" with a smile! This is increasingly important as nursing shortages, inexperienced staff, and the higher acuity of inpatients in hospitals today have created the need for rapid availability of care expertise at the bedside of a needy patient. By creating an RRT, organization can provide patients the care they need when they need it [5].

References

1. Joint Commission Sentinel Event Alert 40, 2008. http://www.jointcommission.org/sentinelevents/sentineleventsalert/sea_40.htm.
2. Mazzocco K, Petitti DB, Fong KT, et al. Surgical team behaviors and patient outcomes. Am J Surg. 2009;197(5):678–85.
3. Fox M, Kilpatrick S, King T, et al. Fetal heart rate monitoring: Interpretation and collaborative management. J Midwifery Womens Health. 2000;45(6):498–507.
4. Vidyarthi AR. Triple handoff. AHRQ WebM&M (ersial online). 2006. Available at: http://www.webmm.ahrq.gov/case/aspx?caseID = 134.
5. Joint Commission Resources. Best practices in Medical Emergency teams: Oakbrook Terrace. Illinois: The Joint Commission; 2006.

Selected Readings

Frankel A, Leonard M, Simmonds T, Haraden C, Vega B. The Essential guide for patient Safety Officers. Chicago: Institute for Healthcare Improvement, Joint Commission Resources; 2009.

Nundy S, Mukherjee A, Sexton JB, et al. Impact of preoperative briefings on operating room delays: a preliminary report. Arch Surg. 2008;143(11):1068–72.

Makary MA, Sexton JB, Freischlag JA, et al. Operating room teamwork among physicians and nurses: teamwork in the eye of the beholder. J Am Coll Surg. 2006;202:746–52.

Leape L, Berwick D, Clancy C, et al. Transforming healthcare: a safety imperative. Qual Saf Health Care. 2009;18(6):424–8.

Edmondson AC. Learning from failure in health care: frequent opportunities, pervasive barriers. Qual Saf Health Care. 2004;13(Suppl II):ii3–9. doi:10.1136/qshc.2003.009597.

Haig KM, Sutton S, Whittington J. SBAR: a shared mental model for improving communication between clinicians. Jt Comm J Qual Patient Saf. 2006;32(3):167–75.

Yates GR, Hochman RF, Sayles SM, et al. Sentara Norfolk General Hospital: accelerating improvement by focusing on building a culture of safety. Jt Comm J Qual Saf. 2004;30(10):534–42.

11. Clinical Care Pathways

Benjamin E. Schneider

Clinical care pathways have been developed to integrate multidisciplinary treatment for a defined diagnosis or treatment. The concept of surgical pathways is not new, with published examples ranging from craniotomy to the treatment diabetic foot ulcers. From the standpoint of the surgical care, such pathways represent an algorithmic approach to patient care beginning with preoperative evaluation and extending through each treatment stage to discharge and follow-up. The components of care are integrated along a timeline with specific treatments outlined in sequence. This outline may serve both provider and patient by aligning expectations for treatment progress and recovery. The goals of the care pathway are to improve the utilization of evidence-based therapies, adopt best practices, and to standardize care. Other anticipated benefits of pathway utilization include, improved documentation, education of house-staff/nurses, improve communication among care providers, improve patient satisfaction, reduce hospital stay, reduce costs, allow for efficient data collection, encourage patient centered care, and improve patient satisfaction.

Conditions or procedures for pathway development generally should be selected with the expectation that they will improve clinical outcomes, costs, or lead to standardization. Procedures that have predictable outcome are high volume, higher cost, or are subject to clinician practice variability may be ideally suited for pathways. Development should begin with a review of current treatment and identify evidence-based best practices that may serve as guidelines for standardization. A multidisciplinary working group should review these guidelines and reconcile with local practice. The pathway itself is oriented along a timeline with categorized aspects of care encompassing preoperative assessment, recovery, and hospitalization to discharge. The care elements may be provider specific but include all aspects of treatment from

D.S. Tichansky, J. Morton, and D.B. Jones (eds.), *The SAGES Manual of Quality, Outcomes and Patient Safety*, DOI 10.1007/978-1-4419-7901-8_11, © Springer Science+Business Media, LLC 2012

infection and thromboembolic prophylaxis, antibiotic usage, catheter and drain management, laboratory studies, XRAY use, as well as other tasks. Best practices should be reviewed periodically with pathways updated accordingly.

While there is evidence to support some claims to improved outcomes, randomized control studies particularly in the area of economic benefits are lacking, as there are obvious difficulties with study design. Most studies are retrospective and subject to secular trends in treatment. More sophisticated analysis such as with deviation cost modeling better account for cost savings attributable to pathway implementation (Figs. 11.1 and 11.2).

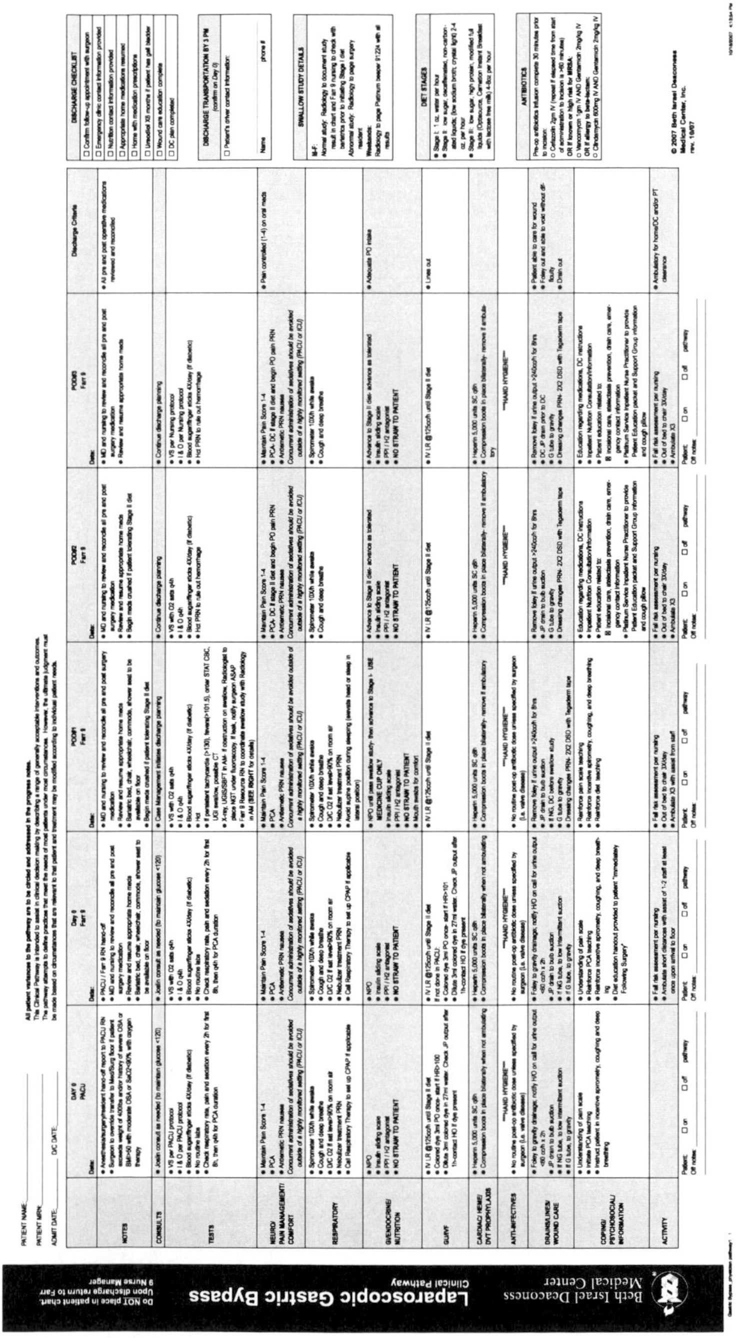

Fig. 11.1. Gastric bypass pathway.

Do NOT place in patient chart. Upon discharge return to Nurse Manager

Colectomy
Clinical Pathway

Beth Israel Deaconess Medical Center

PATIENT NAME: ____________________
PATIENT MRN: ____________________
ADMIT DATE: __________ D/C DATE: __________

Colectomy: ☐ Left ☐ Right ☐ Other: _____

All patient variances to the pathway are to be circled and addressed in the progress notes.
This Clinical Pathway is intended to assist in clinical decision making by describing a range of generally acceptable interventions and outcomes. The pathway attempts to define practices that meet the needs of most patients under most circumstances. However, the ultimate judgment must be made based on circumstances that are relevant to that patient and treatment may be modified according to individual patient needs.

	DAY 0 PACU Date:	Day 0 Farr 9, CC8 Date:	POD#1 Farr 9, CC8 Date:	POD#2 Farr 9, CC8 Date:	POD#3 Farr 9, CC8 Date:	POD#4 Farr 9, CC8 Date:	Discharge Criteria
NOTES	• Anesthesia/surgery/resident hand-off report to PACU RN • Compression boots in place bilaterally	• MD and nursing to review and reconcile all pre and post surgery medication	• MD and nursing to review and reconcile all pre and post surgery medication • Review and resume appropriate home meds	• MD and nursing to review and reconcile all pre and post surgery medication • Review and resume appropriate home meds • **R colectomy home, if foley out, adequate PO and patient had BM**	• MD and nursing to review and reconcile all pre and post surgery medication • Review and resume appropriate home meds • **L colectomy home, if foley out, adequate PO and patient had BM**	• MD and nursing to review and reconcile all pre and post surgery medication • Review and resume appropriate home meds • **L colectomy home, if foley out, adequate PO and patient had BM**	• All pre and post operative medications reviewed and reconciled
CONSULTS		• Consult Ostomy RN for stoma evaluation and pouch fitting • Geriatric consult for patients age>75	• Case Management initiates discharge planning • Ostomy RN stoma evaluation and pouch fitting completed	• Continue Rehab/SNF screenings if appropriate • VNA enterostomal care order through case management	• Continue Rehab/SNF screenings if appropriate	• Continue Rehab/SNF screenings if appropriate	
TESTS	• VS per Nursing protocol • I & O per Nursing protocol • Maintain temporal temperature >96.8F within 1h after leaving OR • Hct, K, Mg	• VS per Nursing protocol • I&O q 8 hours	• VS per Nursing protocol • I&O q 8 hours • CBC • Chem. 10	• VS per Nursing protocol • I&O q 8 hours	• VS per Nursing protocol • I&O q 8 hours	• VS per Nursing protocol • I&O q 8 hours	
NEURO/ PAIN MANAGEMENT/ COMFORT	• Maintain Pain Score 1-4 • Ketorolac 15mg IV q6h • Metoclopramide 10-20mg IV q6h • PCA WITH • Pain pump with ½% bupivacaine OR • Epidural per anesthesia	• Maintain Pain Score 1-4 • Ketorolac 15mg IV q6h • Metoclopramide 10-20mg IV q6h • PCA WITH • Pain pump with ½% bupivacaine OR • Epidural per anesthesia	• Maintain Pain Score 1-4 • Ketorolac 15mg IV q6h • Metoclopramide 10-20mg IV q6h • PCA WITH • Pain pump with ½% bupivacaine OR • Epidural per anesthesia	• Maintain Pain Score 1-4 • Ketorolac 15mg IV q6h • Metoclopramide 10-20mg IV q6h • D/C PCA • D/C pain pump OR epidural	• Maintain Pain Score 1-4 • Ketorolac 15mg IV q6h • Metoclopramide 10-20mg IV/PO q6h	• Maintain Pain Score 1-4 • Ketorolac 15mg IV q6h • Metoclopramide 10-20mg IV/PO q6h	• Pain controlled (1-4) on oral meds
RESPIRATORY	• Spirometer 10X/h while awake • Cough and deep breathe	• Spirometer 10X/h while awake • Cough and deep breathe	• Spirometer 10X/h while awake • Cough and deep breathe	• Spirometer 10X/h while awake • Cough and deep breathe	• Spirometer 10X/h while awake • Cough and deep breathe	• Spirometer 10X/h while awake • Cough and deep breathe	
GI/ENDOCRINE/ NUTRITION	• NPO	• NPO	• Sips as tolerated	• Sips as tolerated	• Sips; advance as tolerated	• Diet as tolerated	• Adequate PO intake • BM
GU/ IVF	• IVF: LR @ 100cc/h	•IVF: LR @ 100cc/hr	• IVF: LR @ 100cc/h • Change to Saline lock when patient tolerates 400cc PO fluids/shift	• IVF: LR @ 100cc/h • Change to Saline lock when patient tolerates 400cc PO fluids/shift	• IVF: LR @ 100cc/h • Change to Saline lock when patient tolerates 400cc PO fluids/shift	• D/C Saline lock	• Lines out
CARDIAC/ HEME/ DVT PROPHYLAXIS		• Heparin 5,000 units SQ q12h beginning evening of surgery • Compression boots in place bilaterally	• Heparin 5,000 units SC q12h • Compression boots in place bilaterally-remove if ambulatory	• Heparin 5,000 units SC q12h • Compression boots in place bilaterally-remove if ambulatory	• Heparin 5,000 units SC q12h • Compression boots in place bilaterally-remove if ambulatory	• Heparin 5,000 units SC q12h • Compression boots in place bilaterally-remove if ambulatory	
ANTI-INFECTIVES	***HAND HYGIENE***	***HAND HYGIENE***	***HAND HYGIENE***	***HAND HYGIENE***	***HAND HYGIENE***	***HAND HYGIENE***	
DRAINS/LINES/ WOUND CARE	• Foley to gravity drainage; notify H/O on call for urine output <60 cc/h x 2h	• Foley to gravity drainage; notify H/O on call for urine output <60 cc/h x 2h	• Remove foley @ midnight except for LAR and IPAA anastomoses • Dressing change by HO • Wound care if infected or open wound • Pouch change for eval of stoma	• If unable to void after 8h or bladder is distended, assess with bladder scan and contact HO • Remove dressing • Wound care if infected or open wound	• Wound care PRN	• Wound care PRN	• Patient able to care for wound • Foley out
COPING/ PSYCHOSOCIAL/ INFORMATION	• Understanding of pain scale • Initiate PCA teaching • Instruct patient in incentive spirometry, coughing and deep breathing	• Understanding of pain scale • Reinforce PCA teaching • Instruct patient in incentive spirometry, coughing and deep breathing	• Reinforce pain scale teaching • Patient education related to: ○ mobility, medications, DC plan, emergency indicators, stoma care • RN education on when to empty pouch • Patient to observe stoma care	• Reinforce pain scale teaching • Patient education related to: ○ mobility, medications, DC plan, emergency indicators, stoma care • Patient to perform stoma care	• Reinforce pain scale teaching • Patient education related to: ○ mobility, medications, DC plan, emergency indicators, stoma care • Patient to perform stoma care	• Reinforce pain scale teaching • Patient education related to: ○ mobility, medications, DC plan, emergency indicators, stoma care • Patient to perform stoma care	• Independent with emptying pouch • Progress with stoma care
ACTIVITY		• Fall risk assessment per nursing • Sit edge of bed as tolerated	• Fall risk assessment per nursing • Out of bed to chair 3X/day • Ambulate X2	• Fall risk assessment per nursing • Out of bed to chair 3X/day • Ambulate X3	• Fall risk assessment per nursing • Independent ambulation and ADLs	• Fall risk assessment per nursing • Independent ambulation and ADLs	• Ambulatory for home/ DC and/or PT clearance
GERIATRIC CONSIDERATIONS (AGE >75)	• Ketorolac is contraindicated in patients with CrCl <50 or in patients with hemodynamic instability • If patient has Parkinsonian features, movement disorders or swallowing problems consider metoclopramide 5-10mg IV q6h	• Ketorolac is contraindicated in patients with CrCl <50 or in patients with hemodynamic instability • If patient has Parkinsonian features, movement disorders or swallowing problems consider metoclopramide 5-10mg IV q6h	• See previous day considerations regarding Ketorolac and metoclopramide • For PO pain medications, consider: • Oxycodone 2.5mg q4-6h if cognitively impaired • Oxycodone 5-10mg q4h if cognitively intact	• See previous day considerations regarding Ketorolac and metoclopramide • For PO pain medications, consider: • Oxycodone 2.5mg q4-6h if cognitively impaired • Oxycodone 5-10mg q4h if cognitively intact	• See previous day considerations regarding Ketorolac and metoclopramide • For PO pain medications, consider: • Oxycodone 2.5mg q4-6h if cognitively impaired • Oxycodone 5-10mg q4h if cognitively intact	• See previous day considerations regarding Ketorolac and metoclopramide • For PO pain medications, consider: • Oxycodone 2.5mg q4-6h if cognitively impaired • Oxycodone 5-10mg q4h if cognitively intact	
	Patient: ☐ On ☐ Off Pathway Off Notes: ______	Patient: ☐ On ☐ Off Pathway Off Notes: ______	Patient: ☐ On ☐ Off Pathway Off Notes: ______	Patient: ☐ On ☐ Off Pathway Off Notes: ______	Patient: ☐ On ☐ Off Pathway Off Notes: ______	Patient: ☐ On ☐ Off Pathway Off Notes: ______	

DISCHARGE CHECKLIST

☐ Follow-up appointment with surgeon made
☐ Ostomy RN appointment set (2-4wks post op)
☐ Home with oral pain medicine
☐ Resume home meds
☐ Wound care/ostomy supplies given and education complete
☐ VNA Enterostomal Therapy consult made
☐ Enterostomal therapy video watched
☐ Home discharge instruction sheet provided
☐ Ostomy product scripts written
☐ DC plan completed

PERI OPERATIVE BETA BLOCKER ADVISORY

Any of the following risk factors:
- History of MI or current angina
- Use of sublingual nitroglycerine
- Positive exercise test results
- Q waves on EKG
- Patients who have undergone PTCA or CABG and have chest pain presumed to be of ischemic origin
- History of TIA
- History of CVA
- DM requiring insulin therapy
- CRI, baseline creatinine level ≥2.0mg/dl
- Compensated CHF

OR Two of the following risk factors:
- Age ≥65
- Hypertension
- Currently smoking
- Serum cholesterol ≥ 240
- DM not requiring insulin therapy
- History of coronary radiation

ANTIBIOTICS

☐ Cefazolin 2gm IV **AND** Metronidazole 500mg IV to be completed within 30 mins prior to incision
OR *If known MRSA colonization or infection:*
☐ Vancomycin 1gm IV **AND** Gentamicin 2mg/kg IV **AND** Metronidazole 500mg IV to be completed within 60 mins prior to incision
OR *If life-threatening cephalosporin/ penicillin allergy:*
☐ Clindamycin 600mg IV **AND** Gentamicin 2mg/kg IV to be completed within 30 mins prior to incision

DELERIUM PREVENTION STRAGETIES

- Frequent re-orientation
- Lights on in daytime & out of bed as tolerated
- Avoid pharmacologic sleep aids
- Wear glasses, hearing aids, dentures (if approp)
- Reference clock and calendar in room
- Use radio, tape recorder, soft lighting (if possible)

DELERIUM MANAGEMENT STRAGETIES

- Appropriate diagnostic workup
- For agitation, calm reassurance, family presence, and/or sitter
- For agitation, if necessary, Haloperidol 0.5mg q4h *If contraindicated, consider lorazepam0.5mg q4h
- Consider geriatrics consult

Fig. 11.2. Colectomy pathway.

Selected Readings

Dy SM, Garg P, Puskal G, et al. Critical pathway effectiveness: assessing the impact of patient, hospital care, and pathway characteristics using qualitative comparative analysis. Health Serv Res. 2005;40(2):499–516.

Campbell H, Hotchkiss R, Bradshaw N, Porteous M. Integrated care pathways. BMJ. 1998;316:133–7.

Vanounou T, Pratt W, Fischer JE, et al. Deviation-based cost modeling: a novel model to evaluate the clinical and economic impact of clinical pathways. J Am Coll Surg. 2007;204(4):570–9.

Pearson SD, Goulart-Fischer D, Lee TH. Critical pathways as a strategy for improving care: problems and potential. Ann Intern Med. 1995;123:941–8.

12. Data Drives Quality: ACS–NSQIP

Matthew M. Hutter

Hospitals, if they wish to be sure of improvement,

Must find out what their results are

Must analyze their results, to find their strong and weak points.

Must compare their result with those of other hospitals…

These words, written by Ernest A. Codman in describing his "End Results" thesis, are just as true today as when they were written in 1917 [1].

Continuous quality improvement requires ongoing data collection and analysis. This chapter will assess the importance of high-quality data to assess the quality of surgical care given, to identify areas for improvement, to assess the effectiveness of quality improvement initiatives, and for ongoing monitoring.

Importance of High-quality data. High-quality data is the key ingredient for quality assessment – without it any subsequent conclusions could be erroneous and potentially dangerous. "Garbage in–garbage out" is a one of the first rules in assessing data, and any limitations of the data collected need to be fully understood before any further analysis can be done. How the data is collected, from what sources, and by whom it is actually collected is critical and will impact the outcome. (Hutter lehman) Specific data definitions and how objective or subjective they might be, will also be important. Inaccurate data will lead to erroneous results. Certain data points might be able to be captured with administrative datasets; however, other data points need to be recorded at the time of care (e.g., in CABG, the pump run time), or need interpretation of clinical data by a clinician or trained data collector to appropriately assess key clinically rich variables.

Need for rigorous statistical analysis, and responsible reporting. High-quality data alone is not sufficient. The data must be analyzed thoughtfully, and interpreted appropriately in order to make responsible conclusions upon which we can determine quality. Identifying significance where none exists or not identifying a difference that does

D.S. Tichansky, J. Morton, and D.B. Jones (eds.), *The SAGES Manual*
of Quality, Outcomes and Patient Safety, DOI 10.1007/978-1-4419-7901-8_12,
© Springer Science+Business Media, LLC 2012

exist can be equally harmful. For example, closing a hospital or a hospital service based on perceived poor quality (where quality of care is actually good or acceptable) has significant impact on those patients who no longer have access to care, as well as to the caregivers. Keeping a hospital open, that does have quality deficiencies, can also cause harm to patients.

CQI (Continuous Quality Improvement) and P-D-C-A (Plan-Do-Check-Act). Highly reliable organizations in any industry continuously monitor data to assure safety and excellence. We as surgeons and healthcare providers need to do the same. Quality control in many of today's high functioning companies are based on P-D-C-A, otherwise known as the "Plan-Do-Check-Act" cycle or the "Deming's Cycle." Central to this hypothesis is the ability to measure new and existing processes, and compare results against the expected results to ascertain any differences. It is an iterative process, and creates an ongoing cycle to improve the quality of care. In Six Sigma programs, this P-D-C-A cycle is referred to as "Define, Measure, Analyze, Improve, Control" (DMAIC). Regardless of the names, the core concept is the ability to accurately measure outcomes, and compare results from one process to another.

Donabedian Principle

Avedis Donabedian described the principles most commonly used today to assess the quality of healthcare. He helped to put a framework on assessing quality by focusing on Structure, Process, and Outcomes.

Structure includes the setting where care takes place and includes not only the bricks and mortar or physical location and resources, as well as the experience of the staff and the coordination of their care. Hospital and surgeon volume have also become a marker for many of these structural factors. Accreditation programs such as the JCAHO, and the Leapfrog Group, rely heavily on such easily captured metrics.

Process measures measure the care that patients actually receive. Examples include patients who are prescribed a Beta blocker after an MI, the measurement of a hemoglobin A1C in diabetics, and in surgery, adherence to the Surgical Care Improvement Program (SCIP) measures like whether or not preoperative antibiotics were given. Although these things are measurable, the direct link to the process and the outcomes are not always clear. Furthermore, few processes that lead to high-quality care have been described.

Outcomes include "the end results" that impact a patient, and are most commonly reported for surgery procedures. Operative mortality, complication rates, readmission rates, length of stay, functional status and patient experience are some variables considered outcomes.

Critical to assessing the quality of surgical care is choosing the right measure to focus on – Structure, Process, or Outcome. John Birkmeyer and colleagues have described a framework to assess the appropriate metrics, based on the procedure volume, and the inherent risk of the procedure. (Fig. 12.1) For high volume procedures, with high inherent risk, such as CABG, assessing an outcome like mortality would be appropriate. For high volume procedures, with low inherent risks, like inguinal hernia repair, then perhaps process measures or patient centered outcomes should be measured. For low volume procedures, with high risk, like esophagectomy, then perhaps a structural metric like hospital volume is most appropriate to assess.

What Is Quality?

Although the Donabedian principle is useful in determining how to measure quality, it does not by itself describe what "quality" really is. I propose a working definition for the quality of surgical care which takes into account many aspects of the surgical decision making process and ultimate care of the surgical patient which need to be considered and assessed (Hutter):

Quality of surgical care means

the right patients,

getting the right operation,

in the right setting,

while minimizing complications and

maximizing clinical effectiveness.

The right patients addresses questions about access to care, as well as appropriateness of care, including medical *versus* surgical treatment.

Getting the right operation addresses the questions of procedure comparisons (procedure A *versus* procedure B), which is where most of surgical outcomes research has historically been focused.

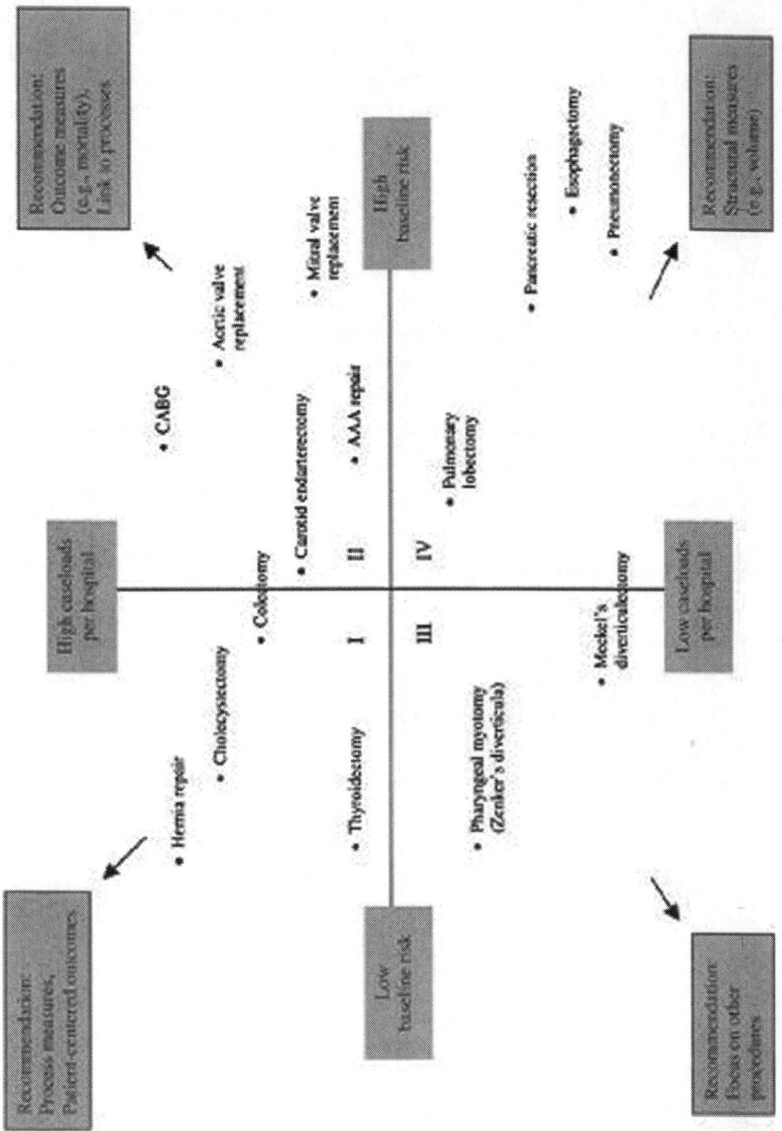

Fig. 12.1. Recommendations for when to focus on structure, process, or outcomes.

In the right setting, has been a recent focus and a direct result of the outcomes research movement, and touches on the issues of hospital volume, surgeon volume, surgeon training, specialization, regionalization, systems, processes, multidisciplinary approaches, and accreditation programs.

While minimizing complications looks at morbidity and mortality of the procedures. Many think that morbidity and mortality are currently well characterized, but in reality we have little standardization of data definitions or of the way that data are captured, infrequent or ineffective risk-adjustment, and data are not universally captured, making comparisons between institutions difficult, if not impossible.

Maximizing effectiveness focuses on disease-free survival, recurrence rates, functional status, reduction in comorbidities, and patient satisfaction. Patient experience, which includes quality of life and satisfaction with the process or receiving care, unfortunately is rarely taken into consideration. Assessing value, which entails accurate assessments of cost as well as quality, is critical. Comparative effectiveness between surgical procedures and their alternatives, as well as compared to the opportunity costs for alternative uses, should be the determinant of how our healthcare dollars are best used. Such data are not currently available.

Data Collection Systems

Perhaps one of the greatest accomplishments of the outcomes research movement is the increased recognition of the inability to define "quality." One of the greatest benefits of this outcomes movement has been the advances in the statistical sophistication and rigid standards of today's research studies and publications. Another benefit has been the development of multi-institutional, prospective, risk-adjusted data collection systems that are based on standardized definitions. These systems were developed due to the need to define quality of care, and as a result of the inherent limitations of administrative and claims data. Outcomes reporting systems were initially developed in the field of cardiac surgery and are now moving into other fields with programs developed by the Society of Thoracic Surgeons, and by the Veteran Affairs Hospitals with the National Surgical Quality Improvement Program (NSQIP). The American College of Surgeons (ACS) has developed the ACS–NSQIP as their platform for quality and safety.

National data collection programs for cancer care, trauma programs, and also for accreditation programs in bariatric surgery have been developed. These reporting systems are now giving us a more objective look at some of the characteristics of "quality." Public reporting of the quality of surgical care is becoming more commonplace – STS is now reporting hospital results for CABG to the public in "Consumer Reports" (Ferris).

ACS–NSQIP

The ACS–NSQIP is a national, validated, risk-adjusted data collection program based on standardized definitions and collected by audited, trained data reviewers. Thirty-day mortality and complication rates following surgical operations are assessed. Real-time, procedure-specific, online reports are available, based on nationally benchmarked data. Multiple risk-adjusted reports are developed two times a year for morbidity, mortality, as well as procedure and complication specific models. The program was initially started in the Veteran Affairs (VA) system, and following an AHRQ funded feasibility study was then expanded to private sector hospitals as the ACS–NSQIP. (Khuri) The program is about to expand into options to include "Essentials", which is a streamlined data collection program to decrease the number of variables, and thereby the costs and burden of data collection, as well as "Procedure Specific", which will allow increased sampling of high risk procedures and will include procedure specific risk-adjustment and outcomes variables (Birkmeyer blueprint).

A bariatric surgery data collection program has been developed for the American College of Surgeons – Bariatric Surgery Center Network (ACS–BSCN) and includes not only bariatric surgery specific variables, but also tracks patients beyond 30-days, to 6-months, 1-year and then yearly thereafter. Data is collected by trained data collectors (lessening the costs of requiring clinical nurse reviewers), and data definitions were chosen to be more objective so as to require less clinical oversight. Data assesses not only morbidity and mortality, but also clinical effectiveness of the procedures including reduction in weight and weight-related comorbidities such as diabetes, hypertension, hypercholesterolemia, gastroesophageal reflux disease, and obstructive sleep apnea. A similar data collection program has been developed by the American Society for Metabolic and Bariatric Surgery/Surgical Review Corporation.

The ACS–NSQIP data collection programs provide high-quality, clinically rich data, with national benchmark comparisons, and risk-adjusted analyses, that can be used as the engine for any surgical quality improvement program. The Bariatric Surgery Data Collection Program demonstrates how such a program can be expanded to assess outcomes longitudinally – beyond 30 days – and to include assessment of clinical effectiveness as well as morbidity and mortality. It also demonstrates how such data can be used to derive accreditation.

Despite this progress, all current data collection programs do not assess all the necessary components to determine the true quality of surgical care – the right patient, getting the right operation, in the right setting, while minimizing complications and maximizing effectiveness. Data about appropriateness, comparative effectiveness of surgical and nonsurgical treatments, the impact of regionalization or accreditation, patient experience, and of course data defining value are noticeably lacking.

Conclusion

High-quality data is the engine that drives continuous quality improvement. Good data, coupled with sound statistics, and thoughtful conclusions can lead to responsible reporting of the quality of care delivered. Such data can inform quality assurance and quality control through the iterative processes of continuous quality improvement. The Donabedian principle of structure, process and/or outcomes is a useful framework for assessing the quality in healthcare. To assess the true quality of care delivered, multiple domains above and beyond measuring morbidity and mortality need to be assessed including appropriateness, comparative effectiveness, the setting such as regionalization or accreditation, patient centered outcomes, and of course value. Though progress has been made in national data collection programs, there is much more we need to measure if we are to truly inform improvements in the quality of healthcare.

Selected Readings

1. Codman EA. A study in hospital efficiency. Oakbrook Terrace, IL: JCAHO; 1996. p. 183.
2. Hutter MM, Jones DB, Riley S Jr M, Snow RL, Cella RJ, Schneider BE, et al. Best practice updates for weight loss surgery data collection. Lehman Center Weight Loss

Surgery Expert Panel. Commonwealth of Massachusetts Betsy Lehman Center for patient Safety and Medical Error Reduction. Obesity. 2009;17(5):924–8.

3. Donabedian A. Evaluating the quality of medical care. Milbank Mem Fund Q. 1966; 44:166–206.

4. Birkmeyer JD, Dimick JB, Birkmeyer NJ. Measuring the quality of surgical care: structure, process, or outcomes? J Am Coll Surg. 2004;198(4):626–32.

5. Hutter MM. Does outcomes research impact quality? Examples from Bariatric Surgery. Am Surg. 2006;72(11):1055–60. discussion 1061–9, 1133–1148.

6. Ferris TG, Torchiana DF. Public release of clinical outcomes data – Online CABG Report Cards. N Engl J Med. 2010;363:1593–5.

7. Khuri SF, Henderson WG, Daley J, Jonasson O, Jones RS, Campbell Jr DA, et al. Principal Investigators of the Patient Safety in Surgery Study. Successful implementation of the Department of Veterans Affairs' National Surgical Quality Improvement Program in the private sector: the Patient Safety in Surgery study. Ann Surg. 2008;248(2): 329–36.

8. Birkmeyer JD, Shahian DM, Dimick JB, Finlayson SR, Flum DR, Ko CY, et al. Blueprint for a new American College of Surgeons: National Surgical Quality Improvement Program. J Am Coll Surg. 2008;207(5):777–82.

13. Clinical Research Improves Patient Care

Alexander J. Greenstein and Bruce M. Wolfe

Introduction

In this chapter, we briefly discuss clinical outcomes research and its effect on minimally invasive surgery and then focus on the recently launched Longitudinal Assessment of Bariatric Surgery (LABS) database as an example of high-quality clinical surgical research. The term "outcomes research" has been used to refer to a wide range of studies, and there is no single definition that has gained widespread acceptance. It encompasses all forms of clinical research that examines the impact of patient, provider, and organizational factors on patients and patient care (function, quality of life, satisfaction, readmissions, costs, etc.), and it has two main applications: assessment of quality of care and study of the effectiveness of a clinical intervention.

Traditionally, surgical outcomes have been assessed in morbidity and mortality conferences which review such issues after the delivery of surgical care. In the past two decades, however, expectations have changed and improvement has come for both the range of outcomes being reported and the quality of the reporting infrastructure. Increasingly, effective resource utilization, cost-effectiveness, and patient-reported outcomes such as quality of life have become important metrics by which to measure surgical success. Outcomes research provides a discussion of these issues by emphasizing health problem-oriented evaluations of care delivered in "real world" settings. Clinical registries and administrative databases are primary sources for studies assessing the quality of surgical care. Their utility in evaluating procedures and determining comparative outcomes has increased greatly relative to the gold standard randomized controlled trial (RCT).

High-quality outcomes research has played a critical role over the last two decades in supporting and substantiating the relative benefits of minimally invasive surgery, often in the face of strong traditional opposition.

D.S. Tichansky, J. Morton, and D.B. Jones (eds.), *The SAGES Manual of Quality, Outcomes and Patient Safety*, DOI 10.1007/978-1-4419-7901-8_13,
© Springer Science+Business Media, LLC 2012

MIS Research

The laparoscopic revolution began in earnest with the introduction of laparoscopic cholecystectomy in the mid-1980s. Despite considerable reservations about the safety of such an approach, the results of a number of RCTs were published, demonstrating the safety and efficacy of laparoscopy in comparison to "mini-laparotomy." Based on this research, laparoscopic cholecystectomy was endorsed as the "procedure of choice" for symptomatic gallstones at a 1992 National Institutes of Health Consensus Development Conference and in the years that followed, multiple high-quality series were produced, helping to expand its application to acute cholecystitis and solidifying its standing. In fact, multiple series with over 1,000 patients were reported, one with a collection of over 77,000 patients [1, 2].

A similar story has been seen with the development of laparoscopic appendectomy. Although first reported in 1983, it was not until the mid-1990s that laparoscopic appendectomy became widely available. Again, it was only because of multiple high-quality RCTs and meta-analyses that the laparoscopic approach gained acceptance by demonstrating shorter hospital stays, less postoperative pain, earlier diet resumption, and fewer wound complications. Unlike with laparoscopic cholecystectomy, results have not been completely uniform between studies, and while there is not complete agreement on the advantages of laparoscopic appendectomy, its advantages are now universally acknowledged in certain target populations such as obese patients, females of childbearing age, and in those patients for whom a diagnosis of appendicitis is unclear [3].

Laparoscopic inguinal herniorrhapy (LIH) is another important setting where clinical research has driven implementation and guidelines. Multiple RCTs and population-based studies have been unable to support LIH for unilateral uncomplicated hernias, but the procedure has proven to be advantageous for recurrent hernias, bilateral hernias, and for patients requiring hernia repairs at the same time as another intra-abdominal procedure. Overall, the data suggests less persistent pain and numbness following laparoscopic repair with a faster return to usual activities, but longer operation times with LIH, and a higher risk of serious complication rate with respect to visceral and vascular injuries [4].

One of the more controversial applications of minimally invasive surgical techniques has been for the treatment of colorectal cancer. The safety and oncologic efficacy of laparoscopy has been demonstrated for colon cancer and confirmed with regards to 5 year results thanks to the Clinical Outcomes of Surgical Therapy Study Group [5]. Laparoscopic resection for rectal cancer, however, remains controversial due to a steep learning curve and technical challenges. Despite several RCTs and a meta analysis demonstrating feasibility, safety and short-term advantages of the laparoscopic approach, long-term data from is lacking with the exception of a recently published comparative study that demonstrates similar survival between groups [6].

Innovation extending laparoscopic/minimally invasive surgical techniques to bariatric surgery has had a major impact on the field, contributing to a several-fold increase in number of procedures performed over the last ten years [7]. A prospective RCT by Nguyen and colleagues demonstrated the safety and multiple physiologic and outcome benefits of laparoscopic compared to open gastric bypass without compromising safety or weight loss [8]. Multiple substudies conducted within this trial demonstrated diminished injury response, induction of a hypercoagulable state, impaired pulmonary function, and more rapid recovery [9–11]. At 3 years, postoperative weight loss was identical, in which the incidence of ventral hernia was greatly reduced (5% vs. 39%) [12]. Having presented an overview of the importance of research to quality of surgical care, we will delve into one excellent example of a surgical outcomes project by focusing on the LABS project.

Introduction to LABS

Since 1991, when first brought to prominence by the National Institutes of Health (NIH) Consensus Conference, a movement has been building to generate a better understanding of bariatric surgery, including its safety and efficacy, risks and benefits, and mechanism of action. Despite multiple independent publications, a knowledge gap has persisted due to a combination of factors, including a lack of standardized data collection methods, procedures, and outcomes assessments. With this in mind, a National Institute of Diabetes and Digestive and Kidney Diseases (NIDDK)-sponsored working Group on research in bariatric surgery was convened in 2002. A consortium of centers with bariatric surgical experience was assembled to create a database and the LABS project was thus conceived. After carefully considering the creation of a RCT, it was concluded that multiple hypotheses regarding important predictors and outcomes could be addressed by an observational trial.

LABS began in 2003 with the funding of six clinical centers and a data coordinating center (DCC). The project was placed under the authority of a steering committee composed of the principal investigators at the clinical centers, the DCC, and the NIH project coordinator. In addition, researchers were recruited to the project from multiple backgrounds including bariatric surgery, obesity research, internal medicine, endocrinology, behavioral science, outcomes research, and epidemiology to collaboratively plan and conduct studies. At the heart of the project is a database consisting of rigorously collected information on patients undergoing bariatric surgery at the participating clinical centers. As an observational study, the vast majority of procedures analyzed are either Roux en-Y gastric bypass (RYGB), laparoscopic and open, or laparoscopic adjustable gastric banding. Less commonly performed procedures performed in the LABS 2 cohort include biliopancreatic diversion with or without a duodenal switch, sleeve gastrectomy, vertical banded gastroplasty, and open adjustable gastric banding. Data points include patient characteristics, surgical procedures, medical and psychosocial outcomes, and economic factors.

Iterations of LABS

The LABS study is organized into three phases: LABS-1, LABS-2, and LABS-3. LABS-1 consists of all patients 18 years of age who underwent bariatric surgery from March 11, 2005, through December 31, 2007, by one of 33 LABS-certified surgeons at participating centers. By the end of 2007 a total of 5,648 patients had agreed to participate in the study, and 4,776 had undergone primary operations. LABS-1 consists of a limited dataset of patient and operative characteristics and was crafted to evaluate the short-term safety of bariatric surgery. Primary endpoints include important adverse outcomes, such as death, operative reintervention, anticoagulation for DVT/PE or continued hospitalization at postoperative day 30.

The primary goal of LABS-2 is to evaluate the longer term safety and efficacy of bariatric surgery and better study patient characteristics as they relate to short- and intermediate-term outcomes. Key groups of non-safety outcomes for LABS-2 include (but are not limited to) weight loss, changes in body composition, functional impairment, psychosocial function (including quality of life), and cardiovascular, metabolic, pulmonary, renal, musculoskeletal, urogynecologic, reproductive, and gastrointestinal outcomes. The sample size for LABS-2 is approximately 2,400 patients, and data collection consists of an array of demographic, anthropometric, clinical, behavioral, surgical, and postoperative care variables. Data is collected before surgery, during surgery, and postoperatively at multiple intervals including 30-day, 6-months, 1-year, and annually thereafter.

LABS-3 involves subsets of patients from the LABS-2 group, and its composition and size has been determined by the subject to be analyzed. These include a detailed study of the relationship of severe obesity, insulin resistance and secretion to gastric bypass-induced weight loss, as well as investigation into the psychosocial and behavioral aspects of obesity. Multiple grants have also been funded annually to study additional subpopulations in detail. Examples include detailed study of physical activity, free fatty acid metabolism, genotype–phenotype relationships, obesity-induced dementia, and bariatric surgery in adolescents.

LABS Publications

Several manuscripts have been published based on LABS and its respective databases. The project was introduced in 2005 with the publication titled *The NIDDK Bariatric Surgery Clinical Research Consortium (LABS)* [13]. This manuscript outlines the genesis of LABS, the primary goals of the consortium, and the structure of the project. More extensive details on the rationale, methodology, risk stratification, and outcome domains are provided in the article *Safety and efficacy of bariatric surgery: Longitudinal Assessment of Bariatric Surgery*, published in 2007 [14]. Of interest, it also provides specific information on the three iterations of LABS as detailed above.

The most influential publication to arise from the LABS database is *Perioperative Safety in the Longitudinal Assessment of Bariatric Surgery*, which was published in the July 2009 issue of the *New England Journal of Medicine (NEJM)* [15]. From a cohort of 3,412 patients with RYGB (87.2% laparoscopic), and 1,198 patients with laparoscopic adjustable gastric banding, 30 day death rate was 0.3%, and major morbidity (defined as anticoagulation for deep-vein thrombosis or venous thromboembolism, reintervention, failure to be discharged by 30 days or death) rate was 4.3%. This composite endpoint occurred in 1.0% of those who underwent adjustable gastric banding, 4.8% of those who underwent laparoscopic RYGB, and 7.8% of those who underwent open RYGB.

A history of deep-vein thrombosis or pulmonary embolus, a diagnosis of obstructive sleep apnea, and impaired functional status were each independently associated with an increased risk of the composite end point, and as were extreme values of body-mass index. Several subtopics based on the LABS dataset have also been explored and published in articles such as *The Relationship of BMI with Demographic and Clinical Characteristics in the Longitudinal Assessment of Bariatric Surgery* [16], the *Relationship between surgeon volume and adverse outcomes after RYGB in Longitudinal Assessment of Bariatric Surgery study* [17], and *Physical Activity Levels of Patients Undergoing Bariatric Surgery in the Longitudinal Assessment of Bariatric Surgery Study* [18].

Future Directions for LABS

LABS is a multisite dataset that comprehensively and consistently captures predictors and outcomes of bariatric surgery. The data being collected by the LABS provides researchers with standardized measurement instruments that can be used across centers. Now that LABS 2 recruitment is complete, the forms and resources are directed to maximizing annual retention (follow up) over as many years as possible. The manuscripts that have already been published represent simply an introduction to the potential breadth and depth of findings that are expected to be garnered from the LABS. In addition to a repository of data, biological specimens for future research are being collected by the centers participating in LABS. There remain for proposal numerous clinical studies to answer questions regarding the impact of surgical procedures on clinical outcomes. Potential examples as presented by the LABS investigative team include study into the impact of bariatric surgery on insulin resistance, mechanisms by which surgery may enhance long-term weight maintenance, or the impact of restrictive versus malabsorptive surgical procedures on hormones presumed to affect weight regulation. Research into the available surgical procedures may provide insights that will lead to new, non-surgical treatments of obesity that mimic the appetite-suppressive effects of surgery.

Extreme obesity affects nearly every organ system and many aspects of the human experience. The goal of the LABS consortium is to accelerate clinical research and progress in understanding the pathogenesis of extreme obesity and its complications, as well as in understanding the risks and benefits of bariatric surgery as a treatment modality. Aspects of the pathophysiology of obesity and obesity-related diseases will be studied, either through substudies or by separately funded ancillary studies. These projects will undoubtedly provide information to assess the broad impact of bariatric operations on both patients and the healthcare system in general. Answers to additional questions regarding the framework of LABS and the process behind project proposal and generation can be found at the LABS website – http://www.edc.pitt.edu/labs/.

Conclusion

Today and in the future, we as surgeons will constantly be assessing the relative clinical advantages of technical options and be forced to balance this with efficient utilization of limited resources and cost-effectiveness. We already have at our disposal a host of clinical studies that have served as the foundation for the validity of laparoscopy and newer endeavors such as LABS as models on which to structure new projects. By moving beyond single center reports of outcomes and rigorous methodology, we will continue to expand our surgical options, improve the overall quality of surgical care, and improve the credibility of surgical research.

Selected Readings

1. Deziel DJ, Millikan KW, Economou SG, et al. Complications of laparoscopic cholecystectomy: a national survey of 4,292 hospitals and an analysis of 77,604 cases. Am J Surg. 1993;165:9–14.
2. Wu JS, Dunnegan DL, Luttmann DR, et al. The evolution and maturation of laparoscopic cholecystectomy in an academic practice. J Am Coll Surg. 1998;186: 554–60. discussion 560–1.
3. Sauerland S, Lefering R, Neugebauer EA. Laparoscopic versus open surgery for suspected appendicitis. *Cochrane Database Syst Rev.* 2004;(4):CD001546.
4. McCormack K, Scott NW, Go PM, et al. Laparoscopic techniques versus open techniques for inguinal hernia repair. *Cochrane Database Syst Rev.* 2003(1):CD001785.
5. Clinical Outcomes of Surgical Therapy Study Group. A comparison of laparoscopically assisted and open colectomy for colon cancer. N Engl J Med. 2004;350:2050–59.
6. Laurent C, Leblanc F, Wutrich P, et al. Laparoscopic versus open surgery for rectal cancer: long-term oncologic results. Ann Surg. 2009;250:54–61.
7. ASMBS, Rationale for the Surgical Treatment of Morbid Obesity. Available at: http://www.asbs.org/Newsite07/patients/resources/asbs_rationale.htm. Accessed 4/20/2010.

8. Nguyen NT, Goldman C, Rosenquist CJ, et al. Laparoscopic versus open gastric bypass: a randomized study of outcomes, quality of life, and costs. Ann Surg. 2001;234:279–89. discussion 289–91.

9. Nguyen NT, Lee SL, Goldman C, et al. Comparison of pulmonary function and postoperative pain after laparoscopic versus open gastric bypass: a randomized trial. J Am Coll Surg. 2001;192:469–76. discussion 476–7.

10. Nguyen NT, Goldman CD, Ho HS, et al. Systemic stress response after laparoscopic and open gastric bypass. J Am Coll Surg. 2002;194:557–66. discussion 566–7.

11. Nguyen NT, Owings JT, Gosselin R, et al. Systemic coagulation and fibrinolysis after laparoscopic and open gastric bypass. Arch Surg. 2001;136:909–16.

12. Puzziferri N, Austrheim-Smith IT, Wolfe BM, et al. Three-year follow-up of a prospective randomized trial comparing laparoscopic versus open gastric bypass. Ann Surg. 2006;243:181–8.

13. Belle S. LABS Consortium. The NIDDK Bariatric Surgery clinical Research Consortium (LABS). Surg Obes Relat Dis. 2005;1:145–7.

14. Belle SH, Berk PD, Courcoulas AP, et al. Safety and efficacy of bariatric surgery: longitudinal assessment of bariatric surgery. Surg Obes Relat Dis. 2007;3:116–26.

15. Longitudinal Assessment of Bariatric Surgery (LABS) Consortium, Flum DR, Belle SH, et al. Perioperative safety in the longitudinal assessment of bariatric surgery. N Engl J Med. 2009;361:445–54.

16. LABS Writing Group for the LABS Consortium, Belle SH, Chapman W, et al. Relationship of body mass index with demographic and clinical characteristics in the Longitudinal Assessment of Bariatric Surgery (LABS). Surg Obes Relat Dis. 2008;4:474–80.

17. Smith MD, Patterson E, Wahed AS, et al. Relationship between surgeon volume and adverse outcomes after RYGB in Longitudinal Assessment of Bariatric Surgery (LABS) study. Surg Obes Relat Dis. 2010;6(2):118–25.

18. King WC, Belle SH, Eid GM, et al. Physical activity levels of patients undergoing bariatric surgery in the Longitudinal Assessment of Bariatric Surgery study. Surg Obes Relat Dis. 2008;4:721–8.

14. National Patient Safety Guidelines

And Strategies to Develop Programs at the Local Level

William Greif and Pascal Fuchshuber

"If the world was perfect, it wouldn't be"

Yogi Berra

Implementing a comprehensive safety program for patients in the perioperative arena involves standardizing and measuring processes based on "Best Practice."

This chapter outlines the main standardized protocol's around this goal:

1. Universal Protocol
2. Culture of Safety in the OR
3. 2010 National Patient Safety Goals
4. Surgical Care Improvement Project (SCIP)
5. OR checklist, time-out and debrief.

Part I: Universal Protocol for Preventing Wrong Site, Wrong Procedure, Wrong Person Surgery

Universal protocol is a process designed by the Joint Commission to prevent wrong site surgeries. In August 1998, the Joint Commission issued a Sentinel Event Alert examining the problem of wrong site surgery, including a review of 15 cases that had been reported to them. The root cause analysis was performed by the hospitals and usually indicated in the majority of cases that the etiology involved a breakdown in communication between surgical team members themselves and/or with the patient or their family [1]. From 1995 through 2005, the Joint

D.S. Tichansky, J. Morton, and D.B. Jones (eds.), *The SAGES Manual of Quality, Outcomes and Patient Safety*, DOI 10.1007/978-1-4419-7901-8_14, © Springer Science+Business Media, LLC 2012

Commission sentinel event statistics database ranked wrong-side surgery as the second of the most frequently reported sentinel events and in a separate survey of orthopedic hand surgeons estimated the lifetime risk of performing a wrong-side surgery as greater than 1 in 5 [2].

The Joint Commission Board of Commissioners originally developed the Universal Protocol for Preventing Wrong Site, Wrong Procedure and Wrong Person Surgery™ in July 2003. In July 1, 2004 it became effective for all accredited hospitals, ambulatory care and office-based surgery facilities. There are three critical elements to Universal Protocol.

- Conduct a pre-procedure verification process (UP.01.01.01)
- Mark the procedure site (UP.01.02.01)
- A time-out is performed before the procedure (UP.01.03.01)

The Joint Commission has emphasized that the Universal Protocol is based on the following principles:

- It applies to all invasive procedures
- Requires active involvement and methods to improve communication among all members of the procedure team for success
- To the extent possible the patient (and family) are involved in the process
- There is consistent implementation

For more detailed information go to: http://www.jointcommission. org/PatientSafety/UniversalProtocol/

The Joint Commission notes that Universal Protocol is *most successfully implemented in hospitals with a culture that promotes teamwork* and where all individuals feel empowered to protect patient safety.

Creating a Culture of Safety in the Operating Room

A first step in creating a culture of safety in the operating room is to understand the perceptions of the safety and teamwork climate from the front line staff in the operating room. As noted in a recent study from John Hopkins, there are considerable discrepancies in perceptions of teamwork in the operating room, with physicians rating the teamwork of others as good, but at the same time, nurses perceive teamwork as mediocre [3] (Fig. 14.1). This same group has developed a Safety

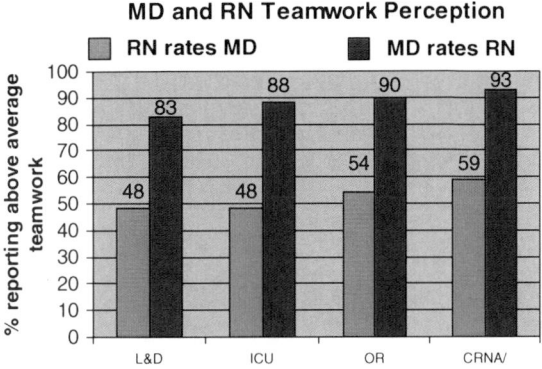

Fig. 14.1. Differences in team perception between physician and nurses based on Safety Attitude Questionnaire (copyright J.B.Sexton and IHI Boston).

Table 14.1. Safety attitude questionnaire (SAQ) categories and examples.

Definitions of factors	Examples
Teamwork Climate: perceived quality of collaboration between staffs	Our doctors and nurses work well together
Job Satisfaction: positivity about work experience	I like my job This is a good place to work
Perception of Management: approval of managerial action	Management is doing a good job
Safety Climate: perception of commitment to safety by the organization	I would feel perfectly safe being treated here
Working Conditions: perceived quality of work environment	Staffing and equipment are adequate
Stress Recognition: is stress recognized as a performance modifier	Excessive work load and fatigue affect my performance and work

Attitudes Questionnaire (SAQ) to quantify perception of safety among different groups of staff and physicians in the operating room which has been administered in over 400 hospitals internationally. It has been validated and has been shown to correlate well with pilot performance in aviation, high speed rail accident rates and outcomes in the medical industry such as length of stay, error rates and nurse turnover rates. [4].

Table 14.1 shows the principal elements of the Safety Attitude Questionnaire.

Exhibit 14.1.

4 step process	95% reliability each step	81% outcome reliability
	99% reliability each step	96% outcome reliability
25 step process	95% reliability each step	28% outcome reliability
	99% reliability each step	78% outcome reliability
50 step process	95% reliability each step	8% outcome reliability
	99% reliability each step	61% outcome reliability

A second step in developing the culture of safety is addressing the areas of concerns once they are identified. One of the most effective methods of teambuilding is through human factors. Human factors are a discipline devoted to studying the interaction of people in communication and teamwork. The approach shifts attention away from the fault of individuals and the framework of human reliability to the larger contributing factors of systemic controls. The core understanding of this discipline is that in complex systems with multiple steps, one can predict mathematically the error rate based on the reliability factor of the process. For example, a process with four steps that are each 95% reliable (the predictable human error rate is 5%) has an overall reliability of only 81%, i.e. an error rate of 19% ($0.95 \times 0.95 \times 0.95 \times 0.95 = 0.81$). One can easily see that with each added complexity of a system the overall reliability decreases and the error rate increases.

Thus the emphasis is designing processes and coordination of efforts to prevent these outcomes rather than sporadically blaming individuals. The Institute for Healthcare Improvement (IHI) has significant training and resources based on well documented strategies for developing safety programs [5]. For further information go to: www.IHI.com

One of the easiest and most effective ways to start the process of team building in the OR is the use of the white board that includes the names of all OR staff. The impact of this small change is enormous as it levels the playing field and sets up the basis for open communication and safety.

Part 2: 2010 National Patient Safety Goals

The Joint Commission created the National Patient Safety Goals (NPSGs) were established in 2002 to promote specific improvements in patient safety. Revised on an annual basis, the goals address problem areas in health care and prescribe evidence-based solutions to promote patient safety and prevent sentinel events. The goals focus on system-wide solutions. NPSGs recently underwent extensive review and revision for 2010. Listed below are the goals for hospitals:

Goal 1 – Two patient identifiers (NPSG.01.01.01) when providing care, treatment and services and to eliminate transfusion errors related to patient misidentification.

Goal 2 – Improve the effectiveness of communication among caregivers: reporting critical values (NPSG.02.03.01).

Goal 3 – Improve safety using medications: label all medications, medication containers, and other solutions on and off the sterile field in perioperative and other procedural settings (NPSG.03.04.01) and reduce harm from anticoagulant therapy (NPSG.03.05.01).

Goal 7 – Reduce risk of health care associated infections with evidence-based medicine practices to:
comply with CDC and/or WHO hand hygiene guidelines (NPSG.07.01.01),
prevent multi-drug resistant organisms (NPSG.07.03.01),
prevent central line associated bloodstream infections (NPSG.07.04.01),
and prevent surgical site infections (NPSG.07.05.01).

Goal 8 – Accurately and completely reconcile medications: additional work is being done to evaluation and refine expectations.

Goal 9, 14, 15 – Reduce risk of Falls (NPSG.09.02.01), prevent health care associated pressure ulcers (NPSG.14.01.01), identify patients at risk for suicide (NPSG.15.01.01) and identify risk with home oxygen therapy and fire (NPSG.15.02.01).

For further information go to: www.jointcommission.org/patientsafety/nationalpatientsafetygoals/

Using Small Test of Change to Promote Compliance with National Patient Safety Goals

The effectiveness of the small test of change model is in the inherent design:

- involvement of front line staff
- small test of change: trial of new process with rapid re-assessment and gradual rollout to larger segments of the institution

- continuous auditing of performance and feedback
- see also: www.ihi.org/IHI/Topics/Improvement/Improvement-Methods/HowToImprove/testingchanges.htm

The Plan-Do-Study-Act (PDSA) cycle is shorthand for testing a change – by planning it, trying it, observing the results, and acting on what is learned. The beauty of this scientific method is that it allows for rapid cycle process improvement.

Part 3: Surgical Care Improvement Project (SCIP)

In early 1999, the Joint Commission collaborated with clinical professionals, health care provider organizations, state hospital associations, health care consumers, performance measurement experts and others to develop core measures for hospitals. These were first launched in 2001 and subsequently the Surgical Infection Prevention (SIP) measure was added in 2003. This was subsequently modified to the Surgical Care Improvement Project (SCIP) developed through a national quality partnership of organizations interested in improving surgical care by significantly reducing surgical complications.

The SCIP goal is to reduce the incidence of surgical complications nationally by 25% by the year 2010. There has been debate as to whether this is attainable. SCIP includes four general process measures for infection prevention – prophylactic antibiotic administration, glucose control, hair removal, and normothermia. These measures are based on studies on who to reduce the rate of surgical site infection [6]. In addition, they are also process measures related to venous thromboembolism prophylaxis. This year a urinary catheter related measure was added and the normothermia measure was revised. These changes were based on studies that (1) demonstrated a direct correlation between the risk of catheter-associated urinary tract infection (UTI) and the duration of indwelling urinary catheterization [7] and (2) found that the incidence of culture-positive surgical site infections among those with mild perioperative hypothermia was three times higher than of normothermic patients [8]. The efficacy of the SCIP process measures has been questioned by a recent study that failed to show a significant change in infection rates in hospital that have adopted SCIP [9].

The following list describes the current SCIP measures:

SCIP INF 1 – Prophylactic antibiotic received within 1 h prior to surgical incision for cardiac, orthopedic hip and knee arthroplasty, colon surgery, hysterectomy, and vascular surgery.

SCIP INF 2   – Prophylactic antibiotic selection from pre-approved list of antibiotics.

SCIP INF 3   – Prophylactic antibiotics discontinued within 24 h after surgery (48 h for cardiac surgery).

SCIP INF 4   – Cardiac surgery patients with controlled 6 AM post-operative blood glucose.

SCIP INF 6   – Surgery patients with appropriate hair removal using clippers and not razors.

SCIP INF 9   – Urinary catheter removed on post-operative day 1 or 2.

SCIP INF 10 – Surgery patients with perioperative temperature management.

SCIP Card 2 – Surgery patients on beta-blocker therapy prior to arrival who received a beta-blocker during the perioperative period.

SCIP VTE 1 – Surgery patients with recommended venous thromboembolism prophylaxis ordered.

SCIP VTE 2 – Surgery patients who received appropriate venous thromboembolism prophylaxis within 24 h prior to surgery to 24 h after surgery.

Use of the Checklist to Develop Consistency in Surgical Care Improvement Project Measures

Dr. Atul Gawande of the Brigham and Women's Hospital speaks eloquently of the first competitive flight of the B-17 bomber the Army Air Corps held on October 30th, 1935 [10]. Created by Boeing, it was called the "flying fortress" because it could carry 5 times as many bombs as other competitive models. After it launched from the runway at this landmark flight, it flew 300 ft and crashed in a fiery explosion and was deemed "too much airplane for one man to fly." The Army Air Corps declared Douglas's smaller design the winner and Boeing nearly went bankrupt.

After further test flights, and with a checklist in hand, the pilots went on to fly the Boeing aircraft a total of 1.8 million miles without one accident. The Army ultimately ordered almost 13,000 of the aircraft, and gained a decisive air advantage in the Second World War.

1 TEAM BRIEFING

There are two parts to the FINAL TIME OUT. The first part is the **team briefing** which occurs prior to anesthesia induction. It occurs in the operating room with the patient awake and participating.

Surgeon
- ☐ **Correct Patient – Name and MRN confirmed by 2 persons**
- ☐ **Correct Procedure – consent visualized**
- ☐ **Side/Site – confirm site marking**
- ☐ **Key equipment / instruments needed – specific implant named**
- ☐ **Position**
- ☐ **Plan for surgery – anticipated issues, bleeding risk**
- ☐ **Relevant images available**

This portion must be <u>repeated</u> when beginning an <u>additional procedure</u> <u>by a different surgeon</u>

Circulator
- ☐ **All names (including patient) on white board and confirm all available (including x-ray tech, vendor, etc.)**
- ☐ **DVT prophylaxis accomplished**
- ☐ **Equipment available and familiar**
- ☐ **Verify all solutions and medications available**

Scrub
- ☐ **Requested instruments available and functioning**
- ☐ **Integrators indicate sterility** (2 person)
- ☐ **All solutions and medications on back table are labeled**

Anesthesia
- ☐ **Anesthesia type**
- ☐ **Allergies reviewed**
- ☐ **Antibiotics plan – correct dose for wt.**
- ☐ **Beta blockade given if required**
- ☐ **Blood available as appropriate**
- ☐ **BMI >50 for x-ray if criteria met**
- ☐ **Normothermia plan**

2 RE-VERIFICATION

The second part of the FINAL TIME OUT is the **re-verification** which occurs after the patient is draped and immediately before incision or invasive procedure:

- ☐ **Circulator: Correct Procedure and Correct Side/Site**
- ☐ **Surgeon: Marking Visible after draping**
- ☐ **Scrub: Confirm Neutral Zone**
- ☐ **Anesthesia: Antibiotics given**

3 POST-OP DEBRIEF

After surgery we perform the **post-operative debriefing.** It occurs at the end of the procedure before the patient has left the room.

Team
- ☐ **Confirm Diagnosis**
- ☐ **Confirm Specimen and correctly labeled**
- ☐ **Confirm Procedure(s) performed**
- ☐ **What went well**
- ☐ **What can be improved**
- ☐ **Special needs for patient post-op**
- ☐ **Next case – confirm what needed**

Fig. 14.2. Surgical Checklist Template.

Through the use of checklists in the World Health Organization's "Safe Surgery Saves Lives" campaign, Dr. Gawande and others have shown that operating rooms in hospitals of all levels of expertise internationally have made strides in safety [11] (Fig 14.2). Numerous studies have shown that the checklist prevents error under stressful conditions in which cognitive function is compromised by fatigue or other factors [12]. The concept of an OR checklist has recently been expanded to include a standardized postoperative debriefing list. The goal is to ascertain correct documentation and gives the team the opportunity to learn from events during the procedure.

Selected Readings

1. Joint commission Sentinel Event Alert, 5 Dec 2001.
2. Seiden SC, Barach P. Wrong-side/wrong-site, wrong-procedure, and wrong-patient adverse events: are they preventable. Arch Surg. 2006;141:931–9.
3. Makary M, Sexon J, Frieshlag J, Holzmueller C, Millman E, Rowen L, Pronovost P. J Am Coll Surg. 2006;202 N5:746–52.
4. The link between safety attitudes and observed performance in flight operations. In: Proceedings of the Eleventh International Symposium on Aviation Psychology, Columbus, OH: The Ohio State University; 2001. pp 7–13.
5. Leonard M, Frankel A, Simmonds T, Vega K. Achieving Safe and Reliable Healthcare strategies and solutions. 2004 Foundation of the American College of Healthcare Executives.
6. Dellinger EP, Hausmann SM, Bratzler DW, Johnson RM, Daniel DM, Bunt KM, et al. Hospitals collaborate to decrease surgical site infections. Am J Surg. 2005;190:9–15.
7. Wald HL, Ma A, Bratzler DW, Kramer AM. Indwelling urinary catheter use in the postoperative period: analysis of the national surgical infection prevention project data. *Arch Surg.* In press.
8. Kurz A, Sessler DI, Lenhardt R. Perioperative normothermia to reduce the incidence of surgical-wound infection and shorten hospitalization. N Engl J Med. 1996;334: 1209–15.
9. G Miller, SCIP's SSI Benchmarks likely unattainable, studies indicate, General Surgery News, V3, 9/2009.
10. The Checklist. If something so simple can transform intensive care, what else can it do? The New Yorker, 10/2007.
11. World Health Organization, Safe Surgery Saves Lives, The Second Global Patient Safety Challenge.
12. Hales B, Pronovost P. The checklist – a tool for error management and performance improvement. J Critical Care. 2006;21:241–35.

Part II
Understanding Error

15. Taxonomy of Errors: Adverse Event/Near Miss Analysis

Dennis L. Fowler

Background

Errors in healthcare delivery received relatively little public attention or scientific scrutiny through most of the twentieth century. Unlike accidents in aviation, nuclear power plants, and chemical processing plants that may result in mass casualties, errors in healthcare tend to affect one individual at a time and, therefore, receive less publicity. Beginning in the 1980s, studies reported the surprisingly high incidence of potentially avoidable errors in healthcare [1, 2]. In 1990, James Reason initiated a sharper focus on the study and analysis of human error in medicine [3], and in 1997 explained the types of human errors and their causes [4].

Despite these publications, most providers had little insight into the degree to which errors harmed patients until the publication of *To Err is Human* by the Institute of Medicine in 1999 [5]. In that publication, the authors based their recommendations for improving patient safety on the premise that human error is inevitable. As Reason suggested years before, healthcare should be delivered in a system designed to prevent harm either by preventing the error itself or by early detection of an error and intervening to prevent harm. Since that publication, there has been an increased focus on patient safety and the need to reduce or eliminate avoidable errors.

Errors usually lead to one of two important outcomes: (1) an adverse event or (2) a near miss. A near miss is an event that had the potential to result in an adverse event. A near miss offers a critical opportunity to intervene before the error recurs and results in an adverse event. A third possible situation involves an error that is of so little consequence that it would never result in harm. The focus of this chapter is on errors that result in an adverse event or a near miss, although much of the work to date to analyze errors in surgery has been based on the analysis of adverse events.

D.S. Tichansky, J. Morton, and D.B. Jones (eds.), *The SAGES Manual*   139
of Quality, Outcomes and Patient Safety, DOI 10.1007/978-1-4419-7901-8_15,
© Springer Science+Business Media, LLC 2012

As a result of a better understanding of error in healthcare, two important concepts should be stressed [6]. First, errors are not character defects, and individuals who have erred should not be treated with discipline and/or education. Second, major consequences of errors are typically the result of a series of errors, often including conditions not previously identified as creating risk. A key to reducing errors and the harm caused by errors is the development of a standardized classification of errors [7]. With this taxonomy, it is easier to report errors. More importantly, analysis of errors reported within a defined system of classification can identify patterns and possible causes, and thereby identify potential solutions.

Definitions (Fig. 15.1)

Error – An error is the failure of a planned action to be completed as intended, or the use of a wrong plan to achieve an aim.

In the case of the failure to execute the plan, the plan may have been adequate to achieve the intended goal, but the actions failed. In the second instance, the plan itself was inadequate. Errors may cause adverse events or result in near misses.

Adverse Event – An adverse event is an event that harms a patient as a result of an error.

For the purpose of this chapter, an adverse event must cause harm to the patient.

Definitions

Error – The failure of a planned action to be completed as intended, or the use of a wrong plan to achieve an aim

Adverse Event – Harm to a patient as a result of an error

Near Miss – An event that had the potential to result in harm to a patient

Fig. 15.1. Definitions.

Near Miss – A near miss is an event that had the potential to harm a patient.

Near misses may fall into two categories. In one case, the error is prevented just prior to its occurrence and the error is narrowly avoided. In the other case, an individual or team actually make an error, but prior to harm, the team identifies the error and prevents or reduces the extent of the harm.

Taxonomy

Errors may be classified in several different ways, depending on the reason for developing the taxonomy. For the purpose of this chapter, we will use with minimal modification the taxonomy described in several publications in the past 10 years by Reason [8–10] and modified by others [11]. Typically in healthcare institutions, the two types of errors fall into two categories: active failure and latent failure (Fig. 15.2).

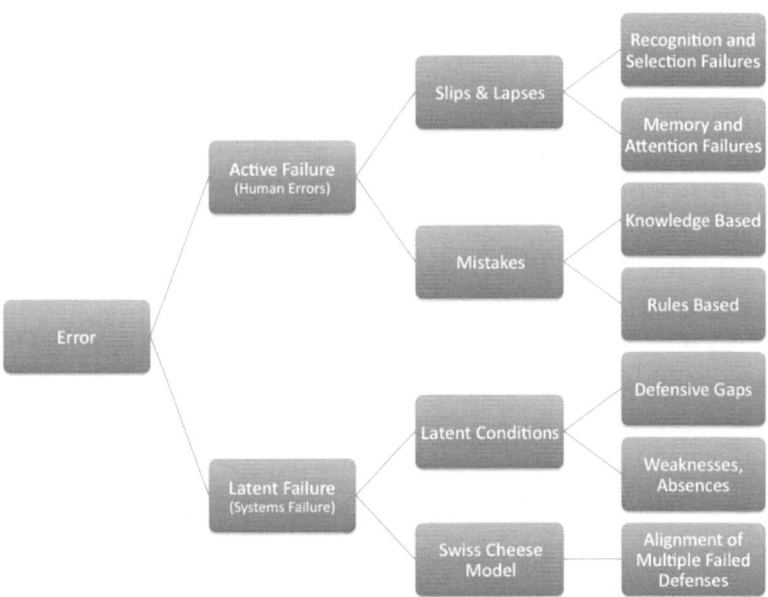

Fig. 15.2. Taxonomy of Errors in Healthcare.

The aspects of active failure and latent failure can be defined in much greater detail. Although the traditional surgical approach to analyzing errors, particularly in mortality and morbidity conferences, has been to focus on active failure by the individual at the point of care, the failure by the individual at the point of care is many times inevitable and should not be the focus for prevention of future similar errors. Modern principles of systems function show that for an organization to be highly reliable, multiple layers of defense against human failure should be in place. Only when multiple layers of defense fail will the active failure by the person at the point of care result in an error that results in an adverse event or a near miss.

Human errors that constitute active failure fall into two categories: (1) slips and lapses and (2) mistakes. Slips are forgetfulness or a failure to recognize something that the individual would usually recognize, and lapses are moments of attention loss. Slips and lapses are errors of execution. The intent of the individual was correct, but because of a slip or a lapse, an error occurred. Mistakes occur because the plan is inadequate. If the plan is in error or otherwise inadequate, the intended outcome will not occur, even with good execution of the plan. Mistakes are errors of intention and are either knowledge-based or rule-based. Knowledge-based mistakes occur when a practitioner encounters a situation outside of his/her knowledge, and he/she must reason what to do. There are many factors leading to failure when this occurs and the incidence of knowledge-based errors in this situation is high. Rule-based errors are different than knowledge-based errors and occur because humans follow rules while doing routine tasks. Although the use of rules results in fewer slips and lapses, when the plan must be changed for any reason, rules-based mistakes occur as a consequence of misapplying a rule or using the wrong rule.

Often, these decisions can be reversed as a result of analyzing adverse events and near misses and thereby identifying the latent failure.

Latent failures are quite different. They are present in systems due to decisions made by people more remote from the point of care, such as designers, builders, procedure writers, and top-level management. Although well intentioned, the decisions by these high-level individuals translate into either error-provoking conditions or result in holes in the defenses against active failure. They may lie dormant in an organization for a long time before a combination of triggering events expose them. They are more often the cause of a harmful outcome than a slip, lapse, or a mistake, and, when exposed, can be modified or reversed to eliminate the latent condition.

Since slips, lapses, and mistakes are inevitable, the best opportunity to reduce the occurrence of harmful errors is by eliminating latent conditions and maximizing the systems in place to prevent and mitigate the consequences of them. Latent conditions should be perceived as weaknesses or absences in the defense against slips, lapses, and mistakes, and may be related to the facility, the policies, the procedures, or other facets of an organization. These failures of design provide the greatest opportunity for improvement. Adverse events are most likely to occur when multiple latent conditions or failed defenses occur in the same situation, and this is called the Swiss cheese model.

Adverse Events

Traditional analysis of errors in the world of surgery has focused on analysis of cases that resulted in an adverse event. Mortality and Morbidity (M & M) conference in most academic departments throughout the twentieth century resulted in a constrained discussion of the causes of an adverse event. The typical M & M discussion focused on the active error of the surgeon or housestaff officer. Less commonly, the discussion included analysis of the conditions surrounding the occurrence of the adverse event. The active failure was often classified as an error of technique or judgment. This approach has resulted in either discipline or education for the individual who committed the error, and almost never resulted in addressing any of the latent conditions that contributed to the error. Additionally, the analysis in M & M Conference rarely included a discussion of how the system failed to prevent or mitigate the consequences of mistakes. Most importantly, until recently, few M & M conferences have included discussion of near misses, despite the fact that they offer the largest opportunity for preventing adverse events.

Near Misses

Although a taxonomy of errors may be helpful by furthering the understanding of the causes of errors, the most critical practical step to using this understanding is to increase the reporting of errors. It is in this area that healthcare has lagged behind other high-risk organizations. Not only is it important to report adverse events, it is even more important to report near misses because near misses outnumber adverse events by a factor of more than 300 [12]. In most cases, there have probably been many more unreported near misses than adverse events involving the same active error or latent condition. Near misses provide a golden opportunity to avoid future, potential adverse events.

Traditionally, surgeons have not had a culture that enabled reporting adverse events and near misses. For many reasons, including lack of time, fear of punishment, loss of reputation, and even a lack of perceived benefit, surgeons have resisted reporting [13]. There are now numerous recent publications documenting the importance of reporting and analyzing not only adverse events, but also near misses [14, 15]. Because there is no adverse outcome caused by a near miss, reporting and reviewing near misses should overcome the resistance to reporting based on risk of medical malpractice litigation or punishment [16].

Summary

The taxonomy of errors presented here describes both active errors and latent conditions that result in adverse events. This taxonomy acknowledges that human error is inevitable and that latent conditions within a system can increase the likelihood that human error will result in an adverse event. With this understanding, latent conditions that pose risk to patients may be modified or eliminated to either prevent human error or mitigate the consequences of human error or both. This has the potential to reduce the incidence and severity of adverse events. Analysis of near misses offers the most promising opportunity to identify and modify latent conditions that pose risk to patients.

Selected Readings

1. Brennan TA, Leape LL, Laird NM, et al. Incidence of adverse events and negligence in hospitalized patients: results from the Harvard medical practice study 1. 1991. Qual Saf Health Care. 2004;13:145–51.
2. Leape LL, Brennan TA, Laird NM, et al. The nature of adverse events in hospitalized patients: results from the Harvard medical practice study II. NEJM. 1991;324:377–84.
3. Reason J. Human error. New York: Cambridge University; 1990.
4. Reason J. Managing the risks of organizational accidents. Hampshire, England: Ashgate Publishing; 1997.

5. Institute of Medicine. To err is human. Kohn LT, Corrigan JM,Donaldson MS, editors. Washington, DC: National Academy Press; 1999.

6. Spencer FC. Human error in hospitals and industrial accidents: Current concepts. JACS. 2000;191:410–8.

7. Zhang J, Patel VL, Johnson TR, et al. Toward an action based taxonomy of human errors in medicine. In: Proc of 24th Conference of Cognitive Science Society; AMIA Annual Symposium Proceedings. 2002:934–938.

8. Reason J. Human error: models and management. BMJ. 2000;320:768–70.

9. Reason J. Beyond the organisational accident: the need for "error wisdom" on the frontline. Qual Saf Health Care. 2004;13(Suppl II):ii28–33.

10. Reason J. Safety in the operating theatre – Part 2: Human error and organisational failure. Qual Saf Health Care. 2005;14:56–61.

11. Brannick MT, Fabri PJ, Zayas-Castro J, et al. Evaluation of an error-reduction training program for surgical residents. Acad Med. 2009;84:1809–14.

12. Cushieri A. Nature of human error implications for surgical practice. Ann Surg. 2006;244:642–8.

13. Leape LL. Reporting of adverse events. N Engl J Med. 2002;347:1633–8.

14. Blendon RJ, DesRoches CM, Brodie M, et al. Views of practising physicians and the public on medical errors. N Engl J Med. 2002;347:1933–40.

15. Bilimoria KY, Kmiecik TE, DaRosa DA, et al. Development of an Online Morbidity, Mortality, and Near-Miss Reporting System to Identify Patterns of Adverse Events in Surgical Patients. Arch Surg. 2009;144(4):305–11.

16. McCafferty MH, Polk HC. Addition of "Near-Miss" Cases Enhances a Quality Improvement Conference. Arch Surg. 2004;139:216–7.

16. Disclosure of Complications and Error

Rocco Orlando III

Communication with patients about medical error is one of the most difficult issues which confront the surgeon. While surgeons strive to care for patients without mistakes, the complexity of the care process allows for the possibility of surgeon error, systems error, or error committed by any member of the care team. Given the complexity of the modern care process, most errors are the result of human rather than technical failures [1]. The current movement to enhance patient safety and improve health care quality will certainly reduce error, but medical error will unfortunately continue to occur. Human fallibility can be limited by robust systems, but will never be completely eliminated.

The definition of error which was adopted by the Institute of Medicine in the seminal report *To Err is Human* [2] was proposed by James Reason in 1990: "occasions in which a planned sequence of mental or physical activities fails to achieve its intended outcome" [3]. This definition includes errors that may not result in an adverse event, the concept of the "near miss." The Harvard Medical Practice Study defined adverse events as "an injury that was caused by medical management (and not the disease process) that either prolonged the hospitalization or produced a disability at the time of discharge or both" [4]. This definition is not only precise, but also includes significant errors which might not result in disability or prolonged hospital stay. These errors may not result in an adverse event but can still be troubling to patients or the health care team.

Toward a Taxonomy of Error

The traditional taxonomy of error employed by most surgeons is the model of the morbidity and mortality conference. This approach recognizes the time-honored concepts of technical error, judgment error,

D.S. Tichansky, J. Morton, and D.B. Jones (eds.), *The SAGES Manual of Quality, Outcomes and Patient Safety*, DOI 10.1007/978-1-4419-7901-8_16, © Springer Science+Business Media, LLC 2012

error of omission, and error of commission [4]. The morbidity and mortality conference analyzes all adverse events on a surgical service – deaths and complications – and the formal structure recognizes that some adverse events are preventable, others are not. This taxonomy of error is incomplete because it is unduly focused on the actions of the surgeon. While the surgeon may, indeed, commit a technical error or make an error in judgment (such as a delay in diagnosis), this approach does not recognize the myriad other kinds of medical error: medication errors, nursing care errors and system errors and latent errors. Latent error refers to the injury which can result from a complex chain of events in the care process – any one of the events might not result in injury, but taken together, an adverse event occurs. A more inclusive categorization of error is useful because it may provide guidance in changing systems of care to prevent future error (Exhibit 16.1).

Reason's definition of error is more broad and helpful as surgeons consider what to disclose to patients when errors occur. From a pragmatic and ethical standpoint, any error which reaches the threshold of the Harvard Medical Practice Study, resulting in prolonged hospital stay, death or disability, must be reported to the patient. However errors recognized by Reason must also be reported at times, specifically those which do not result in injury but may come to the patient's attention. These errors, the "near misses," must be discussed with the patient to avoid a loss in confidence in the caregivers.

Exhibit 16.1. Taxonomy of error.

Traditional surgical paradigm
Technical error
Judgment error
Delay in diagnosis
Error in diagnosis
Error of omission
Error of commission

Practical taxonomy of error
Technical error
Systems error
Latent error
Medication error
Device failure

Regulatory Aspects of Error Disclosure

The modern climate of health care now requires that errors be disclosed. This has resulted from the patient safety movement and increasing demands for transparency and public accountability in health care. In the past, the culture of medicine was to withhold admission of errors. Physicians commonly withheld the disclosure of errors from patients. Errors were only disclosed when the mistake was obvious or significant injury resulted. At times, adverse events were ascribed to the patient's disease rather than to error. The prevailing wisdom was that admission of error would increase the risk of malpractice litigation. Physicians also were embarrassed and unsure of disclosure strategies when confronting error. Patients now expect to be fully informed and involved in their care.

The momentum for the disclosure of error has developed as a result of the patient safety and quality movement. In the United States, the Joint Commission on Accreditation of Healthcare Organizations (the Joint Commission) issued the first nationwide disclosure standard [6]. This standard requires that patients be informed about all outcomes of care including "unanticipated outcomes." The importance of the Joint Commission in the realm of hospital care gave great impetus to the movement to disclose errors. The National Quality Forum (NQF), an organization that operates at the federal level with strong ties to CMS, has developed standards for the disclosure of unanticipated outcomes [7]. The NQF safe practice standards are used by the Leapfrog Group, a coalition of 29 large healthcare purchasing organizations. A total of 1,300 hospitals currently report information about these standards, including disclosure, to the Leapfrog Group.

The Institute for Healthcare Improvement, the Agency for Healthcare Research and Quality, and numerous medical specialty societies have all called for policies of disclosure. Unfortunately, the medical society recommendations for transparent disclosure of error are somewhat vague and lack specificity. The AMA Code of Ethics, for example, states that "a physician should at all times deal honestly and openly with patients" [9].

On the international level, initiatives in Australia and the United Kingdom have been notable. In 2003, Australia initiated an "Open Disclosure Standard" in pilot programs across the country. In the United Kingdom, the "Being Open" initiative has been put in place with an extensive educational campaign. These programs have advocated transparent communication and provided tools for enhancing communication with patients. These efforts have been voluntary and have not specifically addressed poor outcomes which have occurred as a result of medical error [8].

As the regulatory agencies have established standards for the disclosure of error, governmental authorities are beginning to mandate disclosure. Although there are no laws requiring disclosure at the national level, in 2005, Senators Hillary Rodham Clinton and Barack Obama sponsored a bill, the National Medical Error Disclosure and Compensation Act (MEDiC) calling for full disclosure of errors [9]. The bill did not pass, but it linked disclosure, quality and the medical liability system. The recognition at the federal level that issues of quality, openness, and liability are all closely related is important and suggests that these initiatives are likely to continue as health care reform becomes increasingly important as a national issue.

Several states have passed legislation mandating disclosure of serious unanticipated outcomes. Laws are now in effect in Nevada, Florida, New Jersey, Pennsylvania, Oregon, Vermont, and California [8]. The most stringent law is in place in Pennsylvania which requires that hospital notify patients in writing within 7 days of a serious event. The Pennsylvania law also prohibits the use of these communications as evidence of liability. These laws share in common an approach which requires that hospitals develop mechanisms for disclosure, rather than individual physicians. Forty-five states have enacted "apology laws" which protects certain information transmitted in disclosures, especially expressions of regret or other forms of apology [8]. Enforcement of these laws is only stipulated in the Pennsylvania law. Many of the laws are sufficiently vague that regulation of disclosures seems difficult, at best.

Error Disclosure and Risk of Litigation

Physicians have been most concerned that disclosure will increase the likelihood of a malpractice action. These concerns have done much to impede the flow of information to patients and families. Despite this, it is now clear that patients want to know about all errors that cause them harm. A large survey of emergency department patients revealed that 80% wanted to be informed immediately of any medical error. A large majority also supported reporting errors to government agencies, state medical boards, and hospital committees [11]. This study also demonstrated that patients wished to be informed not just about error resulting in injury, but of "near misses" also. A large survey of health plan members reported increased patient satisfaction, trust when presented scenarios in which full disclosure was advocated. The study also indicated that patient felt that they would be less likely to seek legal advice with full disclosure [12].

American and Canadian physicians appear to embrace the soundness of disclosing errors. These attitudes have changed significantly during the last 20 years. In a 1991 survey of house officer, three of four said that they had not reported an error to a patient, largely because of concern about litigation [13]. By 2006, in a survey of 2,637 physicians, 98% supported disclosing serious medical errors to patients. Seventy-four percent thought that disclosing errors would be difficult, and 58% actually reported disclosing a serious error. Physicians who supported disclosing error were more likely to believe that disclosure made patients less likely to sue [14]. Physicians were more likely than hospital risk managers to support providing a full apology for error while the risk managers were more likely to support disclosing error in the first place [15].

The relationship between disclosure and risk of litigation is not at all clear. In 1987, the Veterans Affairs Hospital in Lexington, VA introduced a disclosure program years before any other. An analysis of the results in 1999 showed that the number of claims during the 12-year period was up, but payments made decreased [16]. Nonetheless, there is a paucity of data which relates the likelihood of a lawsuit to a policy of complete disclosure of error. Despite the lack of solid data, most experts believe that disclosure of error and apology likely reduce the risk of litigation. Based upon the University of Michigan experience, Boothman, Campbell et al. have demonstrated that forthright disclosure and a willingness to apologize is associated with a reduced risk of malpractice actions [17].

Strategies for Disclosing Error to Patients

Gallagher and his colleagues have observed that surgeons are more inclined to disclose error than their medical colleagues [14]. This may result in part from the fact that surgical errors are often more clear and unambiguous. In additional work, they documented better ability of surgeons to disclose error using a standardized set of patient scenarios [16]. Surgeons are probably better at disclosing error because of their greater familiarity with transmitting information about complications.

Surgeons tend to be direct in describing adverse events and are good at providing details about the consequences of medical error. However, surgeons are reluctant to state that and adverse event was a "mistake" or "error" [16]. Although surgeons may be better than their colleagues in other specialties, until recently there was very little guidance about how to communicate error. The lack of guidance contributes to the tendency of surgeons to avoid the use of the word error or mistake.

When an error occurs, it is necessary to disclose it forthrightly to the patient. The first decision centers on who should be present when the error is disclosed. This should be discussed prior to meeting with the patient and family. Often, other members of the team should be present to fully address the patient's needs – this may include nursing, hospital administration, risk management, or other physicians, The meeting should take place in a private setting and all participants should be introduced. The conversation with the patient should take place using clear, simple language.

The surgeon must provide all of the facts about the event. The source of the error must be identified, paying particular attention to whether it is a technical error, human error, or system failure. It is entirely appropriate to express regret for the adverse outcome and to offer a formal apology if the outcome is the result of system failure or error. These conversations should be carried out with empathy and sensitivity. It is very important to accept responsibility for the adverse outcome and to avoid the use of the passive voice. During these conversations, it is important to not attribute blame to others or to claim a lack of understanding of the events.

Following a discussion of the error and resulting injury, the surgeon should review its implications with the patient. The consequences of the error should be reviewed and the surgeon should explain what will be done to mitigate the problem. The emotional needs of the patient and family should be remembered at this time and any necessary support should be offered. The patient should also be told what measures will be taken to ensure that a similar error does not occur in the future to another patient.

From an institutional standpoint, the disclosure should be part of a response which includes patient safety and risk management activities – ensuring that a similar event does not occur again and that system problems are addressed. Coaching of physicians in appropriate communication strategies should be available. Given increasing regulatory requirements for disclosure, these events should be tracked using performance improvement tools (see Exhibit 16.2).

Exhibit 16.2. Key elements of the safe practice for disclosing unanticipated outcomes to patients.

Content to be disclosed to the patient
Provide facts about the event
   Presence of error or system failure, if known
   Results of event analysis to support informed decision making by the patient
Express regret for unanticipated outcome
Give formal apology if unanticipated outcome caused by error or system failure

Institutional requirements
Integrate disclosure, patient safety, and risk management activities
Establish disclosure support system
   Provide background disclosure education
   Ensure that disclosure coaching is available at all times
   Provide emotional support for health care workers, administrators, patients
   and families
Use performance improvement tools to track and enhance disclosure

Surgeons have been leaders in the patient safety movement because of a historically longstanding commitment to analyzing and remediating error. Grounded in the tradition of the morbidity and mortality conference, this commitment is no surprise that surgeons are at the forefront of the movement to disclose error.

Selected Readings

1. Cook RI, Woods DD. Operating at the sharp end: the complexity of human error. In: Bogner MS, editor. Human errors in medicine. NJL Erlbaum: Hillsdale; 1994. p. 255–310.
2. Kohn LT, Corrigan JM, Donaldson MS, editors. To err is human. Washington DC: National Academy; 1999.
3. Reason JT. Human error. New York: Cambridge University; 1990.
4. Thomas EJ, Brennan TA. Errors and adverse events in medicine: an overview. In: Vincent C, editor. Clinical risk management. London: BMJ Books; 2001. p. 32.
5. Bosk CL. Forgive and remember: managing medical failure. Chicago: University of Chicago; 1979. p. 36–70.
6. The Joint Commission. Hospital accreditation standards. Oakbrook Terrace, IL: Joint Commission Resources; 2007.
7. Safe practices for better healthcare. Washington, DC: National Quality Forum, 2007. (http://www.qualityforum.org/projects/completed/safe_practices/).

8. Gallagher TH, Studdert D, Levinson W. Disclosing harmful medical errors to patients. NEJM. 2007;356:2713–9.

9. Frangou C. The art of error disclosure. General Surgery News. 2007;34:1–22.

10. Hobogood C, Peck CR, Gilbert B, Chappell K, Zou B. Medical errors-what and when: what do patients want to know? Acad Emerg Med. 2002;9:1156–61.

11. Mazor KM, Simon SR, Yood RA, Martinson BC, Gunter MJ, Reed GW, et al. Health plan members views about disclosure of medical errors. Ann Inter Med. 2004;140:409–18.

12. Wu AW, Folkman S, McPhee SJ, Lo B. Do house officers learn from their mistakes? JAMA. 1991;265:2089–94.

13. Gallagher TH, Waterman AD, Garbutt JM, Kapp JM, Chan DK, Dunnagan WC, et al. US and Canadian physicians attitudes and experiences regarding disclosing errors to patients. Arch Intern Med. 2006;166:1605–11.

14. Loren DJ, Garbutt J, Dunagan WC, et al. Risk Managers, physicians and disclosure of harmful medical errors. Jt Comm J Qual Patient Saf. 2010;36:99–100.

15. Kraman SS, Hamm G. Risk management: extreme honesty may be the best policy. Ann Intern Med. 1999;131:963–7.

16. Boothman RC, Blackwell AC, Campbell DC, Commiskey E, Anderson S. A better approach to medical malpractice claims: the University of Michigan experience. J Health Life Sci Law. 2009;2:125–60.

17. Chan DK, Gallagher TH, Reznick R, Levinson W. How surgeons disclose medical errors to patients: a study using standardized patients. Surgery. 2005;138:851–8.

17. Second Opinion and Transfer of Care

Rocco Orlando III

Surgeons are dedicated to performing technically competent and expert operations: preventing complications wherever possible. Unfortunately, adverse events do occur and must be managed efficiently and effectively. When technical surgical complications occur as a result of an operative procedure, the surgeon must decide when to seek a second opinion and when to consider transfer of the patient for additional care. This chapter will consider second opinions and transfer which may be required as a result of technical surgical complications. Consideration of systemic events such as pneumonia, myocardial infarction, pulmonary embolism, and other medical complications is beyond the scope of this chapter; management of these problems should be carried out in accordance with the capabilities of the hospital.

When an adverse event occurs, in most instances the surgeon will be able to develop a clear approach to manage the situation. However, when the approach to decision making is controversial, a second opinion is advisable. A second opinion is primarily beneficial by providing a fresh and unbiased evaluation of the problem. The consulting surgeon may suggest a treatment which was not anticipated by the primary surgeon. More importantly, the dialogue may offer additional insight into the management of this problem. The consulting surgeon should be experienced with the procedure. In the event that there is not another surgeon with a solid track record with the procedure at the hospital, the case should be reviewed via telephone with a surgeon at another institution.

The consultation which follows a complication should be formal with a written request to consult. Many surgeons obtain a "curbside" consult which is undocumented. In the event of future litigation, this lack of documentation may be problematic in defending the case. When a surgeon gets an informal "curbside," he or she should document with whom they discussed the case and the recommendations that were made.

D.S. Tichansky, J. Morton, and D.B. Jones (eds.), *The SAGES Manual of Quality, Outcomes and Patient Safety*, DOI 10.1007/978-1-4419-7901-8_17, © Springer Science+Business Media, LLC 2012

Intraoperative consultation is an important aspect of managing complications. When a complication is recognized during surgery, the additional input from an experienced surgeon afford the patient the best possible chance at effective management. This intraoperative evaluation should be documented in the record with a dictated report; the consulting surgeon should not simply be listed as a surgical assistant. This aspect of documentation may assist in the event that litigation follows. As a matter of policy at many hospitals, dictated notes are required when a surgeon from another specialty scrubs into a case or when a surgeon scrubs to assist with the management of a complication. In general, intraoperative consultation should be sought when the complication is outside of the usual scope of practice of the primary surgeon. For example, a vascular consultation should be obtained in the event of major vascular injury, especially when reconstruction rather than simple ligation or repair is required. When a surgeon views the operative findings without scrubbing and offers advice, the primary surgeon may choose to document this in the operative note.

From the stand point of the patient and family, a second opinion may be affirming. Since complications of minimally invasive surgery are relatively uncommon, the patient may question the surgeon's experience in managing the complications. Statements made by the surgeon such as "this is a rare complication" or "I've never seen this before" may threaten the patient's confidence in the surgeon. A second opinion may bolster the patient's belief in the surgeon. In addition, patient and family appreciate knowing that all of the expertise of the hospital has been brought to bear in helping with their problem. In dealing with complications in my own patients, I routinely tell them that I will involve my colleagues in assessing the situation. Most patients and their families are reassured by this approach.

In addition to same-specialty consultation, GI consultation can often be helpful in managing the complications of a minimally invasive surgical procedure. This is particularly true of the complications of biliary and bariatric surgery.

When the surgeon does not have experience in the management of a complication, particularly its operative management, consultation should be obtained. The surgeon at the institution who has the best skills to manage the situation should be involved whenever possible. If the surgeons at a hospital lack the experience to manage a complication, particularly a technical complication, transfer to a referral center should be considered. Ideally, the operating surgeon should be aware of regional resources available for referral. For example, a surgeon performing laparoscopic cholecystectomy who does not routinely perform hepaticojejunostomy should be aware of the regional center with experience in biliary reconstructive surgery.

When transfer to a tertiary center is desired, the operating surgeon must contact the surgeon at the referral facility. In this era of evolving health systems, many community hospitals will have a referral relationship with a tertiary center which is part of the system. Some hospitals have formal transfer agreements in place to facilitate a step-up in the level of care. Increasingly, many tertiary centers have transfer centers to facilitate the movement of patients [1]. When the referring surgeon identifies the receiving surgeon and institution, the transfer should be arranged. It is imperative that all documentation at the initial facility including operative reports, images, and laboratory studies be sent with the patient. When transfer is contemplated, it should be performed early in the course of treatment. Transfers to a higher level of care are associated with a higher mortality rate and greater likelihood for a need to intensive care [2].

Patient dissatisfaction with care may also lead to a decision to transfer to a tertiary care center. The patient's and family's relationship with the physician and the community hospital have a strong impact on the desire to consider transfer. When patients and their surrogates request transfer, it is most often because of a perception of medical error or because communication has been suboptimal [3].

Technical complications of certain minimally invasive procedures with a higher likelihood of serious consequences and resulting litigation include laparoscopic cholecystectomy, bariatric surgery, and incisional hernia repair. When common bile duct injury occurs or is suspected, referral to a center should be considered if there is not an experienced biliary reconstructive surgeon at the hospital. If the injury is recognized intraoperatively, and expert help is not immediately available, a drain should be left in place. The gallbladder need not be removed since its presence may assist the reconstructive surgeon in defining the anatomy. There should be no attempts to repair the duct. If the injury is to the common bile duct, the duct should be intubated with a catheter and placed to external drainage. If the injury is to the common hepatic duct, the duct should be intubated as atraumaticly as possible and without ligatures so as not to shorten the duct and make reconstruction technically more difficult. Injuries to the hepatic duct confluence are the most difficult to treat and are prone to complications of stricture, sepsis, and portal hypertension [4].

When the injury is recognized postoperatively, percutaneous placement of a subhepatic catheter may limit toxicity to the patient if interventional radiology is available. However, these interventions should not delay transfer of the patient if the definitive repair is not to take place at the primary hospital. Delay in the diagnosis of bile duct injury is a frequent cause of litigation. With delayed diagnosis, transfer to a tertiary center should be strongly considered unless there is a high degree of expertise [5, 6].

Certain complications of bariatric procedures may also warrant transfer to larger centers if experience is lacking. These include esophageal injury and at time of surgery if the surgeon is not experienced in thoracotomy, esophagectomy, and esophageal repair. Anastomotic leak in patients undergoing gastric bypass may warrant transfer if sepsis occurs and taxes the abilities of the intensive care unit. Some techniques such as endoscopic stenting for perforation or leak may not be available at a community hospital and warrant transfer.

Intestinal perforations are a well-known complication of laparoscopic incisional hernia repair, occurring in about 1% patients. When recognized promptly, this complication can be readily handled at the primary hospital. However, in a number of cases the diagnosis is delayed and the patient presents with sepsis. In the event of respiratory failure, renal failure, or hemodynamic instability, transfer to a tertiary care center or an institution with dedicated critical care resources should be considered.

Sepsis and intestinal fistula are two conditions which may result from complications where transfer may be indicated. In-hospital mortality is known to be higher for these complications and has been correlated with delays in transfer after the onset of complications [7]. Those patients who are transferred have a higher severity of illness and resource consumption than patients who enter an ICU at the initial treating hospital [8].

Selected Readings

1. Southard PA, Hedges JR, Hunter JG, Ungerleider RM. Impact of a transfer center on interhospital referrals and transfers to a tertiary care center. Acad Emerg Med. 2005;12:653–7.
2. Hill AD, Vingilis E, Martin CM, Hartford K, Speechely KN. Interhospital transfer of critically ill patients: demographic and outcomes comparison with non-transferred intensive care unit patients. J Crit Care. 2007;22:290–5.
3. Dy SM, Rubin HR, Lehmann HP. Why do patients and families request transfers to tertiary are? A qualitative study. Soc Sci Med. 2005;61:1846–53.

4. Jarnigan WR, Blumart LH. Operative repair of bile duct injuries involving the hepatic duct confluence. Arch Surg. 1999;134:769–75.

5. Alkhaffaf B, Decadt B. !5 years of litigation following laparoscopic cholecystectomy in England. Ann Surg. 2005;251:682–5.

6. Carroll BJ, Birth M, Phillips EH. Common bile duct injuries during laparoscopic cholecystectomy that result in litigation. Surg Endosc. 1998;12:310–3.

7. Wong K, Levy RD. Interhospital transfers of patients with surgical emergencies: areas for improvement. Aust J Rural Health. 2005;13:290–4.

8. Golestanian, E, Scruggs JE, Gangon RE, Mark RP, Wood KE. Effect of interhospital transfer on resource utilization and outcomes at a tertiary care referral center.

18. Morbidity and Mortality Conference

Chirag A. Dholakia and Kevin M. Reavis

> We believe it is the duty of every hospital to establish a follow-up system, so that as far as possible the result of every case will be available at all times for investigation by members of the staff, the trustees, or administration, or by other authorized investigators or statisticians.
>
> Ernest Amory Codman

Morbidity and mortality (M&M) conferences are a vital component of the peer review process exercised by surgical services at academic and private medical centers. The backbone of the M&M conference is founded in the process in which the errors made and resultant complications during the care of patients are scrutinized and discussed by students, residents, colleagues, and mentors [1]. The modern day objectives of M&M conference are to learn from those complications and errors, to modify behavior and judgment based on previous experiences, and to prevent repetition of errors leading to further complications. The conferences are designed to be nonpunitive and focus on the goal of improved patient care. They take place with regular frequency, often weekly, biweekly, or monthly, and highlight recent patient encounters and identify areas of clinical and systems improvement such as outdated policies, changes in patient identification procedures, and mathematic errors.

Origins

M&M conferences have long been part of the practice of medicine. The origins of which are difficult to trace but many report having originated in the early 1900s with the publication of the Flexner report regarding the state of American medical education [2], the creation of the American College of Surgeons, and in part due to the contributions

D.S. Tichansky, J. Morton, and D.B. Jones (eds.), *The SAGES Manual of Quality, Outcomes and Patient Safety*, DOI 10.1007/978-1-4419-7901-8_18, © Springer Science+Business Media, LLC 2012

of Dr. Ernest Codman at the Massachusetts General Hospital. Dr. Codman embraced the concept of "End Result Cards" which were documents he used to record demographic data on every patient treated, along with the diagnosis, the treatment he rendered, and the outcome of each case. Each patient was followed up on for at least 1 year to observe long-term outcomes. It has been almost 100 years since Dr. Codman attempted to institute the first of these plans and conferences to evaluate clinician competence in 1914. His actions were seen as disruptive to the cultural status quo at the time and ultimately prompted his colleagues at the Massachusetts General Hospital to banish him from the institution. His efforts were not in vain, however, as the wheels of progress had been set in motion. Dr. Codman's ideas contributed to the standardization of hospital practices – including a case report system that ascribed responsibility for adverse outcomes – by the American College of Surgeons in 1916 [3]. As the medical profession evolved, physicians grew accustomed to discussing their errors at mortality conferences, where autopsy findings were presented, and subsequently published in case reports. By 1983, the ACGME began requiring that accredited residency programs conduct a weekly review of all complications and deaths [4, 5].

Philosophy

…the golden hour of surgical education
…the short can outwit the tall, the not so intelligent can outwit the intelligent, and…the resident can outwit the attending.

Leo Gordon [6]

The conference should facilitate the open discussion of medical/surgical error, without the institutions of hierarchy, public embarrassment, and fear of punishment. The type of error reviewed should be one from which others can learn; cases should not be chosen to demonstrate gross mismanagement. The manner in which the error is reviewed should be for the improvement of the clinician and patient care outcomes [7].

Implementation: Since the ACGME mandate, M&M conference has been in place at accredited programs. There is, however, no standardization of the process involved. The reporting process, process of examination and discussion, and educational component are highly variable, related to the leadership and importance placed on the conference.

Definition: The basis of M&M conference should be designed to identify medical errors in order to learn from them to improve medical practice.

A well-organized M&M conference should:

- Identify the events that resulted in the adverse patient outcomes
- Create an environment that facilitates the discussion of adverse events
- Identify and disseminate information and insights about patient care that are drawn from experience and literature review
- Constructively assign accountability
- Create a forum in which physicians acknowledge and address reasons for mistakes without the fear of punishment or mockery

Case selection: All serious adverse patient outcomes should be identified for discussion and presented in a timely manner at M&M conference. Attendees should have an understanding of how cases are screened and chosen. These cases should be discussed prior to presentation with the attending physician to elucidate the errors, the etiology for their occurrence, and to facilitate conference discussion.

Moderator: The creation of an educational and supportive atmosphere is the role of the moderator. The moderator should call on one or more prepared discussants, whose comments represent a middle ground of the topics and cases being discussed. The moderator and/or senior members of the staff should be encouraged recount relevant errors that they have made and the lessons/benefits that they have learned by reflecting on these scenarios.

Attendance: The entire surgical service should be present within reason of clinical care, from the chief of the service to student or intern, and from all relevant departments, especially the treating team of the patient cases being presented. The treating physician(s) should be given the opportunity (but not be required) to present the case, the circumstances leading to the outcome, and the lessons they have drawn. The conference should be conducted with a tone that would be appropriate for the treating physician(s) to hear, whether or not they are actually present.

Conclusions: The moderator should summarize the conference patient case and systems learning points [8]. Follow up and subsequent changes should be reported at later M&M conferences.

Selected Readings

1. Thompson JS, Prior MA. Quality assurance and morbidity and mortality conference. J Surg Res. 1992;52(2):97–100.
2. Flexner A. Medical education in the United States and Canada. From the Carnegie Foundation for the Advancement of Teaching, Bulletin Number Four, 1910. Bull World Health Organ. 2002; 80(7): 594–602. Epub 2002 Jul 30.
3. Proceedings of conference on hospital standardization. Joint session of committee on standards. Bull Am Coll Surg. 1917; 3: 1.
4. Orlander JD, Barber TW, Fincke BG. The morbidity and mortality conference: the delicate nature of learning from error. Acad Med. 2002;77(10):1001–6.
5. ACGME Program Requirements for Graduate Medical Education in Surgery. Chicago, IL: Accreditation Council for Graduate Medical Education; 2008. http://www.acgme. org/acWebsite/downloads/RRC_progReq/440_general_surgery_01012008.pdf. Accessed June 3, 2008.
6. Gordon LA. Gordon's guide to the surgical morbidity and mortality. St. Louis: Hanley & Belfus; 1994.
7. Harbison SP, Regehr G. Faculty and resident opinions regarding the role of morbidity and mortality conference. Am J Surg. 1999;177(2):136–9.
8. Hamby LS, Birkmeyer JD, Birkmeyer C, Alksnitis JA, Ryder L, Dow R. Using prospective outcomes data to improve morbidity and mortality conferences. Curr Surg. 2000;57(4):384–8.

Part III
Preoperative Risk Assessment

19. Preoperative Risk Assessment: Anesthesia

Grant R. Young and Stephanie B. Jones

Goals of Preoperative Testing

The goal of preanesthetic evaluation and assessment is to educate the patient, organize necessary resources for perioperative care, and formulate appropriate plans for intraoperative management, postoperative care, and perioperative pain management. Preanesthetic assessment should also seek to determine any comorbid conditions that may require further evaluation or treatment prior to surgery. Factors to be considered include assessment of surgical necessity, timing of surgery, and the impact of surgery on underlying diseases. Additionally, preoperative testing seeks to evaluate the need for further testing if it is not possible to adequately quantify the patient's health from previous healthcare records, consultations, and tests.

The American Society of Anesthesiologists Physical Status (ASA PS) classification system was initially created to classify the overall physical state of a patient prior to selecting the anesthetic or performing surgery. The ASA PS was designed for recordkeeping, uniform statistical tracking, and communicating between colleagues but was not originally intended to predict overall perioperative outcome. However, ASA PS class III and IV have been shown to confer a higher risk of postoperative complications.

Airway Considerations

Always on the forefront of the anesthesiologist's mind is the ability to manage the surgical patient's airway. A history of difficult intubation with previous surgery should be communicated to the anesthesiologist. Many studies have provided tools for predicting difficult intubation

D.S. Tichansky, J. Morton, and D.B. Jones (eds.), *The SAGES Manual of Quality, Outcomes and Patient Safety*, DOI 10.1007/978-1-4419-7901-8_19, © Springer Science+Business Media, LLC 2012

Table 19.1. Preanesthetic assessment of difficult intubation.

Physical exam component	Predictors of less difficult intubation	Predictors of more difficult intubation
Mallampati classification	• Class I and II: visualize soft palate, uvula, fauces +/− tonsillar pillars	• Class III and IV: visualize only hard palate +/− soft palate and base of uvula
Dentition	• Normal dentition • Dentures/edentulous (note: this may make patients *more* difficult to mask ventilate)	• Protruding upper incisors • Cosmetic veneers • Loose teeth
Mouth opening	• >3 cm	• <3 cm • Narrow mouth • High arched palate
Jaw subluxation/ protrusion	• Freely able to sublux mandible anteriorly relative to upper teeth	• Significant overbite • Receding mandible (retrognathia) • Limited ability to protrude mandible • TMJ dysfunction
Hyomental distance	• >3 cm from hyoid to chin	• <3 cm from hyoid to chin
Thyromental distance	• >6 cm from thyroid cartilage to chin with neck extended	• <6 cm from thyroid cartilage with neck extended
Neck range of motion	• Free range of motion on extension and flexion	• Limited extension (i.e., arthritis, previous cervical spine surgery) • Excessive posterior neck soft tissue/fat deposits

based on physical exam. Prior to surgery, the patient should have a complete airway exam including assessment of Mallampati classification, dentition, range of motion on neck extension, thyromental and hyomental distances, and jaw subluxation and protrusion. The implications of these physical exam findings on prediction of difficult intubation are described in Table 19.1. Prediction of difficult intubation is an important consideration as it allows the anesthesia provider to plan for appropriate airway management procedures and equipment on the day of surgery.

Although endotracheal intubation is often considered the gold standard for airway management, equally important is the ability to mask ventilate a patient. The ability to successfully mask ventilate a patient obviates an airway emergency should intubation be difficult. Given the importance of mask ventilation, patients should also be assessed for difficulty with mask ventilation. Kheterpal et al. demonstrated that a history of neck irradiation, male gender, obstructive sleep apnea (OSA), Mallampati III or IV airway, and the presence of a beard were independent predictors of impossible mask ventilation. In this same study, 25% of the patients with impossible mask ventilation were also difficult to intubate.

Cardiac Considerations

The American College of Cardiology and American Heart Association (ACC/AHA) Guidelines for noncardiac surgery provide guidance for risk stratification and management for patients with cardiac disease undergoing noncardiac surgery and are reviewed elsewhere. General guidelines for perioperative beta-blockade should be followed as well in patients undergoing either open or laparoscopic procedures.

Laparoscopic surgery presents several unique challenges to normal cardiovascular physiology. Establishment of pneumoperitoneum can have a myriad of effects on the cardiovascular system. Insufflation of CO_2 induces hypercapnia which can result in sympathetic nervous system activation and cause an increase in blood pressure, heart rate, myocardial contractility, and arrhythmias leading to an added cardiac stress load. Insufflation also increases the intra-abdominal pressure (IAP) and can cause an initial rise in preload from compression of splanchnic vessels. IAP > 15 mmHg can cause caval compression and decrease venous return reducing cardiac output. This can be compounded with reverse Trendelenberg positioning. Patients who are preload dependent to maintain their cardiac output such as those with aortic stenosis may suffer cardiovascular compromise. Consideration should be given to pre-op volume loading to prevent this complication in patients who can tolerate it.

Pulmonary Considerations

In all patients, it is important to assess history of and current tobacco use as cigarette use confers a 26% increased risk of postoperative pulmonary complications. Support for smoking cessation should be initiated very early in the preparation for elective surgery.

Patients with obstructive lung disease such as COPD and asthma pose a unique challenge to laparoscopic surgery using carbon dioxide insufflation. There may be significant impairment in the ability to adequately eliminate the absorbed CO_2 resulting in hypercapnia and acidosis. In the setting of severe COPD or poorly controlled asthma, the use of an alternate insufflation gas such as helium, argon, or xenon should be entertained. In patients with decreased pulmonary compliance due to obesity, scoliosis, or other restrictive lung pathology, there may be undesirably high peak airway pressures with difficulty adequately oxygenating the patient after establishment of pneumoperitoneum.

Neurological Considerations

Consideration should be given to evaluating patients, as part of a history and physical, for any preexisting neuropathies. These may be exacerbated during the perioperative period by direct surgical trauma near the operative site or from patient positioning intraoperatively. The most commonly injured nerve as a result of positioning is the ulnar nerve which can become compressed with supine positioning. The brachial plexus can be injured from upper extremity traction, such as when securing a patient's arms to arm boards if they are incorrectly positioned. Lower extremity nerves including the lateral femoral cutaneous, obturator, sciatic, or common peroneal nerves can be injured with lithotomy positioning. This risk increases in proportion to the time the patient remains in the lithotomy position. Lateral positioning such as for laparoscopic adrenalectomy or nephrectomy can damage the neurovascular structures of the axilla (such as with an improperly placed axillary roll) or the suprascapular or long thoracic nerves. A careful assessment of any preexisting neuropathies will allow for conscientious or alternate positioning in the perioperative period.

Preoperative Medication Management

An important component of preanesthetic assessment is the management of medications in the perioperative period. Patients should be counseled regarding continuation or discontinuation of outpatient medications prior to surgery. While a complete review of preoperative medication management is beyond the scope of this chapter, some of the major considerations are summarized below.

Beta-blockers should be continued through the perioperative period in patients already taking them. Patients not currently taking beta-blockers should not necessarily be started on them immediately preoperatively as this has been shown to increase the risk of intraoperative hypotension, bradycardia, and stroke. Patients with an indication for beta-blocker therapy should have beta-blockade carefully titrated to achieve effective heart rate control while avoiding frank hypotension or bradycardia.

Angiotensin-converting enzyme (ACE) inhibitors and angiotensin II receptor blockers (ARB) should be held the day of surgery in patients undergoing general anesthesia, lengthy procedures, or those with expectations of large blood loss or fluid shifts. These medications can exacerbate hemodynamic lability intraoperatively. Similarly, phosphodiesterase (PDE) inhibitors (sildenafil/Viagra®, tadalafil/Cialis®, etc.) should be held 24 h prior to surgery as the vasodilatory effects can exacerbate hypotension.

Monoamine oxidase inhibors (MAOIs) should be considered for discontinuation at least 2 weeks prior to surgery due to the potential for severe intraoperative drug interactions including hypertension, hypotension, hyperpyrexia, hyperreflexia, and convulsions. However, these interactions are significant in only a small number of patients and discontinuation of MAOIs perioperatively may result in exacerbation of severe depression. In all cases, MAOI usage should be communicated to the anesthesia provider preoperatively so that drug interactions can be minimized.

Diabetic patients require specific instructions on medication management preoperatively. Generally, oral hypoglycemic agents should be held the day of surgery as mandatory NPO status preoperatively can result in severe hypoglycemia. Long-acting insulin doses should be reduced to one-third or one-half the usual dose in the NPO patient. Blood glucose should be checked regularly to prevent complications from hypoglycemia or hyperglycemia.

Patients taking medications affecting coagulation, platelet function, and clot formation should also be given specific instructions on when or if to discontinue these agents. Aspirin, clopidogrel (Plavix®), and warfarin should be carefully considered in the context for which each is indicated in the patient and the nature of the planned surgical procedure.

Preoperative Diagnostic Testing

Laboratory testing should be ordered selectively in patients based on an individual's detailed preoperative history and physical. Generally, if there has been no clinical change in the patient's health, test results within 4–6 months are acceptable. Routine testing of every patient should be avoided as this confers significantly increased cost, increased risk if invasive testing is used to pursue false-positive results, and may increase legal liability if test results are obtained and ignored, as opposed to never having been done at all. Additionally, selective testing is widely supported by multiple studies.

Suggested testing guidelines are offered below, but as mentioned above, should be clinically correlated with the patient's history and physical.

- *Hemoglobin/hematocrit*: Indicated if the planned procedure could result in significant blood loss or history is concerning for severe anemia. A medical history of profound fatigue, anemia, malignancy, or renal insufficiency could warrant testing.
- *BUN/creatinine*: Renal insufficiency is increasingly recognized as a significant perioperative risk factor. The recently revised ACC/AHA guidelines on perioperative cardiac evaluation indicate that renal insufficiency confers risk equivalent to mild angina, previous MI, compensated CHF, and diabetes. Consider testing renal function in all patients with a substantial likelihood of renal insufficiency undergoing major surgery including patients >50 years of age, and those with diabetes, hypertension, known cardiac disease, or using medications that may alter renal function such as ACE inhibitors and NSAIDs.
- *Serum electrolytes*: Routine testing is appropriate for patients with baseline renal insufficiency, CHF, or taking diuretics, digoxin, ACE inhibitors, or other medications that can significantly alter electrolytes.
- *Coagulation studies*: Patients with a history of a bleeding disorder, chronic liver disease, malnutrition, or chronic antibiotic use who may develop clotting factor deficiencies are a reasonable population to screen. However, in patients without this history, routine PT and PTT testing has not been shown to predict perioperative bleeding risk nor prove reassuring that bleeding would not occur.

- *Serum glucose*: Known diabetics or patients suspected of having previously undiagnosed diabetes should have preoperative glucose measured. However, multiple studies have demonstrated a low incidence of unsuspected, clinically occult diabetes (0.5%) among patients preparing for surgery and there is a lack of evidence that identification and treatment of these patients improves perioperative outcomes.
- *Liver function tests*: Patients with known liver disease should undergo testing of transaminase and alkaline phosphatase levels. In other patients, hepatic enzyme determinations have not been shown to change perioperative management. In a meta-analysis, only 0.4% of routine preoperative LFTs were abnormal and only in 0.1% was management changed by canceling surgery or pursuing further diagnostic testing. Serum albumin levels have been shown in multivariate analysis to be the single strongest predictor of postoperative morbidity and mortality. In one study by Gibbs et al., postoperative mortality was 1% for serum albumin of 4.6 g/dL compared with 28% with albumin <2.1 g/dL. Low serum albumin should trigger a re-evaluation of the need for the planned surgery.
- *Chest radiography*: Routine chest radiography is rarely useful and infrequently changes perioperative management. However, radiography is useful to establish a baseline in patients undergoing video-assisted thoracoscopic surgery (VATS) or extensive upper abdominal surgery and in patients with severe COPD or unstable cardiac disease.
- *Electrocardiogram*: Recommended for patients whose age and medical comorbidities increase the likelihood of occult coronary artery disease including men >40 years old, women >50 years old, and patients with diabetes, hypertension, tobacco use, or obesity.
- *Pregnancy test*: Indicated in female patients of child-bearing age who have not undergone sterilization, though institutional policies and practice patterns may influence the necessity of this test.
- *Urinalysis*: Urinalysis is indicated if a patient has symptoms consistent with a urinary tract infection or if a urological procedure is planned. There is little data to support routine urinalysis in other clinical settings based on poor predictive value and unnecessary costs.

Postoperative Planning

Certain factors predict the need for longer postoperative monitoring and may influence the decision to provide care in an inpatient setting versus ambulatory surgery center. Patients with OSA are at increased risk of postoperative respiratory complications and longer PACU monitoring is to be expected. Preoperatively, some consideration should be given regarding postoperative pain management. This should take into account the surgical procedure to be performed, expected recovery time, preoperative pain management issues of the patient including chronic pain and comorbid conditions (i.e., OSA patients with increased sensitivity to opioids, renal insufficiency precluding the use of NSAIDs, etc.). For many patients, postoperative multimodal analgesia may be appropriate including the use of epidural analgesia, NSAIDs, tramadol (Ultram®), opioids, acetaminophen, gabapentin (Neurontin®), pregabalin (Lyrica®), ketamine, clonidine, or dexamethasone. This is most effectively accomplished when discussed with the perioperative care team prior to surgery.

Suggested Readings

1. El-Orbany M, Woehlck H. Difficult mask ventilation. Anesth Analg. 2009;109(6): 1870–80.
2. Fleischmann KE, Beckman JA, Buller CE, Calkins H, Fleisher LA, Freeman WK, et al. 2009 ACCF/AHA focused update on perioperative beta blockade: a report of the American College of Cardiology Foundation/American Heart Association Task Force on Practice Guidelines. J Am Coll Cardiol. 2009;54:2102–28.
3. Gerges F, Kanazi G, Jabbour-khoury S. Anesthesia for laparoscopy: a review. J Clin Anesth. 2006;18:67–78.
4. Gibbs J, Cull W, Henderson W, et al. Preoperative serum albumin level as a predictor of operative mortality and morbidity. Arch Surg. 1999;134:36–42.
5. Henny CP, Hofland J. Laparoscopic surgery. Surg Endosc. 2005;19:1163–71.
6. Kheterpal S, Martin L, Shanks A, Tremper K. Prediction and outcomes of impossible mask ventilation. Anesthesiology. 2009;110:891–7.
7. Pasternak LR, Arens JF, et al. Practice advisory for preanesthesia evaluation: a report by the American Society of Anesthesiologists task force on preanesthesia evaluation. Anesthesiology. 2002;96:485–96.
8. Qaseem A, Snow V, Fitterman N, et al. Risk assessment for and strategies to reduce perioperative pulmonary complications for patients undergoing noncardiothoracic surgery: a guideline from the American College of Physicians. Ann Intern Med. 2006;144:575–80.

9. Richman D. Ambulatory surgery: how much testing do we need? Anesthesiol Clin. 2010;28:185–97.
10. Saidha S et al. Spectrum of peripheral neuropathies associated with surgical interventions; a neurophysiological assessment. J Brachial Plex Peripher Nerve Inj. 2010;5:9.
11. Silverman D, Rosenbaum S. Integrated assessment and consultation for the preoperative patient. Med Clin N Am. 2009;93:963–77.
12. Smetana G, Macpherson D. The case against routine preoperative laboratory testing. Med Clin N Am. 2003;87:7–40.
13. Warner M, Warner D, Harper CM, et al. Lower extremity neuropathies associated with lithotomy positions. Anesthesiology. 2000;93:938–42.
14. Wolters U, Wolf T, Stützer H, Schröder T. ASA classification and perioperative variables as predictors of postoperative outcome. Br J Anaesth. 1996;77:217–22.

20. Preoperative Cardiac Considerations in General Surgical Patients

Jadd Koury, Pinckney J. Maxwell, and David S. Tichansky

Introduction

As medical technology and care have advanced, patients are living longer and more often present with general surgical disease in the presence of multiple chronic comorbid conditions. Despite these advances, coronary artery disease (CAD) is still the number one killer of men and women in the United States. The prevalence of CAD increases with age, especially in patients older than 65, and this is the age group in which the largest number of surgical procedures is performed. It is, therefore, critical to obtain a thorough preoperative evaluation on elderly patients who have chronic medical conditions and who may have or are known to have CAD. This evaluation helps to optimize surgical outcomes and ensures a smooth postoperative course.

Initial Preoperative Evaluation

A thorough preoperative evaluation is critical to obtaining optimal surgical results. It begins with a history and physical exam focusing on various risk factors for cardiac disease. The depth of investigation and work up required during a preoperative assessment varies based upon the patient's history, current symptoms, and nature of the procedure (elective vs. emergent). Patients with a known history of CAD or with new onset of signs or symptoms consistent with CAD require a baseline cardiac assessment. Asymptomatic patients who are 50 or older require an extensive evaluation as much of the derived cardiac risk indices

D.S. Tichansky, J. Morton, and D.B. Jones (eds.), *The SAGES Manual of Quality, Outcomes and Patient Safety*, DOI 10.1007/978-1-4419-7901-8_20, © Springer Science+Business Media, LLC 2012

were derived from studying this patient population. A limited evaluation is necessary in patients undergoing emergent surgery and may include assessment and optimization of the vital signs, volume status, hematocrit, electrolytes, renal function, and ECG evaluation. A more thorough evaluation can be done after the acute surgical emergency has been addressed. Noninvasive stress testing should be reserved for patients who present for elective surgery and are candidates for revascularization should treatable lesions be found. Expert consultation with a primary care provider and/or cardiologist should be obtained in patients at high risk for CAD based on the initial preoperative history and physical exam.

History

Obtaining a thorough history is crucial in appropriately risk stratifying patients and discovering cardiac and/or comorbid diseases. Patients should be asked specifically about serious cardiac conditions such as arrhythmias, unstable coronary syndromes, prior angina, recent or past MI, decompensated heart failure (HF), and severe valvular disease. One should also ascertain a complete surgical history inquiring about prior revascularizations with stents or bypass, or the need for a pacemaker or implantable cardioverter defibrillator. Risk factors for coronary disease should be recorded and evidence of associated diseases such as peripheral vascular disease, cerebrovascular disease, diabetes, renal impairment, and chronic pulmonary diseases should be noted. Patients with a cardiac history must be asked about new or recent symptoms or changes in their symptoms. All medications, especially cardiac specific ones, must be recorded accurately including the correct dosing.

Assessing preoperative functional capacity is also very important in risk stratifying patients scheduled for general surgical procedures. A person's capacity to perform their daily tasks has been shown to correlate well with maximum oxygen uptake by treadmill testing. Patients who are deemed high risk because of age or known CAD but who are asymptomatic and highly active (i.e., they run for 30 min daily) may not need further evaluation. In contrast, a sedentary individual without a history of cardiovascular disease but with risk factors that suggest increased operative risk may need a more extensive preoperative evaluation.

Physical Exam

A complete physician exam with special focus on the cardiovascular system can be very informative and help guide and further needed work up. Assessment of the blood pressure, pulse, and auscultation of the heart and lungs are requisite. Aside from these standard evaluations, one should pay special attention to the following.

The general appearance of a patient can provide invaluable insight into their overall status. For example, cyanosis, pallor, dyspnea occurring during conversation or with minimal activity, poor nutritional status, obesity, tremor, and anxiety can lead an astute clinician to suspect underlying CAD. In patients with chronic HF, many of the signs seen with acute HF (i.e., rales, chest X-ray with pulmonary congestion, etc.) are absent. Reliable indicators of hypervolemia in these patients include an elevated jugular venous pressure or a positive hepatojugular reflux, both of which are more sensitive signs of hypervolemia in patients with chronic HF. A thorough evaluation of peripheral pulses is also essential as peripheral vascular disease makes the likelihood of occult CAD more likely. Cardiac auscultation is an important adjunct to the vascular exam as valvular heart disease-associated murmurs are critical to detect. Of note, finding aortic stenosis preoperatively and working this up appropriately is very important as this lesion poses a higher risk for noncardiac surgery.

Clinical Predictors of Perioperative Risk (Comorbid Diseases)

When a patient presents for preoperative evaluation, it is important to understand that many comorbid medical conditions may be present. The presence of these conditions can heighten the risk of anesthesia and may complicate the intraoperative and postoperative cardiac management. It is important to obtain appropriate consultation for medical evaluation for the most common of these conditions to minimize this risk.

Patients with pulmonary disease are at increased risk for developing perioperative respiratory failure and complications. Both obstructive and restrictive pulmonary disease places patients at increased risk for hypoxemia, hypercapnia, acidosis, and increased work of breathing perioperatively. This can be a severe problem and lead to further deterioration in those with already compromised cardiopulmonary systems. Suspected pulmonary disease should be worked up with an assessment of functional capacity, response to bronchodilators, and/or evaluation for the presence of carbon dioxide retention via arterial blood gas analysis. If an underlying pulmonary infection is suspected or found, appropriate antibiotics are critical.

Diabetes mellitus is the most common metabolic disease accompanying cardiac disease, and its presence should heighten suspicion of CAD since myocardial ischemia and CAD are more likely in these patients. In fact, the need for insulin therapy is a significant risk factor for perioperative cardiac morbidity. Older patients with diabetes more readily develop HF postoperatively than nondiabetics even when adjustments are made for treatment with angiotensin-converting enzyme inhibitors. Meticulous medical management and perioperative blood sugar control is essential and may reduce the morbidity associated with some common general surgical procedures (i.e., wound infection).

Renal failure and azotemia is commonly seen in patients with cardiac disease and puts them at increased risk for cardiovascular events. Intravascular volume status determination and maintenance in these patients can be very challenging especially in the setting of chronic HF. One may exacerbate an increase in blood urea nitrogen (BUN) and creatinine (Cr) if excessive diuresis of HF patients is done along with the initiation of ACE inhibitors. Careful attention to fluid status is also critical since preexisting renal disease (i.e., Cr 2 mg/dL or higher) is a risk factor for postoperative renal dysfunction and increased long-term morbidity and mortality compared to those without renal dysfunction.

Preoperative anemia in patients with cardiac disease can exacerbate myocardial ischemia and aggravate HF. In patients with known CAD and/or HF, preoperative transfusion to a hematocrit of no less than 28% may reduce perioperative cardiac morbidity. In fact, hematocrits below 28% are associated with an increased incidence of perioperative ischemia and postoperative complications in patients undergoing prostate and vascular surgery. In a VA study, mild degrees of preoperative anemia (Hct <39%) or polycythemia (Hct >51%) were associated with an increased risk of 30-day postoperative mortality and cardiac events in older, mainly male veterans undergoing noncardiac surgery.

Which Patients Require Ancillary Testing?

A common clinical conundrum involves deciding which patients would benefit from further cardiac specific testing prior to elective noncardiac surgical procedures. Typically, this question is approached from the perspective of risk stratification based on clinical risk factors. Major cardiac clinical conditions which would lead to postponement and/or cancellation of elective procedures include unstable coronary syndromes (unstable/severe angina, recent M.I.), decompensated HF, significant arrhythmias, and severe valvular heart disease. These patients require workup and management according to the American College of Cardiology (ACC) and American Heart Association (AHA) guidelines. Patients with a recent M.I. should have a complete cardiac evaluation and treatment and elective surgery should be delayed for 4–6 weeks.

In patients without major active conditions, one must use the presence or absence of specific clinical risk factors to decide whether further testing is necessary. These clinical risk factors include a history of ischemic heart disease, a history of compensated or prior HF, a history of cerebrovascular disease, diabetes mellitus, and renal insufficiency. The current clinical guidelines recommend that noninvasive stress testing is reasonable for patients undergoing vascular surgery who have three or more of these clinical risk factors and poor functional capacity. Noninvasive testing should be considered for patients with at least 1–2 risk factors and poor functional capacity requiring intermediate risk surgery or vascular surgery. In this setting, procedures considered to be of intermediate risk include intraperitoneal and intrathoracic procedures, orthopedic surgery, and prostate surgery. Patients with no clinical risk factors do not benefit from noninvasive testing prior to intermediate-risk noncardiac surgery. These guidelines are important to consider but other factors are used to decide which patients benefit from preoperative assessment of left ventricular (LV) function.

Looking at LV function can be very important in select patients. Several studies, both retrospective and prospective, have been done and show a positive correlation between decreased preoperative ejection fraction and postoperative mortality or morbidity. Consequently, the following recommendations have been made regarding the use of preoperative assessment of LV function prior to noncardiac surgery. It is reasonable for patients with dyspnea of unknown origin to have their preoperative LV function assessed. In those with current or prior HF who are having worsening dyspnea or other change in clinical status to undergo an LV function evaluation if one has not been performed within the past 12 months. The routine evaluation of LV function preoperatively is not recommended.

Patients with a known history of CAD may need no further testing depending on their current status and prior evaluations. Specifically, patients without symptoms and who have had a normal cardiac stress test within the past 2 years or who have had a coronary artery bypass graft (CABG) in the last 5 years need no further assessment. Clinically stable patients who underwent a percutaneous coronary intervention (PCI) 6 months to 5 years previously do not need any further testing.

Preoperative Cardiac Interventions and Their Role

The ultimate goal of any preoperative cardiac assessment is to limit morbidity and mortality and optimize outcomes. At times, patients will require preoperative interventions either with a procedure of change in medications. With respect to cardiac interventions, the current guidelines are as follows. Invasive cardiac interventions (CABG or PCI) are generally only recommended preoperatively for those patients who would otherwise have benefited regardless of the need for surgery. This presumes that these patients have a significant cardiac risk regardless of the planned, noncardiac surgery and this risk would lead to significant morbidity or mortality.

An often simple and life-saving preoperative intervention in patients with known CAD involves the use of aspirin and beta-blocker therapy. These patients should be continued on their antiplatelet therapy if possible as it can reduce perioperative cardiac events. Recently, the data regarding the use of preoperative beta-blocker therapy has been questioned; however, some patients do appear to benefit from their use. Current guidelines stipulate that beta-blockers should be continued in patients undergoing surgery who are receiving beta-blockers to treat angina, symptomatic arrhythmias, or hypertension. Beta-blockers should probably be used for patients in whom preoperative assessment identifies coronary heart disease or high cardiac risk as defined by the presence of more than one clinical risk factor who are undergoing intermediate risk or vascular surgery.

Summary

It is clear that a preoperative evaluation involving a thorough history and physical exam plays a critical role in risk stratification and preoperative cardiac assessment. The information garnered from this evaluation can and is used to guide any further testing. This strategy not only appropriately selects patients for preoperative interventions that can be life saving, but it is also cost effective in that it minimizes unnecessary testing and the potential sequelae of unrecognized or inadequately treated heart disease.

Selected Reading

1. Fleisher L, Beckman JA, Brown KA. Hugh Calkins, et al. ACC/AHA 2007 Guidelines on perioperative cardiovascular evaluation and care for noncardiac surgery: a report of the American College of Cardiology/American Heart Association Task Force on Practice Guidelines (Writing Committee to Revise the 2002 Guidelines on Perioperative Cardiovascular Evaluation for Noncardiac Surgery). Circulation. 2007;116:e418–500.

21. Pulmonary Effects of Obesity and Assessment for Bariatric Surgery

Bernadette C. Profeta

Obesity can profoundly alter lung function and exert adverse effects on respiratory muscle function, mechanics, lung volumes, exercise capacity, and gas exchange. Most morbidly obese patients show some degree of exertional dyspnea and many may have significant impairment of measurable pulmonary function, while showing few symptoms. Fortunately, the detrimental effects of morbid obesity can be improved or reversed with weight loss. Postoperative pulmonary complications play an important role in the morbidity and mortality of major abdominal surgery and this amplified by obesity. The key to a clinically valuable preoperative assessment is to identify which risk factors allow for intervention that will improve postoperative outcomes.

The anatomy of obesity has been shown to significantly alter lung mechanics. The increased weight of the chest wall and the increased intra-abdominal pressures can translate into decreased lung volumes and functional reserve, which can lead to rapid desaturation during induction of anesthesia. Increases in airway resistance and decreases in chest wall and lung compliance increase the work of breathing. The increased girth of the neck tissue and collapse of the pharyngeal musculature can lead to sleep apnea. Chronic hypoxia during the apneic episodes or from the baseline low lung volumes can create the cascade of hypercarbia, pulmonary vasoconstriction, pulmonary hypertension, and subsequent arrhythmias or heart failure. Failure to anticipate the potential pitfalls can lead to significant pulmonary complications precipitated or exacerbated by surgery, general anesthesia, and the use of perioperative narcotics [1].

D.S. Tichansky, J. Morton, and D.B. Jones (eds.), *The SAGES Manual of Quality, Outcomes and Patient Safety*, DOI 10.1007/978-1-4419-7901-8_21, © Springer Science+Business Media, LLC 2012

Obstructive Sleep Apnea

Sleep apnea has been recognized as one of the most underdiagnosed conditions in the morbidly obese population. Numerous studies identify its presence in more than 75% of morbidly obese patients, although some argue that the incidence increases with the increasing BMI, while others have not shown this association [3, 4]. There is repetitive pharyngeal collapse (partial or complete) during sleep due to a combination of muscular relaxation during various phases of sleep and the weight of the surrounding fatty tissue in the neck. Airway obstruction causes cessation of airflow (apnea) or shallow breaths (hypopnea). This leads to hypoxia, with associated hypercarbia, and this stimulates repeated arousals from sleep to reestablish breathing. The disrupted sleep produces daytime somnolence. Prolonged untreated sleep apnea, with chronic hypoxia and hypercarbia, can stimulate pulmonary vasoconstriction, pulmonary hypertension, and significant arrythmias or eventual heart failure. Secondary polycythemia can occur after prolonged hypoxia and this can predispose a patient to blood clots.

A thorough clinical investigation for the signs of sleep apnea should be elicited from the patient or his family with regards to loud snoring, abnormal breathing patterns during sleep, and daytime somnolence. Screening questionnaires, such as the STOP-BANG, the Epworth Sleepiness Scale, or the American Society of Anesthesiologist checklist, have been validated with high sensitivity for identifying sleep apnea [5]. There is an increased prevalence in patients with central obesity, increased neck circumference, males, older patients, and diabetics.

With the high prevalence of OSA noted, routine overnight polysomno-graphy is recommended for all patients being evaluated for bariatric surgery. Sleep cycle phases, respiratory effort, pulse oximetry, ECG, and snoring are all monitored, recorded, and correlated. Apneas and hypopnea lasting at least 10 s are counted and OSA is defined as the apnea–hypopnea index (AHI) of greater than or equal to 5 per hour. As the AHI increases, so does the severity of the sleep apnea. The majority of hypoxia occurs during REM sleep, which is then disrupted by the arousal stimulus to breath [6]. Identification of sleep apnea can aid with perioperative management decisions with regards to intubation/extubation protocols, perioperative narcotic use, and telemetry monitoring after surgery.

OSA can be effectively treated with the nocturnal use of Continuous Positive Airway Pressure (CPAP). CPAP delivers oxygen at an individual titrated pressure to maintain airway patency during sleep and minimize the number of apneas. This will reduce the hypoxemia and break the cycle of pulmonary vasoconstriction and improve cardiac function. Regular CPAP use for at least 1–2 months preoperatively is recommended and patients are instructed to bring their own machines for ease of use and comfort during their hospital course. In the postoperative period, CPAP use can help offset the cumulative adverse effects that anesthesia, narcotics, and supine positioning can have on the obese patient. Also, preserving adequate oxygenation postoperatively helps to minimize wound infections.

Obesity Hypoventilation Syndrome

Obesity hypoventilation syndrome (OHS) occurs when poor breathing mechanics lead to daytime hypoxia and hypercarbia. The exact cause is unknown, but it is believed to be the combined result of a defective mechanism in the central control breathing and the excess weight against the chest wall, which leads to impaired breathing (shallow breaths). Central obesity, with increased visceral fat, causes elevation of the diaphragm. Hypoxia and hypercarbia are the end result, with associated pulmonary hypertension and similar cardiac effects, as described in the previous section.

Many patients with OHS also have sleep apnea. On questioning, they can also describe excessive daytime sleepiness, increased accidents or decreased mental alertness, and depression. On clinical exam, they also can display a thickened neck, cyanosis of the fingers, toes, and lips, and signs of right heart failure, with peripheral edema. Polycythemia is also common with this condition and increases the risk of blood clots and possible pulmonary embolism. An arterial blood gas and spirometry with lung volumes can make the diagnosis. Prophylactic vena cava filters should be considered in patients with OHV who display polycythemia, severe pulmonary hypertension, and an extreme BMI [1].

Treatment options depend on the severity of the syndrome and include, in the order of increasing acuity, the use of nasal cannula oxygen, a Bilevel Positive Airway Pressure (BiPAP) device, or a ventilator. BiPAP is usually used at night and provides a higher level of positive pressure during inspiration and a lower level during expiration. A patient with severe OHS requiring a ventilator would not be a surgical candidate. OHS and the associated conditions are reversible with weight loss.

Pulmonary Function

A significant percentage of morbidly obese patients have abnormal pulmonary function tests and morbid obesity exacerbates many pulmonary conditions, including asthma, COPD, and restrictive lung disease. However, many studies have failed to show a correlation between abnormal preoperative spirometry testing and postoperative complications after bariatric surgery [1, 7, 10]. Spirometry indirectly measures airway resistance in the medium bronchi. The largest percentage (50%) of abnormalities identified on routine testing was obstructive, with the majority being mild. These patients were usually identified as having mild asthma. Nine percent showed restrictive abnormalities and these could be correlated with and predicted by increased age, BMI, and sleep apnea. Therefore, it was felt that the routine use of spirometry on all patients did not provide clinically relevant information that would alter perioperative care in most patients preparing for weight loss surgery [7].

Lung volumes are commonly reduced in the obese patient due to multiple factors including impaired lung mechanics and increased intra-abdominal pressure, and this can manifest in the form of atelectasis, apnea, and hypoxia. The decrease in functional reserve capacity (FRC) can translate into rapid desaturation [1]. Nguyen et al. showed that there is a 40% transient reduction in lung volumes and pulmonary function after laparoscopic bariatric surgery, and that is increased to 50% after open procedures. Recovery of function begins approximately 24 h after surgery, but before that patients with significant preoperative impairment may be at high risk for profound hypoxia during emergence from anesthesia/extubation [8]. When anticipated, this potential problem can be offset with the use of BiPAP in the recovery room. Selective use of spirometry and lung volume measurements in patients with known pulmonary issues, significant clinical dyspnea, or higher BMIs may be beneficial to identify patients who may be at highest risk and have their conditions adversely exacerbated in the perioperative period.

Smoking

Tobacco use at the time of surgery is a known risk factor for peri- and postoperative pulmonary complications after anesthesia. Those risks decrease with the cessation of smoking at least 4 weeks and preferably 8 weeks before surgery [9]. Smoking is also known to impair healing and many programs insist on abstinence from tobacco use for at least 1 month prior to surgery. Pharmacologic treatments, counseling, hypnosis, and other various means may be utilized to achieve abstinence. Nicotine blood tests can be used to test for compliance and it is recommended that surgery be delayed until the tests are negative.

Conclusion

The deleterious pulmonary effects of morbid obesity are reversible with weight loss. Patients can show significant improvement in lung function, even with small amounts of weight loss, and complete resolution is seen in many by the end of one year. The purpose of a preoperative workup is to identify modifiable risk factors that will allow for anticipation and possible prevention of postoperative complications. Many pulmonary tests can be utilized in the preparation of a morbidly obese patient for bariatric surgery, including spirometry, lung volume measurement, arterial blood gas measurement, polysomnography, and nicotine testing. It is universally agreed that all morbidly obese patients who are being evaluated for weight loss surgery should undergo an assessment for sleep apnea, have a routine ABG performed to identify resting hypoxia, and stop smoking before surgery. Most programs, however, have opted for selective spirometry and lung volume testing based on clinical assessment to further characterize the degree of pulmonary impairment in patients with known disease, significant pulmonary symptoms, or BMI greater than 60. Data suggests that the only components of the preoperative pulmonary assessment that provide any clinical perioperative benefit are polysomnograms, ABGs, nicotine tests (to confirm tobacco cessation compliance) in all patients, and spirometry and lung volume measurements selectively for patient optimization [11].

References and Selected Readings

1. Davis DG, Bessler M. Patient selection and preoperative assessment. In: Inabet W, DeMaria E, Ikramuddin S, editors. Laparoscopic bariatric surgery. Philadelphia: Lippincott; 2005;32–37.
2. Shafazand S. Perioperative management of obstructive sleep apnea: Ready for prime time? The Cleveland Clinic Journal of Medicine. Audio transcript of lecture from The 4th Annual Perioperative Medicine Summit. 2009.

3. Hallowell PT, Stellato TA, Schuster M, et al. Potentially life threatening sleep apnea is unrecognized without aggressive evaluation. Am J Surg. 2007;193:364–7.

4. O'Keefe T, Patterson EJ. Evidence supporting routine polysomnography before bariatric surgery. Obes Surg. 2004;14:23–6.

5. Chung F, Yegneswaran B, Liao P, et al. Validation of the Berlin questionnaire and the American society of Anesthesiologist checklist as screening tools for obstructive sleep apnea in surgical patients. Anesthesiology. 2008;108:822–30.

6. Dixon JB, Schacter LM, O'Brien PE. Polysomnography before and after weight loss in obese patients with severe sleep apnea. Int J Obes. 2005;29:1048–54.

7. Ramaswamy A, Gonzalez R, Smith CD. Extensive preoperative testing is not necessary in morbidly obese patients undergoing gastric bypass. J Gastrointestinal Surg. 2004;8:159–65.

8. Nguyen NT, Lee SL, Goldman C, et al. Comparison of pulmonary function and postoperative pain after laparoscopic versus open gastric bypass: a randomized trial. Am J Surg. 2001;192:469–77.

9. Bluman LG, Mosca L, Newman N, Simon DG. Preoperative smoking habits and postoperative pulmonary complications. Chest. 1998;113:883–9.

10. Crapo RO, Kelly TM, Elliott CG, Jones SB. Spirometry as a preoperative screening test in morbidly obese patients. Surgery. 1986;99:763–7.

11. Deitel M, Gagner M, Dixon JB, Himpens J, Madan AK. Respiratory function and pulmonary assessment for bariatric surgery. Handbook of obesity surgery. Toronto: FD Communications; 2010.

22. Contraindications to Laparoscopy

Brandon Williams

With improvements in technology and surgeon expertise, most situations once considered contraindications to laparoscopy are now only relative contraindications or not contraindications at all. This chapter will review settings where laparoscopy should be used cautiously and the considerations that should be taken into account when deciding to proceed with a laparoscopic approach.

Surgeon Expertise

Patient demand has been a major driving force in the increased use of laparoscopy despite the fact that the laparoscopic approach to a given operation may not yet be proven to produce better outcomes. Indeed, surgeons without much training or experience in laparoscopy may feel compelled to adopt new techniques and must find ways to gain comfort and expertise with those techniques. Surgeons must hold themselves accountable and honestly consider whether performing an operation laparoscopically will be of the greatest benefit to the patient.

Surgical Team Expertise

Laparoscopic operations often depend on special OR equipment, surgical instruments, and a team of assistants familiar with them. A highly skilled laparoscopic surgeon can find even a simple laparoscopic operation nearly impossible when forced to work with inadequate equipment or with a team having little to no experience with laparoscopy. The surgeon must take these matters into consideration when determining whether the laparoscopic approach will be best for the patient.

D.S. Tichansky, J. Morton, and D.B. Jones (eds.), *The SAGES Manual*
of Quality, Outcomes and Patient Safety, DOI 10.1007/978-1-4419-7901-8_22,
© Springer Science+Business Media, LLC 2012

Peritoneal Access

The ability to gain access to the peritoneal cavity can limit the safe application of a laparoscopic approach. The peritoneal cavity is typically accessed via an open cut-down method (Hasson technique), blind puncture with a trocar or Veress needle, or introduction of an optical trocar. Recent review articles on laparoscopic entry have not shown a superiority of one technique over the others [1, 2].

Accessing the peritoneal space can particularly be hazardous in patients with a history of prior abdominal operations, as the bowel may be adherent to the anterior abdominal wall. In general, selecting a site for abdominal entry well away from previous incisions seems prudent. Classically, the left upper quadrant (Palmer's point) has been advocated as a safer site for peritoneal entry in patients with suspected periumbilical or midline adhesions [1, 3]. Also, staying away from the midline should reduce the chance of major vascular injury.

If using the Veress needle technique some practical tips include: (1) avoid wagging the needle from side to side after peritoneal penetration as it could worsen a puncture injury. (2) Initial insufflation pressure from the Veress needle should be less than 10 mmHg and is a useful indicator of correct intraperitoneal placement. (3) Elevation of the anterior abdominal wall does not help avoid vascular or visceral injury [1].

Bladeless optical trocars offer the advantages of being fast, providing excellent visualization of passage through the layers of the abdominal wall, and minimizing the risk of port-site bleeding or hernia. Several recent large series have reported very low complication rates with optical trocar entry in morbidly obese patients and those with previous abdominal operations [4–7].

Obliterated Peritoneal Space

Adhesions

Patients who have had prior abdominal operations may present hazards not only with accessing but also developing a peritoneal work space. Compromised laparoscopic visualization of bowel within dense adhesions can increase the risk of inadvertent bowel injury while at the same time make such injuries less apparent at the time of the operation. Also, an extensive laparoscopic adhesiolysis may significantly increase operative time and thereby decrease the safety of the operation. Patients with prior intraperitoneal prosthetic mesh are more likely to have adhesions which may be quite dense. Preoperatively determining the size, location, and type of mesh placed may be helpful in predicting the extent of adhesions and likelihood of requiring an open operation.

Bowel Obstruction

Diffusely dilated small bowel can dramatically diminish the peritoneal work space, and the distended bowel wall is more susceptible to injury with manipulation. However, laparoscopy by well-trained surgeons has been shown to be safe in the management of acute small bowel obstruction, with a high percentages of cases successfully treated laparoscopically [8–10]. The laparoscopic approach offers the advantage of decreased incidence of wound infection, incisional hernia, and postoperative pneumonia and a faster return of bowel function thereby reducing hospital stay [11]. As the laparoscopic approach is generally less likely to result in additional adhesion formation, excellent long-term results with few recurrent episodes of bowel obstruction can be expected [12].

Liberal use of operative table tilting can facilitate exposure with gravity-assisted bowel retraction, so patients should be well secured to the table. If steep reverse Trendelenberg is anticipated a foot board should be placed. It may also be helpful to run the bowel from distal to proximal, starting with the decompressed terminal ileum if possible.

Pregnancy

The gravid uterus in the late third trimester markedly limits the peritoneal space, making laparoscopic operations difficult if not impossible. Moreover, pregnancy presents a contraindication to any elective operation in the first trimester due to the possible teratogenicity of anesthetic agents and in the third trimester due to the risk of preterm labor. The second trimester (13–26 weeks) is considered relatively safe for abdominal operations. A recent review article on laparoscopic appendectomy during pregnancy reported a low rate of intraoperative complications in all trimesters but a higher rate of fetal loss compared to open appendectomy [13]. However, several other reports of laparoscopic appendectomy during all trimesters show it to be as safe as an open operation in terms of perinatal complications [14–16]. A report of laparoscopic appendectomy and cholecystectomy during pregnancy also showed these operations to be as safe as their respective open operations [17].

Morbid Obesity

Massive hepatomegaly and excessive visceral fat can also diminish the peritoneal space to the point of making laparoscopic operations very difficult, though rarely impossible. Some bariatric surgeons require preoperative weight loss or put patients on a strict diet immediately before surgery. A very low calorie preoperative diet has been proven to significantly reduce liver size and visceral fat, with most of the reduction occurring in the first 2 weeks [18]. Additionally, a very thick abdominal wall in the obese patient can make trocar manipulation difficult. Trocars should be placed in a trajectory so as to minimize the angulation that must be applied to perform the operation. Re-angulation of trocars for different parts of the operation may be helpful.

Cirrhosis and Portal Hypertension

In cirrhotic patients, abdominal wall varices should be carefully avoided in trocar placement. Ascites may need to be drained prior to peritoneal insufflation as it can become frothy and obscure the work space. Cholecystectomy is particularly hazardous in the setting of portal hypertension due to fragile engorged collateral vessels in the liver hilum. Great care must be used when dissecting in this area and it is prudent to have open instruments readily available should prompt conversion be required.

Cancer

Laparoscopic resection of colon cancer has been well studied. Prospective trials comparing laparoscopic and open resections for colorectal carcinoma have shown no significant difference in disease recurrence and death rates [19–21]. Based on these results, laparoscopy is being increasingly used for tumor staging and resection of other intra-abdominal cancers.

Shock/Congestive Heart Failure

Patients with severe heart failure may not tolerate the decreased cardiac venous return caused by increasing peritoneal pressure. Invasive blood pressure monitoring may provide crucial information with these patients when laparoscopy is attempted. If hypovolemic shock cannot be corrected before an urgent operation, laparoscopy is not recommended.

Conclusion

There are several important factors that must be considered before proceeding with laparoscopy, including issues related to the patient, surgeon, and surgical team. The question is not whether the operation can be performed laparoscopically but if that approach is in the best interest of the patient from a standpoint of quality, outcomes, and safety.

Selected Readings

1. Vilos GA, Ternamian A, Dempster J, et al. Laparoscopic entry: a review of techniques, technologies, and complications. J Obstet Gynaecol Can. 2007;29(5):433–65.
2. Ahmad G, Duffy JMN, Phillips K, et al. Laparoscopic entry techniques. Cochrane Database Syst Rev. 2008;(2):CD006583.
3. Granata M, Tsimpanakos L, Moeity F, et al. Are we underutilizing Palmer's point in gynecologic laparoscopy? Fertil Steril. 2010;94(7):2716–9.
4. String A, Berber E, Foroutani A, et al. Use of the optical access trocar for safe and rapid entry in various laparoscopic procedures. Surg Endosc. 2001;15(6):570–3.
5. Thomas MA, Rha KH, Ong AM, et al. Optical access trocar injuries in urological laparoscopic surgery. J Urol. 2003;170(1):61–3.
6. Berch BR, Torquati A, Lutfi RE, et al. Experience with the optical access trocar for safe and rapid entry in the performance of laparoscopic gastric bypass. Surg Endosc. 2006;20:1238–41.
7. McKernan JB, Finley CR. Experience with optical trocar in performing laparoscopic procedures. Surg Laparosc Endosc Percutan Tech. 2002;12(2):96–9.
8. Kirshtein B, Roy-Shapira A, Lantsberg L, et al. Laparoscopic management of acute small bowel obstruction. Surg Endosc. 2005;19(4):464–7.
9. Zerey M, Sechrist CW, Kercher KW, et al. Laparoscopic management of adhesive small bowel obstruction. Am Surg. 2007;73(8):773–8. discussion 778–9.

10. Grafen FC, Neuhaus V, Schöb O, et al. Management of acute small bowel obstruction from intestinal adhesions: indications for laparoscopic surgery in a community teaching hospital. Langenbecks Arch Surg. 2010;395(1):57–63.

11. Szomstein S, Lo Menzo E, Simpfendorfer C, et al. Laparoscopic lysis of adhesions. World J Surg. 2006;30(4):535–40.

12. Wang Q, Hu ZQ, Wang WJ, et al. Laparoscopic management of recurrent adhesive small-bowel obstruction: long-term follow-up. Surg Today. 2009;39(6):493–9.

13. Walsh CA, Tang T, Walsh SR. Laparoscopic versus open appendicectomy in pregnancy: a systematic review. Int J Surg. 2008;6(4):339–44.

14. Lemieux P, Rheaume P, Levesque I, et al. Laparoscopic appendectomy in pregnant patients: a review of 45 cases. Surg Endosc. 2009;23(8):1701–5.

15. Kirshtein B, Perry ZH, Avinoach E, et al. Safety of laparoscopic appendectomy during pregnancy. World J Surg. 2009;33(3):475–80.

16. Sadot E, Telem DA, Arora M, et al. Laparoscopy: a safe approach to appendicitis during pregnancy. Surg Endosc. 2010;24(2):383–9.

17. Corneille MG, Gallup TM, Bening T, et al. The use of laparoscopic surgery in pregnancy: evaluation of safety and efficacy. Am J Surg. 2010;200(3):363–7.

18. Colles SL, Dixon JB, Marks P, et al. Preoperative weight loss with a very-low-energy diet: quantitation of changes in liver and abdominal fat by serial imaging. Am J Clin Nutr. 2006;84(2):304–11.

19. Franklin ME, Kazantsev GB, Abrego D, et al. Laparoscopic surgery for stage III colon cancer: long-term follow-up. Surg Endosc. 2000;14(7):612–6.

20. Patankar SK, Larach SW, Ferrara A, et al. Prospective comparison of laparoscopic vs. open resections for colorectal adenocarcinoma over a ten-year period. Dis Colon Rectum. 2003;46(5):601–11.

21. Champault GG, Barrat C, Raselli R, et al. Laparoscopic versus open surgery for colorectal carcinoma: a prospective clinical trial involving 157 cases with a mean follow-up of 5 years. Surg Laparosc Endosc Percutan Tech. 2002;12(2):88–95.

Part IV
Common Complications and Management

23. Common Complications and Management

David Earle, Elsa B. Valsdottir, and John Marks

Access

The performance of a laparoscopic procedure requires access to the peritoneal cavity. The initial access and placement of subsequent or secondary portals of entry have unique features that make it helpful to consider them separately in terms of issues related to complications. The primary goal of both initial and subsequent port placement is to gain safe access to the peritoneal cavity that allows the surgeon and assistant(s) to work in an ergonomically favorable position. Good ergonomics are an often neglected topic, but will enhance patient safety by maximizing the capability of the surgeon to consistently perform fine motor movements. Complications related to access include:

Bleeding from the abdominal wall
Injury to the G.I. tract
Bleeding from the omentum or mesentery
Injury to the spleen or liver
Injury to retroperitoneal vessels
Injury to the surgeon
Injury to adjacent structures at the operative site due to suboptimal port
  placement and poor ergonomics

Options for initial (primary) access include "blind" and "direct visualization" techniques. Both types of techniques may be safely performed, and should be individualized based on the clinical scenario in the surgeon's experience [1]. Blind techniques are those that gain access to the peritoneal cavity without direct visualization of the point of entry. These include Veress needle placement or direct trocar placement with or without a retractable shield. Placing a Veress needle first will allow for the establishment of pneumoperitoneum prior to placing the primary trocar and port [2, 3]. Pneumoperitoneum will lift the abdominal wall up,

D.S. Tichansky, J. Morton, and D.B. Jones (eds.), *The SAGES Manual of Quality, Outcomes and Patient Safety*, DOI 10.1007/978-1-4419-7901-8_23, © Springer Science+Business Media, LLC 2012

and lower the risk of injury to the intraabdominal and retroperitoneal structures. When placing the primary trocar without first establishing a pneumoperitoneum is important to lift the abdominal wall during placement. This technique should only be performed if the surgeon has extensive experience with the safe performance of this technique. Direct visualization techniques include the utilization of optical trocars and standard open surgical techniques [4]. Optical trocars allow the laparoscope to be placed within the trocar so that the clear tip is being continuously monitored while it is being passed through the abdominal wall and into the peritoneal cavity. This may be performed with or without establishing a pneumoperitoneum with a Veress needle. The surgeon should be aware of the manufacturers recommendations regarding use of optical trocars, and use them according to his/her experience and judgment. Standard open surgical techniques can be utilized as primary access, and usually require sutures to anchor the port in place, as the opening in the tissues is typically too large to maintain a proper seal to prevent loss of pneumoperitoneum without sutures.

While an injury may occur with any of the above techniques, it may be more readily detected with the direct visualization techniques. It is also important to note that when using the blind techniques, the first order of business after establishing pneumoperitoneum should be to inspect the area where the Veress needle or first port was placed for any evidence of injury. This would include inspecting for excess intraperitoneal blood, hematoma within the mesentery, omentum, and retroperitoneum, presence of G.I. contents in the peritoneal cavity, or enterotomy of the G.I. tract. If an injury is identified, the appropriate action should be taken, and this may vary with surgeon experience and among clinical scenarios. Because there will always be a rate of access related injury, albeit low, minimizing morbidity and mortality require prompt recognition and appropriate management.

Overall Primary Access-Related Injuries (Table 23.1)

Table 23.1. Incidence of access related injuries in current literature.

Author/year	Type of study	Nr of patients	Occurrence
Sasmal (2009)	Single center	15,260	0.41%
Azevedo (2009)	Review	696,502	0.23%
Moberg (2005)	Single center	4,363	0.11%

Pneumoperitoneum

Complications related to the peritoneum used in laparoscopy are related to both chemical and pressure effects.

Alterations of the cardiac rhythm include sinus tachycardia, bradycardia, and premature ventricular contractions. Additionally, decreased cardiac output is common, and there is a risk for varying degrees of hypotension due to the combination of the cardiovascular effects of pneumoperitoneum [5]. These changes are most significant within the first 15–20 min after the establishment of pneumoperitoneum, may be exacerbated by existing cardiac disease, hypovolemia and patient position, and vary among individuals. It is for these reasons that it is important to monitor cardiac rate and rhythm, blood pressure, end-tidal CO_2, and oxygen saturation throughout the procedure.

Respiratory problems that may arise during pneumoperitoneum include decreased pulmonary compliance, decreased functional residual capacity (FRC), and increased peak airway pressures [6]. These pressure effects along with the peritoneal absorption of CO_2 will result in hypercarbia, typically dealt with by increasing minute ventilation. These pulmonary changes are also most significant within the first 15–20 min after the establishment of pneumoperitoneum, are exacerbated by existing pulmonary disease, volume status, and patient position, and vary among individuals [7].

Renal changes related to pneumoperitoneum include decreased renal blood flow and glomerular filtration rate manifest by low urine output. It is for this reason that urine output may not be a reliable indicator of volume status during a laparoscopic procedure. Renal physiology rapidly resumes after pneumoperitoneum is evacuated, and urine output typically is normal or increased during the early postoperative recovery period [8].

Risk of venous thromboembolic events (VTE) is present with any procedure requiring the patient to remain still, particularly those performed with general anesthesia. In addition to lowering venous return, the pneumoperitoneum also seems to induce a mild hypercoagulable state. It does not appear, however, that laparoscopic procedures have a higher risk for VTE compared to open surgical procedures [9]. Nonetheless, appropriate prophylactic therapy based on individual risk stratification should be undertaken to avoid VTE. Risk factors include those related to the operation and those related to the patient. In general, longer and more complex procedures are at higher risk than their counterparts. Patient risk factors include age, immobility, history of VTE, varicose veins, malignant disease, severe infection, chronic renal failure, more than three pregnancies, current pregnancy, early postpartum period, congestive heart failure, history of myocardial infarction, inflammatory bowel disease, female hormone replacement therapy, oral contraceptive use, obesity, inherited or acquired thrombophylias (e.g., protein C or S deficiency, factor V Leiden, antithrombin deficiency), and a strong family history of VTE. Strategies for prophylactic therapy will depend on the risk factors, and can be seen in detail in the SAGES publication, Guidelines for Deep Venous Thrombosis Prophylaxis during Laparoscopic Surgery (www.SAGES. org). In general, the more risk factors that are present, the more aggressive the prophylactic therapy is.

Intraoperative hypothermia and postoperative pain are also potential complications from pneumoperitoneum. Hypothermia is rarely a significant clinical problem specifically related to the pneumoperitoneum. Strategies to avoid hypothermia are the same as an open surgery and include warmed IV fluids, forced air body surface warmer, warm room temperature, and warm irrigation fluid. Postoperative pain related to pneumoperitoneum is due to the chemical effects of carbon dioxide on the peritoneal lining as well and has stretch of the peritoneum and diaphragm. This pain is often referred to the shoulder and may last for 1–3 days [10]. Utilizing a low flow rate to establish pneumoperitoneum and lower pressures during the operation should improve postoperative pain. The use of warmed and humidified gas has not been shown to have any clinically significant impact to avoid intraoperative hypothermia or postoperative pain.

Gas Emboli

Clinically significant gas embolism during laparoscopic surgery is a rare event, occurring in less than 1% of cases [11]. Studies with continuous transesophageal echocardiography during laparoscopic surgery suggest that clinically insignificant gas bubbles appear in the right heart chambers much more commonly. While rarely clinically significant, the manifestation of significant gas embolism is usually sudden cardiovascular collapse due to severely impaired venous return to the heart. This will be clinically apparent by the presence of severe hypotension, tachycardia, jugular venous distension, and possibly a characteristic mill wheel murmur. Treatment should consist of abrupt cessation of insufflation, evacuation of pneumoperitoneum, and positioning the patient into the left lateral decubitus position with the head down, to prevent the embolus from entering the right ventricular outflow tract. Rapid placement of a central venous catheter into the right atrium and ventricle may break up or allow aspiration of the gas embolus and restore normal cardiac blood flow.

Enterotomy

Enterotomy during laparoscopic surgery is only considered a complication if it is unintentional. The issues related to enterotomy during laparoscopic surgery are no different than during traditional open surgical procedures. It is important to realize that an unrecognized enterotomy poses a potentially life-threatening condition. Unintentional enterotomy may occur during primary access to the peritoneal cavity or secondary port placement [12]. To minimize the risk of an unrecognized enterotomy after primary access to the peritoneal cavity, the area underneath the access site should be inspected carefully for this complication regardless of the technique. This inspection is easy, and does not significantly add to the time of the procedure, but may identify and unintentional injury. To avoid unrecognized enterotomy during secondary port placement, the ports should be placed under direct visualization. The surgical team should have a low threshold to inspect the area underneath secondary port insertion sites for evidence of injury. Unintentional enterotomy may also occur during the course of the operative procedure due to direct injury during adhesiolysis, traction injury during manipulation of the G.I. tract, or during instrument exchanges. When releasing adhesions that are near the bowel is important to inspect the bowel carefully once the adhesiolysis is complete. It is also important to note that only sparing use of an energy source that is clearly away from the G.I. tract should be utilized during the adhesiolysis to avoid thermal injury which may not be immediately apparent and result in a delayed enterotomy. The surgeon should have a low threshold to repair any questionable area. Additionally, if an enterotomy occurred away from the field of vision during manipulation of the G.I. tract or an instrument exchange, it may not be readily apparent. To avoid missing an enterotomy that occurred away from the field of vision, a brief inspection of the abdominal cavity for evidence of an enterotomy at the conclusion of the procedure may be prudent, particularly for technically difficult cases, or those requiring extensive adhesiolysis involving bowel.

Intestinal Injury

Table 23.2. Incidence of laparoscopy related intestinal injury in current literature.

Author/year	Type of study	Nr of patients	Occurrence
Tinelli (2010)	Multicenter	194	0.01%
Azevedo (2009)	Review	696,502	0.004%
Sasmal (2009)	Single center	15,260	0.07%
Moberg (2005)	Single c enter	4,363	0.09%
Molloy (2002)	Meta-analysis	NA	0.7/1,000
Catarci (2001)	Questionnaire	12,919	0.06%
Bonjer (1997)	Review	501,779	0.05–0.08%

Vascular Injury

Vascular injury may occur within the abdominal wall, the omentum, the retroperitoneum/mesentery, or at the operative site [13]. Vascular injury may be a complication of access to the peritoneal cavity or the operation itself. This complication may be related to trocar insertion, operative dissection, or a thermal injury from the use of an energy source [14]. Significant vascular injury as a result of trocar insertion may not be readily apparent, particularly if it occurs in the retroperitoneum and is obscured by overlying bowel [15]. This underscores the importance of a visual inspection of the area under the primary port, and placement of secondary ports under direct visualization. The differential diagnosis of hypotension early in the course of the procedure should include significant vascular injury. In the absence of another identifiable cause, prompt investigation for this problem laparoscopically or via laparotomy should occur. Significant vascular injury as a result of operative dissection is no different during laparoscopic surgery than with traditional open surgical techniques. Unique to laparoscopic surgery, however, is the fact that the instruments go through a port, thus have a fulcrum on which the instruments are manipulated. If there is excessive torque, loss of fine motor movement will occur, and it will be increase risk for inadvertent organ injury, including vascular injury. It is also important to note that if an energy source is being utilized for hemostasis, the tip of the instrument will often retain an elevated temperature even after the energy source has been turned off. If the heated instrument tip then touches an adjacent vessel, either immediate or more worrisome delayed, vascular injury may occur. Vascular injury at or near the operative site may also be not readily apparent due to the fact that the surgeon's attention is at a location other than where the bleeding is occurring. Because of patient positioning and a relatively narrow field of view, the blood may pool away from the operative field. It is for this reason that a brief inspection of the abdominal cavity at the conclusion of the procedure may be prudent, particularly in the dependent portions of the abdomen that are away from the immediate field of view. Vascular injury of the abdominal wall may not be readily apparent until after the ports are removed. It is for this reason that the ports should be removed with direct laparoscopic visualization to look for any bleeding in the peritoneal cavity that may not be readily apparent from the skin incision. Removal of the final port will require a bit more careful inspection from the skin incision because there is no laparoscope available for viewing the peritoneal portion. Bleeding into the peritoneal cavity should be included in the differential diagnosis of postoperative hypotension, and the surgeon should have a low threshold to return to the operating room for a diagnostic laparoscopy or laparotomy in the absence of other causes of the hypotension (Tables 23.2 and 23.3).

Vascular Injury

Table 23.3. Incidence of major and minor vascular injuries related to laparoscopy.

Author/year	Type of study	Nr of patients	% occurrence
Tinelli (2010)	Multicenter	194	Major 0%
			Minor 0.03%
Sasmal (2009)	Single center	15,260	0.14%
Moberg (2005)	Single center	4,363	Major 0%
			Minor
Molloy (2002)	Meta-analysis	NA	Major 0.4/1,000
Catarci (2001)	Questionnaire	12,919	Major 0.05%
			Minor 0.07%
Bonjer (1997)	Review	501,779	0–0.075%

Selected Readings

1. Ahmad G, Duffy JM, Phillips K, Watson A. Laparoscopic entry techniques. Cochrane Database Syst Rev. 2008, Issue 2. Art. No.:CD006583. DOI:101002/14651858. CD006583.pub2.

2. Sasmal PK, Tantia O, Jain M, Khanna S, Sen B. Primary access-related complications in laparoscopic cholecystectomy via the closed method: experience of a single surgical team over more than 15 years. Surg Endosc. 2009;23(11):2407–15.

3. Azevedo JL et al. Injuries caused by Veress needle insertion for creation of pneumoperitoneum: a systematic literature review. Surg Endosc. 2009;23(7):1428–32.

4. Moberg AC, Montgomery A. Primary access-related complications with laparoscopy: Comparison of blind and open techniques. Surg Endosc. 2005;19(9):1196–9.

5. O'Malley C, Cunningham AJ. Physiologic changes during laparoscopy. Anesth Clin N Am. 2001;19(1):1–19.

6. Bardoczky GI et al. Venitaltory effects of pneumoperitoneum monitored with continuous spirometry. Anaesth. 1993;48:309–11.

7. Frazee RC et al. Open versus laparoscopic cholecystectomy. A comparison of postoperative pulmonary function. Ann Surg. 1991;213:651–3.

8. Yao FSF. Anesthesiology: problem oriented patient management. Philadelphia: Lippincott; 2003.

9. Milic DJ. Coagulation status and the presence of postoperative deep vein thrombosis in patients undergoing laparoscopic cholecystectomy. Surg Endosc. 2007;21(9):1588–92.

10. Alexander JI. Pain after laparoscopy. Br J Anaesth. 1997;79:369–78.

11. Ikegami T et al. Argon gas embolism in the application of laparoscopic microwave coagulation therapy. Surg Endosc. 2009;16(3):394–8.

12. Tinelli A, Malvasi A, Istre O, Keckstein J, Stark M, Mettler L. Abdominal access in gynaecological laparoscopy: a comparison between direct optical and blind closed access by Verres needle. Eur J Obstet Gynecol Reproductie Biology. 2010;148:191–4.

13. Molloy D et al. Laparoscopic entry: a literature review and analysis of techniques and complications of primary port entry. Aust N Z J Obstet Gynaecol. 2002;42(3):246–54.

14. Catarci M et al. Major and minor injuries during the creation of pneumoperitoneum: a multicenter study on 12,919 cases. Surg Endosc. 2001;15(6):566–9.

15. Bonjer HJ et al. Open versus closed establishment of pneumoperitoneum in laparoscopic surgery. Br J Surg. 1997;84(5):599–602.

24. Common Endoscopic Complications: Recognition and Management

Scott Melvin and Jeffrey Hazey

General Considerations/Complications, Recognition, and Management

Patients undergoing flexible endoscopic procedures including esophagogastric duodenoscopy (EGD), total colonoscopy (TC), and endoscopic retrograde cholangiopancreatography (ERCP) must be evaluated prior to the procedure to determine potential risks associated with not only the procedure but also conscious sedation, monitored anesthesia care (MAC), or general anesthesia. A thorough history and physical exam are essential to determine possible risks. A patients' history of prior flexible endoscopic procedures, previous surgical procedures, past medical and surgical history, current medications, and allergies may guide the endoscopist to provide quality care and avoid potential complications. Comorbidities may contribute to these risks, increasing a patients' risk of nonprocedure or procedure-related complications. Continuous monitoring of the patient with electrocardiography (ECG), blood pressure, and pulse oximetry are an important part of recognition, treatment, and/or avoidance of complications. Similarly, all patients require intravenous access for intravenous fluid administration, sedation and potential reversal of anesthesia.

D.S. Tichansky, J. Morton, and D.B. Jones (eds.), *The SAGES Manual of Quality, Outcomes and Patient Safety*, DOI 10.1007/978-1-4419-7901-8_24, © Springer Science+Business Media, LLC 2012

Nonprocedure-Related Complications

Conscious Sedation/Anesthesia

Patients undergoing EGD or TC often are treated with conscious sedation. ERCP can be performed under conscious sedation or more commonly MAC/general anesthesia. Overall, complication rates with conscious sedation vary and are dependent upon the criteria used to determine what constitutes a complication. The use of fentanyl and versed is common in conscious sedation as meperidine has fallen out of favor due to its high complication rates. Meperidine should not be used in patients with liver disease (over sedation due to inadequate metabolism/clearance), if they are taking monoamine oxidase inhibitors or have an element of renal insufficiency (normeperidine accumulation). Over sedation may require reversal with narcan (narcotic reversal) and/or romazicon (benzodiazepine reversal) but care must be taken to closely monitor patients as the reversal agents may be eliminated more rapidly than the sedation agents causing patients to return to a state of over sedation.

Close monitoring is essential to avoid cardiopulmonary complications during sedation/anesthesia. Continuous EKG monitoring and pulse oximetry are required. Carbon dioxide monitoring may be used as an adjunct as hypercarbia is sensitive for hypoventilation and is present prior to hypoxia.

Cardiopulmonary

Cardiopulmonary complications comprise just under 50% of all serious complications during endoscopy. Cardio respiratory events as defined by Thompson et al. as oxygen saturation <90%, heart rate <50 or >100, and blood pressure <100 systolic occurred in 67.7% of patients. As a result of instrumentation or dilation of the stomach or colon, bradycardia can develop. Treatment may be as simple desufflation or atropine administration. Patients may develop hypotension in addition to bradycardia or independent of cardiac arrhythmias that may require intervention. The fluid status (complicated by the fact that all patients are npo in preparation of the procedure or have undergone a bowel preparation) may contribute to hypotension. Intravenous access and fluid administration is essential and may be required to treat hypotension.

Rarely vasoactive medications are required with conscious sedation. Additionally, conscious sedation or MAC may be associated with hypoxia. Up to 15% of patients undergoing upper endoscopy will have pulse oximetry below 85%. Administration of narcotics and benzodiazepines together may lead to hypoventilation and hypercarbia, hypoxia, or obstruction of the airway in patients prone to airway obstruction. Treatment includes oxygen administration and potential reversal of narcotics with narcan or benzodiazepines with romazicon. In extreme situations, airway support with an oral airway, nasal trumpets, mask, or intubation is required.

Infectious

Endoscopes are generally considered "clean" instruments but not sterile. Guidelines for cleaning and care of endoscopes are well documented and should be meticulously followed. Endoluminal passage of an endoscope transorally or transrectally can expose the patient to a small but measureable risk of contamination/infection from previous users of these instruments. Transient bacteremia (especially with dilation) can lead to endocarditis or infectious seeding of a prosthesis. Viral transmission is exceedingly rare. Bacterial colonization of water bottles and circuits has been documented with transmission to patients thus changing of the water bottle is recommended. Current ASGE recommendations for antibiotic prophylaxis for endoscopic procedures are limited to patients with prosthetic valves, a history of endocarditis, a systemic-pulmonary shunt, or a synthetic vascular graft under the age of 1. Antibiotic prophylaxis is recommended only if they are to undergo stricture dilation, variceal sclerosis, or ERCP for biliary obstruction.

Upper Endoscopy/Esophagogastro Duodenoscopy (EGD)

Overall complication risk of upper endoscopy is 0.28% in early studies and 0.008% in more recent studies with a mortality of 0.004%. Diagnostic upper endoscopy carries the lowest risk, while complication rates increase with therapeutic interventions.

Diagnostic

Diagnostic upper endoscopy is generally thought to be safe with few complications. Perforations of the esophagus, stomach, or duodenum are rare events occurring 0.03% of the time with a mortality of 0.001%. Perforation rates increase in the presence of abnormal pathology and therapeutic maneuvers (see below). Risks of esophageal perforation, especially perforation of the cervical esophagus, include the use of a rigid endoscope, blind passage of the endoscope, cervical rib, stricture, web or zenker's diverticulum.

Perforation of the lower esophagus can occur as a result of webs, pathology (distal esophageal cancer), strictures, or variable anatomy (paraesophageal hernia). The use of over tubes may increase the risk of perforation in the presence of an abnormality and also may decrease risks associated with multiple passages of the endoscope.

The presence of chest or neck pain and crepitus should alert the clinician to a possible perforation. If there is any concern for perforation, the patient should be admitted and kept npo. Plain X-ray of the neck, chest, and abdomen should be ordered with broad spectrum antibiotic coverage. In the absence of hard signs (peritonitis, mediastinitis, or pleural effusion/pneumothorax), a contrast study/swallow should be ordered to evaluate and confirm the site of possible perforation. Contained perforations (especially in the cervical esophagus) in a hemodynamically stable patient may be treated non-operatively. There should be no delay in operative treatment of a patient who is unstable, has a free perforation or has failed conservative management. Options include exploration, +/– repair, drainage, and enteral access. Morbidity and mortality of a cervical esophageal perforation is lowest, if the mediastinum is not contaminated and treatment is limited to cervical drainage. Mid- and distal esophageal perforations with mediastinal/pleural contamination carry the highest morbidity and mortality and require prompt, aggressive surgical treatment in the form of drainage and/or resection.

Intubation of the esophagus can cause local trauma to a patient's oropharyngeal cavity causing dislodgement of teeth, lacerations, and a sore throat.

In an attempt to intubate the esophagus, unintended tracheal intubation and aspiration can occur. This can result in transient hypoxia and an increase in the risk of aspiration pneumonia. Occasionally, emesis and aspiration of gastrointestinal contents can further complicate a diagnostic EGD and require a chest X-ray, hospitalization, and antibiotics.

Therapeutic

Therapeutic endoscopic interventions carry an increase in the rate of complications by their very nature. Once the endoscopist has decided to intervene with a therapeutic maneuver such as biopsy, polypectomy, endoscopic mucosal resection (EMR), dilation, energy delivery, or placement of a stent, they need to be sensitive to the potential for complications.

Biopsy

When removing tissue at upper endoscopy for diagnosis as in a biopsy or polypectomy, patients are at risk for developing bleeding from the biopsy site and/or perforation. Biopsies can be performed with "hot" biopsy forceps to ablate tissue and decrease the risk of bleeding after biopsy. Polypectomy typically is performed with a snare and energy application to cauterize the stalk or base of the lesion with its feeding vessels. Bleeding complications are best managed expectantly. One should avoid patients with a bleeding diathesis or on medications that inhibit formation of clot (coumadin, heparin, antiplatelet therapy, etc.). Correction of clotting parameters and/or availability of medications and/or blood products should be made prior to an endoscopic procedure where therapeutic maneuvers may be necessary. The endoscopist should be familiar with equipment (energy sources) and their settings (different settings for different lesions and locations in which hemostasis is desired) before embarking on a therapeutic maneuver that may cause bleeding. One should also be aware that the application of energy for cauterization of bleeding [monopolar and bipolar energy application and argon plasma coagulation (APC)] increases the risk of perforation. Familiarity with other therapies such as epinephrine, clips, and sclerotherapeutic agents should also be in the armamentarium of the endoscopist. If bleeding cannot be controlled endoscopically, intervention may be necessary in the form of angiographic embolization of the offending/feeding vessel or surgery in extreme circumstances.

EMR

As with biopsy and polypectomy, EMR poses a unique risk of perforation of the esophagus, stomach, and duodenum. This advanced technique involves submucosal injection and suction/snare resection or free needle-knife resection of mucosal-based lesions. The size of the lesion and location of the lesion are proportional to the risk of perforation with the large lesions in the esophagus stratified as the highest risk lesions. Prompt recognition and treatment is the hallmark. Contrast studies are often more sensitive than endoscopic evaluations when assessing a patient for possible perforation. Treatment of perforations can range from close monitoring with antibiotics to surgical drainage and/or repair/resection. The treatment must be tailored to the location and extent of the perforation and clinical presentation.

Bleeding is a less common complication of EMR and typically can be managed locally with endoscopic techniques outlined above. Delivery of energy, injection of hemostatic agents, or clips often will control bleeding from mucosal surfaces and edges. Rarely embolization or surgical hemostasis is necessary.

Dilation

The method of sedation (conscious, deep, or anesthesia) is important in facilitating patient comfort and avoidance of complication. Airway management may also facilitate serial bougie dilation that may not be tolerated in patients otherwise. Additionally, knowledge of patient anatomy (as in a postoperative patient) and location of the stricture are important. Balloon dilation allows for stricture management typically in a single passage of the endoscope. The use of a guide wire to traverse tight strictures and guide either balloon dilation or savary dilation will decrease the incidence of perforation. Proximal strictures high in the esophagus/neck are not amenable to balloon dilation and must be approached with a bougie, whereas distal esophageal strictures are amenable to both balloon and bougie dilation. The utilization of fluoroscopy to visualize the area in question and ensure passage of a guide wire and/or bougie beyond the site of narrowing may help the clinician guide therapy. Similarly, under fluoroscopy, injection of contrast within the balloon in patients undergoing balloon dilation allows the clinician to visualize the "waist" imparted on the balloon at the site of stricture and guide therapy. Overall perforation rate in patients undergoing esophageal dilation is 0.2%. The risk of perforation is independent of the technique (both wire and non-wire-guided bougie dilation or wire and non-wire-guided balloon dilation) but dependent upon the pathology causing stricture formation (Table 24.1). Bleeding is an uncommon

Table 24.1. Perforation risk as a function of stricture type in patients undergoing endoscopic dilation.

Type of stricture	Perforation risk (%)
Peptic	0.1–0.3
Malignant	9–24
Radiation	0 –3.6
Anastamotic	1
Achalasia	0–6.6
Caustic	0–15.4 (0.8%/dil)

complication of dilation although one must be sensitive to its possibility. Hematemesis will occur in 1–1.5% of patients but is often self-limited.

Bacteremia will occur in up to 50% of patients undergoing dilation of a stricture. Rates are so significant, ASGE recommends antibiotic prophylaxis for any patient with a prosthetic valve or history of endocarditis should they undergo endoscopic dilation.

Stent

Endoluminal stenting of strictures whether they be benign or malignant is generally considered safe. Many of the complications can occur with dilation or passage of a guide wire across the area of narrowing and include perforation and bleeding (see dilation). Complications unique to stenting include stent migration and restenosis after stenting. Endoluminal stenting for benign lesions typically with removable plastic stents may allow healing/closure of a fistula or act as a scaffold across a scarred anastomosis. Migration of a stent may present as a recurrence of symptoms that are a result of the area of stricture that is no longer effectively stented. Treatment is unique to the individual patient but should involve removal of the dislodged foreign body and retreatment of the stenosis whether it be endoscopic or with surgical maneuvers. Most endoluminal stenting takes place as palliation of a malignant lesion to allow patients to take oral fluid and/or nutrition. In this scenario, permanent metal stents can migrate and may cause obstruction. Again, treatment is tailored to the patient and the stage of disease for which palliation was administered. Restenosis of an endoluminal metal stent may be managed with recanalization within the lumen of the previously placed stent and deployment of a second stent.

Energy Delivery

The delivery of monopolar, bipolar, APC, or radiofrequency (RF) energy to the lumen of the esophagus, stomach, or duodenum can result in perforation or stricture. Perforation rates are highest with monopolar energy and least with APC or RF energy as in Stretta or Barrx. Prompt recognition and treatment is essential. After delivery of energy, the presence of pain, fever, and leukocytosis should prompt the clinician that a perforation may have occurred. Evaluating the patient with a CT scan and/or contrast study is more sensitive than repeat endoscopy. Treatment should involve at least admission to the hospital, nothing by mouth (consider nasogastric decompression) and intravenous antibiotics. This is appropriate if the perforation is contained with minimal contamination and the patient remains stable. Significant contamination or hemodynamic instability mandates a more aggressive approach with prompt surgical intervention.

Varices

Endoscopic treatment of varices carries an unusually high complication rate and deserves special notice. Stricture, perforation, and bleeding rates from variceal banding or sclerotherapy are high. Placement of variceal bands carries a 0.07% perforation rate, 2.6–7.8% bleeding rate, and 1% mortality rate. Chest pain from esophageal spasm is not uncommon after banding. Injection of sclerosant can have a 20–40% complication rate. Strictures will develop in 11.8%, perforation in 4.3%, bleeding in 12.7%, pneumonia in 6.8%, and a mortality of 2%. Bacteremia, chest pain, the development of pulmonary infiltrates, or effusions will occur in up to 50% of these patients.

Lower Endoscopy/Total Colonoscopy (TC)

Overall complication risk of lower endoscopy is 0.02% with mortality of 0.001%. Diagnostic lower endoscopy has the lowest risk of complications but similar to upper endoscopy, complication rates increase with therapeutic interventions such as polypectomy and delivery of energy.

Diagnostic

Perforation of the colon during diagnostic colonoscopy is less than 0.005% with rates doubling in patients who have a history of previous abdominal surgery, diverticulitis, intra-abdominal adhesions, or if therapy (polypectomy or lesion ablation) is delivered during colonoscopy. Causes of perforation during a diagnostic procedure include barotrauma from over insufflation of the colon or direct trauma from the colonoscope. The cecum is most susceptible to barotrauma, whereas the sigmoid colon, splenic, and hepatic flexures are susceptible to direct trauma and sheer forces applied by loops formed during colonoscopy. Avoidance of over insufflation and distension of the colon can prevent many perforations. Deep sedation prevents patients from alerting the endoscopist to significant pain with potentially dangerous maneuvers. Locking the handles of the endoscope providing rigidity to the end of the colonoscope may also contribute when advancing or withdrawing the scope especially when the lumen cannot be visualized. Free perforations into the peritoneum mandate prompt surgical repair or resection depending on the location and extent of the injury. Perforations of the rectum and retroperitoneum may be managed nonoperatively if the patient has minimal or no contamination, a clean bowel prep, minimal or no pain, and a CT scan showing the perforation as being limited to the retroperitoneum. Nonoperative management should be undertaken with IV antibiotics and serial abdominal exams. Peritoneal signs mandate surgical intervention.

Occasionally during diagnostic colonoscopy lesions are missed and this should be considered a complication. A poor bowel prep and inattention to detail are the most likely contributing factors. The endoscopist must be sure that they have traversed the entire colon with visualization of the cecum confirmed by identification of the ileocecal valve, appendiceal orifice, transillumination of the right lower quadrant or intubation of the small bowel. Even in experienced hands, the cecum is not adequately visualized in 5–10% of cases. Slow, methodical withdrawal of the colonoscope with appropriate distension, and visualization of the entire mucosa is essential. Attention to detail at points of flexure or angulation is important to ensure no polyps/lesions are hidden behind mucosal folds.

Therapeutic

Biopsy/Polypectomy

Bleeding is the most common complication after colonoscopy. Typically, it is due to inadequate hemostasis after tissue sampling (biopsy or polypectomy of lesions >15 mm), trauma to the hemorrhoid veins or mucosal erosions. Intraperitoneal hemorrhage can occur as a result of direct trauma to the splenic capsule resulting in splenic rupture as the endoscope loops at the splenic flexure. Control of bleeding using endoscopic techniques such as injection of hemostatic agents, energy delivery, or clips is often successful and surgery is rarely required. Angiographic embolization although utilized for bleeding in the upper GI tract is not routinely recommended for bleeding after colonoscopy as compromise of blood supply to the colon can result in transmural ischemia.

Perforation can occur after biopsy when the colon is distended and the wall thin. Special consideration should be made when a biopsy is taken in the cecum especially when energy is applied increasing the risk of perforation. Perforation can occur immediately or may be delayed as the area of ischemia may not perforate for 12–72 h. If the site is on the mesenteric border, a "contained" perforation may occur presenting simply as pain and a leukocytosis. Plain films of the abdomen or chest may not reveal free air, but a CT scan may identify the site of perforation and its containment. This scenario is treated similar to diverticulitis without intraperitoneal contamination. Admission to the hospital, broad spectrum antibiotics with gram negative and anaerobic coverage and serial abdominal exams are appropriate treatments. Should the patient develop peritonitis or clinical decompensation, prompt surgical intervention is indicated.

Polypectomy at colonoscopy carries a 0.36% complication rate and 0.06% perforation rate. At the time of polypectomy, specimens may be lost or unable to be retrieved for definitive pathologic examination. Control of any specimen resected with knowledge of available tools that aid the endoscopist with specimen retrieval will prevent such an occurrence. A suction trap can aid the removal of small specimens. Clearance of fecal material to allow for visualization can be helpful as well. When retrieval is essential and cannot be accomplished endoscopically, the patient can be instructed to "screen" his/her stool over the next 48 h in an effort to retrieve the specimen.

Dilation

Strictures of the colon are treated in a similar fashion to those of the upper gastrointestinal tract. Benign strictures can occur at the site of an anastomosis, as a result of ischemia or as a result of inflammation (diverticulitis or colitis from inflammatory bowel disease). Dilation of benign strictures can result in bleeding and perforation. Often, strictures are dilated only to allow for stent placement and an adequate bowel preparation in anticipation of surgical resection. Morbidity from a perforation can be quite high because of bacterial overgrowth in a proximal colon with partial obstruction. It is for this reason dilation should be only enough to allow for safe passage of a stent.

Stent

Stenting of the lower GI tract for palliation and as a bridge to surgery is generally safe with good results. Results are best when stenting the rectum and the more distal bowel. Perforation, stent migration, and restenosis highlight potential complications. Perforations are treated similar to those occurring with instrumentation of the colon. Treatment of stent migration is dependent on the indications for stent placement. Should migration result in obstruction, removal of the stent endoscopically is difficult with high complication rates thus surgery is often required. Restenosis can be treated with recanalization of the previously placed stent and deployment of a new stent within the lumen of the obstructed stent.

Endoscopic Retrograde CholangioPancreatography (ERCP)

Overall complication risk of ERCP is 6.85% with mortality of 0.33%. Diagnostic ERCP carries a slightly lower risk of complications, whereas complication rates increase significantly with therapeutic interventions, specifically endoscopic sphincterotomy (ES).

Diagnostic and Therapeutic

Perforation at ERCP can be due to the passage of the endoscope, manipulation of the sphincter of oddi and/or instrumentation of the biliary tree. Overall, perforation rates from ERCP should be at or below 0.03% but have occurred in up to 0.6% of patients in larger series. Perforations resulting from endoscopy can occur when passing the side viewing endoscope in the neck (cervical perforation), the esophagus, stomach, or passage through the duodenum. Recognition and management are similar to the perforation complications noted with traditional upper endoscopy. Duodenal perforation may be confined to the retroperitoneum and managed medically. Patients may present with abdominal or back pain, fever, and/or leukocytosis and should have an upright KUB/chest X-ray looking for free air. Free air mandates abdominal exploration. In the absence of free air, an abdominal CT scan is required to make the diagnosis of a retroperitoneal perforation. If it is contained, with minimal contamination in an otherwise stable patient, broad spectrum antibiotic with serial abdominal examinations is appropriate. Patients should be kept npo with a nasogastric tube in place. Prompt surgical intervention is indicated should the patient's condition change or deteriorate and may require retroperitoneal drainage alone or combined with more aggressive approaches, should the injury to the duodenum be extensive (pyloric exclusion and duodenal diverticularization). Perforation during manipulation of the sphincter of oddi may occur as well. Perforation at ERCP is unusually occurring in less than 1.1% of patients undergoing ES at the time of ERCP. This may be prevented by using a short cutting wire and limiting the extent of the sphincterotomy such that it does not go beyond the duodenal fold. These perforations may be confined to the retroperitoneum or freely perforate spilling duodenal contents and/or bile into the peritoneum. Perforations of the bile duct itself independent of the duodenum and sphincterotomy may occur during instrumentation of the biliary tree. Passage of wires, balloon, and extraction of stones or biopsies of the bile ducts can cause perforation and bile to spill into the retroperitoneum or freely in the abdomen. Prompt recognition during ERCP limits the morbidity but occasionally it is not recognized until sometime after the procedure. A HIDA scan should identify a perforation. Placement of a stent in the biliary tree across the ampulla at the time of ERCP or once the bile duct perforation is recognized will promote antegrade flow of bile and healing. This must be done in conjunction with external drainage of any biloma that may have accumulated as a result of the injury. Rarely surgical intervention is required to promote external drainage. Perforations limited to the bile duct typically do not require Roux-en-y biliary reconstruction as they do not involve more than 50% of the circumference of the bile duct. In extreme circumstances where the bile duct has been completely destroyed, Roux-en-y hepaticojejunostomy may be required.

Pancreatitis as a result of ERCP is one of the more common complications occurring in 3–5% of patients undergoing ERCP. Risks include a history of pancreatitis, young age, injection of the pancreatic duct, ES, ERCP for sphincter of oddi dysfunction, and instrumentation of the bile/pancreatic duct (stone removal, stenting, and manometry). Efforts to minimize this risk of post-ERCP pancreatitis have included temporary pancreatic duct drainage in the form of a temporary pancreatic duct stent. The resulting pancreatitis usually is limited to a 24–72 h period of abdominal pain and elevated amylase and lipase. Treatment of uncomplicated post-ERCP pancreatitis is limited to inpatient admission, bowel rest, intravenous fluids, and nasogastric decompression if the patient has emesis. This should abate in 24–72 h with close clinical observation. Occasionally, conversion to complicated pancreatitis can occur in the form of pancreatic phlegmon, pseudocyst formation, and/or pancreatic necrosis. These complications will require hospital admission and treatment.

Bleeding after ERCP and specifically as a result of ES occurs in just under 2.5% of patients. Patients with liver dysfunction and/or jaundice may be coagulopathic and require vitamin K or fresh frozen plasma to correct clotting parameters prior to ERCP and ES. This risk has decreased over the years with the introduction of slow, pulsed and blended cutting with sphincterotomes. Minimization of the size of the sphincterotomy with little tension on the cutting wires and tailoring the size of the sphincterotomy to the therapeutic maneuver can mitigate this risk. Treatment includes conversion of the sphincterotome to a pure coagulation mode and applying energy to the bleeding site. Injection of 1:10,000 epinephrine and balloon tamponade with a biliary dilating balloon at the time of ERCP can also halt bleeding. Rarely, angiographic embolization or surgery in the form of duodenotomy and suture ligation of the bleeding vessel is necessary to stop ongoing bleeding unresponsive to endoscopic maneuvers.

Cholangitis after ERCP can occur in up to 1.4% of patients and usually will present in patients with an obstructed biliary tree. Prevention is the hallmark with pre-procedural antibiotics (piperacillin is excreted and concentrated in the bile) and biliary drainage via an endoscopic stent. If stenting is unsuccessful, prompt percutaneous or surgical drainage may be required.

More unusual complications during ERCP include stone and/or basket impaction. In an effort to remove stones from the bile duct, a stone basket may engage the stone but not be able to be removed from the bile duct. This occurs in less than 0.2% of patients. In rare events, the basket must be cut and the endoscope removed. A lithotripter may be used to fracture the stone/basket to facilitate removal endoscopically, but if unsuccessful, surgical extirpation is necessary.

The use of biliary and pancreatic stents poses a unique risk to patients. Stents may occlude and contribute to cholangitis/pancreatitis or migrate. Biliary stents of various sizes range from 7 to 10 French and 11.5 French. Small stents (7 Fr) have patency rates ranging from 4 to 6 weeks, while larger stents (10 and 11 Fr) will have patency rates up to 12 weeks and longer. Uncovered metal stents maintain patency rates up to 6 months with covered metal stents approaching 1 year. Metal stents should only be used in malignant non-operative obstructions. Occlusion requires replacement (as in a plastic stent) or recanalization (as in a metal stent) with another metal stent or plastic stent as appropriate. Stent migration presents a challenge to the endoscopist when it migrates into the biliary or pancreatic ductal system. Endoscopic removal with forceps is recommended and on rare occasions surgical removal is required.

Selected Readings

1. Arrowsmith J, Gerstman B, Fleisher D, et al. Results from the American Society for Gastrointestinal Endoscopy/U.S. Food and Drug Administration collaborative study on complication rates and drug use during gastrointestinal endoscopy. Gastrointest Endosc. 1991;37:421–7.
2. ASGE recommendations for antibiotic prophylaxis for endoscopic procedures. Gastrointest Endosc. 1995;42(6):630.
3. Marks J. Esophagogastroduodenoscopy. In: Ponsky J, editor. Complications of endoscopic and laparoscopic surgery. prevention and management. Philadelphia, PA: Lippincott-Raven; 1997. p. 13–28.
4. Silvis S, Nebel O, Rogers G, et al. Endoscopic complications. Results of the 1974 American Society of Gastrointestinal Endoscopy Survey. JAMA. 1976;235:928.
5. Reed W, Kilkenny J, Dias C, et al. A prospective analysis of 3525 esophagogastroduodenoscopies performed by surgeons. Surg Endosc. 2004;18:11–21.
6. Bokemeyer B, Bock H, Huppe D, et al. Screening colonoscopy for colorectal cancer prevention: results from a German online registry on 269000 cases. Eur J Gastroenterol Hepatol. 2009;21:650–5.
7. Rathgaber S, Wick T. Colonoscopy completion and complication rates in a community gastroenterology practice. Gastrointest Endosc. 2006;64:556–62.

8. Lqbal C, Chun Y, Farley D. Colonoscopic perforations: a retrospective review. J Gastrointest Surg. 2005;9:1229–35.

9. Freeman M. Adverse outcomes of endoscopic retrograde cholangiopancreatography: avoidance and management. Gastrointest Endosc Clin North Am. 2003;13:775–98.

10. Freeman M. Understanding risk factors and avoiding complications with endoscopic retrograde cholangiopancreatography. Current Gastroenterol Rep. 2003;5:145–53.

11. Freeman M, Nelson D, Sherman S, et al. Complications of endoscopic biliary sphincterotomy. N Engl J Med. 1996;335:909–18.

12. Andriulli A, Loperfido S, Napolitano G, et al. Incidence rates of post-ERCP complications: a systematic survey of proscpective studies. Am J Gastroenterol. 2007;102:1781–8.

25. Energy and Energy Safety in the Operating Room

Jonathan E. Efron

Since Cushing and Bovie introduced the use of the electricity to facilitate coagulation in 1926 [1], the use of energy has become a vital component of modern-day operating. This is particularly true in laparoscopic surgery, where our quest to eliminate incisions, while improving efficiency, has led to the development of a variety of energy devices that can seal and divide tissue. These devices are now available for both open and minimally invasive surgical procedures. The benefit of these devices is a decrease in blood loss and operative time, however, the use of energy is not without risks. Therefore, the role of this summary is to describe currently available energy devices for use in the operating room and how to use them ensuring minimal risk to the patient and surgeon.

Patient and equipment positioning is always essential to ensure a tension-free and smooth operation. All energy devices require a generating unit that is generally positioned at the head or foot of the bed. When using these devices in laparoscopic surgery, there are many other cords that will come off of the patient and having all the cords drape to one side is beneficial. It helps prevent "trapping" the surgeon and avoids the potential for tripping on the cords if the surgeon has to move from one side of the patient to the other during the operation. The cords that attach the instruments to the generators also must be inspected for breaks in the insulation.

Whenever using energy devices, the surgeons want to maximize the ability to coagulate and divide tissue with minimal damage to other structures. Being constantly aware of other structures near the device is fundamental and often requires keeping the active portion of the instrument in view at all times. Injuries may occur from direct use of the instrument on a structure such as a blood vessel, nerve, or piece of intestine. Triangulating the tissue under tension helps open planes and prevents direct injury from electrical current. While direct injury is a

D.S. Tichansky, J. Morton, and D.B. Jones (eds.), *The SAGES Manual*
of Quality, Outcomes and Patient Safety, DOI 10.1007/978-1-4419-7901-8_25,
© Springer Science+Business Media, LLC 2012

possibility, arcing of the electrical current may also occur. This refers to the current jumping from the instrument to another structure near the area of dissection. Using the minimal effective settings helps avoid arcing. Finally, lateral spread of heat may result in indirect injury and the degree of spread varies according to the instrument used.

Electrocautery

The first diathermy unit that bears his name was built by William Bovie and used by Harvey Cushing at the Peter Bent Brigham Hospital in 1926 to resect a vascular myeloma [1]. The diathermy device has gone through various changes since 1926, but is still based on the same principles. The electrocautery passes current through the patient's tissue resulting in division or cauterization. The electrocautery changes its desired effect by modulating the voltage and waveform delivered. There are two extremes of these variations, the cut mode and the coagulation mode. When using the diathermy in the cut mode the generator provides a lower voltage, with continuous current output. In the coagulation mode, the generator has a higher voltage current output, which is interrupted. Most modern diathermy generators also provide various combinations of the two extremes [1].

Tissue effects of the electrocautery include cutting, fulgarization, and desiccation [1]. In addition to the continuous or interrupted current, the desired effect varies according to where the electrode is held with respect to the tissue. Use of the coagulation mode with the electrode in close proximity, but not touching the tissue, will result in fulgarization of the tissue. Using the cut mode and direct contact on the tissue results in division or cutting of tissue, while direct contact from the electrode and the tissue in the coagulation mode results in desiccation and therefore coagulation [1].

The safe use of the electrocautery requires that the surgeon keep constant vigilance as to the tissue being treated, the mode and level of the diathermy, and the surrounding tissue. Table 25.1 lists common injuries occurring from the use of the electrocautery. Current may be passed from the tip and edge of the electrode being used. Minimizing tissue exposure and keeping other pieces of tissue or organs out of harms way prevents inadvertent and undetected injury that may result in complications. In open surgery, this is managed by retracting mobile tissue away from the operating field with the use of self-retaining retractors or packs.

Table 25.1. Common electrocautery injuries.

Direct tissue injury from contact
Direct tissue injury from arcing
Indirect injury from associated heat generation
Unknown pacemaker or AICD implant resulting in implanted device
   malfunction
Off site burn form poorly attached grounding pad

Laparoscopic procedures require the use of gravity by correctly positioning the table to keep mobile structures away from the area of dissection. The inadvertent delivery of energy to tissue may result in significant harm in the form of immediate perforation or division of the injured structure. Delayed perforation or scarring and subsequent stricturing may also occur and not be detected until well in the postoperative period.

The advent of laparoscopic surgery has resulted in significant instrument innovations that utilize diathermic energy. These instruments are by necessity much longer than open diathermy electrodes and are often reusable. This results in a large surface area that must be adequately insulated. The shorter the area of exposed metal on these devises, the lesser the chance of inadvertent injury to intrabdominal structures. Any instrument that will deliver electrical energy either during a laparoscopic or open procedure must be carefully inspected to ensure that there is no violation of the insulation on the device prior to use, so as to reduce the risk of inadvertent injury.

Safety in the operating room begins prior to making an incision. Most energy devices use electrical energy and this electrical energy may influence previously implanted devices in the patient. When taking a patient history, it is vital to determine if the patient has had any implanted device. Knowledge of the presence of an implanted pacemaker, AICD, or artificial joints is essential. This knowledge should be obtained by the surgeon, anesthesiologists, and the operating room nurses who will be caring for the patient during the procedure. Pacemaker and AICD issues should be discussed and resolved by the OR team before bringing the patient into the room. Likewise, the placement of the grounding pads should be discussed and approved by all members of the team. This information and the final results of these discussions are often reviewed in the pre-procedure briefing or "time out" that takes place prior to incision. Pacemakers should be programmed to be set at a constant rate during the procedure, while AICDs often require deactivation if electrical energy is to be used during the surgery to prevent inadvertent activation of the device. Appropriate monitoring with the placement of temporary defibrillator pads at secure locations on the patient is then required in the event of a cardiac arrhythmia. After the procedure, the devices must be interrogated and reactivated, a process often performed in the recovery room.

All electrical energy devices require grounding and the grounding pads placed on the patient must not be in close proximity to artificial joints. The pads are generally placed on the patient's thigh, but can be placed on the back when necessary. A smooth, dry, surface free of hair allows for an adequate seal to the skin. This helps prevent a loss of contact between the skin and the pad during surgery which can cause an offsite burn at the grounding pad site. Incomplete coupling between the grounding pad and skin does not allow for sufficient dispersion of the current at that site. This allows build up of current at one point between the pad and the skin and may result in a significant burn. If the grounding pads get wet they may also lose coupling, and therefore the pad should be kept well away from any operative field to avoid soaking from either skin preparation liquids or body fluids.

Vessel Sealing Devices

Vessel sealing devices have started to be used routinely in all forms of surgery from thyroidectomies to hemorrhoidectomies. These devices are used in both open and laparoscopic surgery and can be used specifically for vessel ligation or generalized tissue division. There are both 5 and 10 mm devices available. These devices use either electrical current or ultrasound to coagulate, thereby "sealing" blood vessels. They may help to reduce blood loss and significantly reduce the length of an operation which has been well documented in a variety of surgeries, such as hemorrhoidectomy [2]. Clearly, one must be aware of the limitations and potential complications that may occur with these new tools. A list of the commercially available devices is listed in Table 25.2 [3].

The harmonic scalpel is available in 5 mm size and is approved by the FDA for ligation of blood vessels up to 5 mm. It utilizes ultrasonic energy generating heat in an effort to establish hydrogen bonds between tissue proteins [4]. In doing so, it seals the vessels. While approved only for sealing vessels 5 mm in diameter, the lateral spread from the energy source is significantly smaller than that of the devices that utilize electrical current to coagulate and cut [5].

Table 25.2. Commercially available vessel sealing devices.

Harmonic Scalpel
Surg RX Enseal
Ligasure V
Force Triad
PKS Cutting Forceps
Plasma Trisector

The other commonly available commercially devices (Ligasure, Force Triad, and Enseal) all utilize varying methods of applying bipolar energy. These instruments are impedance controlled and their generators release the energy in a pulsatile fashion [4]. They are approved for the sealing of vessels up to 7 mm in diameter. The Ligasure and Force Triad devices vary in their generator technology. The Force Triad generator measures the impedance created during delivery of the energy, thereby allowing a non-pulsatile delivery of energy which significantly reduces the time to seal [4]. The Enseal device uses nanotechnology to measure temperature and current delivered during sealing [6]. In a direct comparison study the vessel sealing time for vessels 7 mm or less was found to be greatest for the Enseal device and shortest for the force triad device [4]. Failure rates between the commonly available instruments did not significantly differ when comparing data on sealing vessels 6–7 mm in size [4]. Calcified blood vessels do not seal well with the bipolar energy devices. An alternate method of sealing and dividing should be used when calcified vessels with a large amount of atherosclerotic plaque are suspected, for example, in patients with known carotid or peripheral vascular disease. Other options in this situation include dividing with a vascular stapler or hemoclips.

All the devices have some element of lateral energy spread which must be kept in mind. The extent of peripheral energy spread varies with each device and is related to the maximum temperature generated and the length of time the tissue is exposed to that temperature [4]. Being aware of this energy spread is vital to ensuring closely associated structures are not injured. A summary of bursting pressure, sealing time, and energy spread of the Ligasure, Force Triad, Enseal device, and the Harmonic Scalpel is found in Table 25.3. When using these devices it is best to keep them at least 5–8 mm away from structures that may be harmed by lateral energy spread such as blood vessels, nerves, intestine, or the ureters.

Table 25.3. Comparison of Enseal, Harmonic Scapel (HS), Ligasure, and Force Triad (FT) energy sealing devices for 7 mm vessels [4, 5].

Device	Bursting pressure (mmHg)	Sealing time (s)	Energy spread
Enseal	720	6.4	N/A
HS	532	5.1	1.5 mm
Ligasure	645	6.1	6.3 mm
FT	369	3.1	N/A

Some recommendations for the safe division of large vessels −5 to 7 mm − with the energy sealing devices are as follows. Always ensure that the vessel being divided is completely grasped in the jaws of the devices. This often requires skeletonizing the vessel and will avoid incomplete vessel transection and uncontrolled bleeding. There is a certain failure rate with all of these devices [4] and, therefore, proximal control of the blood vessels is also recommended prior to attempted division. Complete mobilization of the blood vessels from all medial and lateral structures will avoid inadvertent injury of structures not in view. Finally, making sure the full length of the device's jaws is visualized when in use is essential.

Electrical energy has revolutionized surgical technique allowing larger operations to be conducted faster and with lower morbidity and mortality. However, the use of energy devices does not come without a cost, and care must be taken to ensure injury does not occur to the patient or the surgeon when using devices from the simple Bovie to the Enseal vessel sealing device. Constant vigilance and following some basic safety rules will minimize the potential for costly injuries.

Selected Readings

1. Massarweh NN, Cosgriff N, Slakey DP. Electrosurgery: history, priniciples, and current and future uses. J Am Coll Surg. 2006;202(3):520–30.

2. Nienhuijs S, de Hingh I. Conventional Versus LigaSure hemorrrhoidecotmy from patients with symptomatic hemorrhoids. Cochrane Database Syst Rev. 2009;21(1): CD006761. Review.

3. Newcomb WL, Hope WW, Schmelzer TM, Heath JJ, Norton HJ, Lincourt AE, et al. Comparison of blood vessel sealing among new electrosurgical and Ultrasonic devices. Surg Endosc. 2009;23:90–6.

4. Harrell AG, Kercher KW, Heniford BT. Energy sources in laparoscopy. Semin Laparosc Surg. 2004;11:201–9.

5. Hruby GW, Franzo CM, Durak E, Collins SM, Pierorazio P, Humphrey PA, et al. Evaluation of Surgical Energy devices for vessel sealing and peripheral energy spread in a porcine model. J Urolog. 2007;178(6):2689–93.
6. Denes B, de la Torre RA, Krummel, TM, Oleson LSM. Evaluation of a vessels sealing system in a porcine model. In 21st Worl Congress of Endourology, Moderated poster session, Endourology/Laproscopy: Laboratory and teaching montreal, Canada.

26. Laparoscopic Cholecystectomy: Complications and Management

Nathaniel J. Soper and B. Fernando Santos

Background

Since the first reports of cholecystectomy appeared in the latter half of the nineteenth century, cholecystectomy has become the mainstay of treatment for a variety of gallbladder diseases, most commonly symptomatic cholelithiasis. For more than 100 years, open cholecystectomy was the primary technique performed. However, laparoscopic cholecystectomy, first performed in 1985 by Mühe in Germany, very quickly became the accepted standard of care, and revolutionized surgical practice by ushering in the laparoscopic era. The utilization of a laparoscopic approach to cholecystectomy has increased dramatically in the USA since its introduction, increasing from approximately 52% of cases in 1991 to approximately 87% in 2006, of an estimated 500,000–600,000 cholecystectomies performed each year [1–3].

Safety of Laparoscopic Cholecystectomy

The adoption of laparoscopic cholecystectomy occurred rapidly, initially driven largely by public demand and commercial pressure, before its benefits or safety had formally been compared with the open approach through large, prospective series. Nevertheless, subsequent studies have shown it to be a generally safe procedure, performed with low overall rates of morbidity and mortality. A prospective analysis of 1,518 consecutive laparoscopic cholecystectomies by the Southern Surgeons Club in 1991 showed a low rate of major complications and mortality (Table 26.1) [4]. A distinct "learning curve" was demonstrated, however, with more bile duct injuries occurring early in a surgeon's

D.S. Tichansky, J. Morton, and D.B. Jones (eds.), *The SAGES Manual of Quality, Outcomes and Patient Safety*, DOI 10.1007/978-1-4419-7901-8_26, © Springer Science+Business Media, LLC 2012

Table 26.1. Complications of Laparoscopic Cholecystectomy in 1,518 patients, as reported by the Southern Surgeons Club [4].

Minor Complications	Incidence (%) 3.26	Major Complications	Incidence (%) 1.74
Superficial wound infection	0.9	Bile duct injury	0.5
Ileus	0.4	Bleeding requiring reoperation	0.3
Urinary retention	0.4	Bowel injury	0.3
Retained stones	0.4	Bleeding requiring transfusion	0.2
Subcutaneous emphysema	0.3	Bile leak	0.2
Unexplained abdominal pain	0.17	Pulmonary edema	0.1
Deep wound infection	0.1	Empyema	0.07
Fever	0.1	Pneumonia	0.07
EKG changes	0.07		
Gastritis	0.07	Mortality[a]	0.07
Peptic ulcer	0.07		
Pancreatitis	0.07		
Cautery burn	0.07		
Drug reaction	0.07		
Pleuritic pain	0.07		

[a]One patient died from a ruptured abdominal aortic aneurysm postoperatively

experience. Subsequent larger studies have reported similar rates of major complications and mortality.

While laparoscopic cholecystectomy is generally performed with an acceptable safety profile, it is important to recognize the types of injuries and complications that are responsible for most of its potential major morbidity and mortality. Deziel et al. in 1993 performed a retrospective survey of surgical department chairs, collecting data on 77,604 cases at 4,292 hospitals in the USA, to more closely examine major complications and mortality [5]. These investigators found a major complication rate of 2%, including a 0.61% rate of bile duct injuries, 0.25% vascular injuries, and 0.14% bowel injuries, and a 0.04% rate of mortality. An important finding of this study was that injuries to the bile ducts, intestines, or major vessels, were associated with a significant mortality of 1.6%, 4.5%, and 8.8%, respectively. Vascular and bowel injuries tended to occur during Veress needle or trocar insertion, dissection in the porta hepatis, or from electrocautery and retraction injuries, with a tendency towards delayed diagnosis in the case of bowel injuries. Additional non-technical causes of mortality accounting for about half of the mortality observed in this study included myocardial infarction, pulmonary embolism, pneumonia, ischemic bowel, respiratory failure, necrotizing fasciitis, and sepsis.

The Problem of Bile Duct Injury

While the overall morbidity and mortality of laparoscopic cholecystectomy was seen to be less than that of open cholecystectomy, it was soon realized, however, that laparoscopic cholecystectomy was associated with higher rates of bile duct injury compared with the open approach. A retrospective analysis of a large single-institution series of 3,051 cholecystectomies during the "open era" compared with 1,630 subsequent laparoscopic cholecystectomies reported a bile duct injury rate of 0.6% and 0.95% for each approach, respectively [6]. Similarly, an analysis of 34,490 cholecystectomies using a state-wide database from Connecticut showed an increase in the rate of bile duct injuries from 0.04% to 0.41% from 1989 to 1990 during the transition from open cholecystectomy to laparoscopic cholecystectomy [7]. Since the introduction of laparoscopic cholecystectomy, however, the rate of major bile duct injuries requiring operative repair appears to have decreased and leveled off to around 0.1% from 1991 to 2000 [1]. Nevertheless, bile duct injury remains a major source of morbidity and mortality as well as a source of increased health care costs and litigation. Savader et al. estimated that laparoscopic cholecystectomy-related bile duct injuries were associated with an additional $50,000 in cost, 32 days of inpatient hospitalization, 378 days of chronic biliary intubation, and 4% mortality per case [8].

Prevention of Bile Duct Injuries

Given the significant morbidity and mortality of bile duct injuries, it is critical to understand the risk factors leading to their occurrence, and strategies for their prevention. While learning curve effects are important and have been shown to influence the rate of bile duct injuries early in a surgeon's experience, these complications continue to occur even beyond

200 cases, suggesting that a learning curve is not the only explanation for injuries [9]. Demographic and clinical factors play a role, as patients of older age, male gender, and with a prolonged duration of symptoms have been found to have higher rates of bile duct injury during laparoscopic cholecystectomy [10, 11]. Anatomic variants such as low-lying aberrant right hepatic ducts, cystic ducts draining directly into a right hepatic duct or a right sectoral duct, as well as a parallel configuration of the cystic duct – common hepatic duct junction may predispose to injury by bringing normally remote biliary structures into the area of dissection. More commonly, however, the anatomic factors that play a role in increasing the risk of bile duct injury are those which make dissection in the hepatocystic triangle (formed by the edge of the liver and common hepatic duct, the cystic duct, and the gallbladder wall) more difficult, including acute cholecystitis, chronic inflammation, and impacted gallstones in the neck of the gallbladder. A difficult dissection, coupled with improper operative techniques, increases the risk of bile duct injuries.

It is important to define improper dissection techniques, as the danger of relying on them does not become evident to many surgeons until after a bile duct injury has occurred. These surgical techniques, which work the majority of the time but are prone to critical failures in certain situations, have become known as "error traps," first described by Strasberg [12]. The first of these error traps is the infundibular technique. This technique for identifying the infundibulum of the gallbladder begins by following the putative cystic duct until it funnels out circumferentially. This flaring of the duct is used to identify the infundibulum of the gallbladder, after which the putative cystic duct is clipped and transected. This technique is prone to critical failure, however, when there is acute or chronic inflammation in the hepatocystic triangle, bringing the common bile duct in close opposition to the infundibulum of the gallbladder. In these situations, the widening of the cystic duct – common hepatic duct junction is misinterpreted as the flaring of the infundibulum and leads to common bile duct injury. Another improper technique and error trap associated with bile duct injuries is the fundus-down technique. In this technique, a difficult dissection in the hepatocystic triangle is averted by beginning at the fundus and dissecting the gallbladder off the liver bed, heading towards the porta hepatis. The goal of the technique is to leave the infundibulum of the gallbladder attached by only the cystic duct and artery. Again, this technique may be effective in most cases, but in the setting of severe inflammation or chronic scarring of the hepatocystic triangle it may lead to severe vasculo-biliary injuries, as the plane of dissection between the gallbladder and porta hepatis becomes obliterated and the dissection often proceeds into the portal structures. Another error trap worth mentioning which is relevant to the current practice of laparoscopic cholecystectomy, applies to the use of intra-operative cholangiography (IOC). While routine IOC (or intraoperative ultrasound) has been widely championed as aiding in the identification of intraoperative bile duct injuries, or even decreasing the incidence of bile duct injuries, improper interpretation of an IOC may lead to missed injuries while providing a false sense of security [13, 14]. The most common errors of interpretation of IOC occur when only the common bile duct is visualized, or when right- or left-sided ductal branches fail to opacify. The first situation is easier to spot, and should alert to surgeon to a potential occlusion or transection of the common hepatic or common bile duct. The second situation should alert the surgeon to a potential injury of the right or left hepatic duct system. It is essential for the surgeon to recognize these risk factors and error traps in order to minimize the occurrence of bile duct injuries.

In contrast to the previous techniques described, establishment of the "critical view of safety" has become recognized as the preferred technique for increasing the safety of laparoscopic cholecystectomy and the prevention of bile duct injuries [15]. This technique is performed by meticulously clearing the hepatocystic triangle of its fibrous and lymphatic tissues, beginning above the presumed infundibulo-cystic junction on the gallbladder wall, well away from the common hepatic duct. In addition, the lateral and medial peritoneal attachments of the gallbladder near the infundibulum are incised to elevate the infundibulum away from the liver bed. The critical view of safety is achieved only when the base of the liver bed is exposed and there remain only two structures leading to the gallbladder (the cystic duct and artery). Ligation of any structures prior to achieving the critical view of safety risks misidentification and vasculo-biliary injury.

Even when using a proper technique for laparoscopic dissection and definitive identification of biliary structures, however, it is important to know how to proceed when faced with intraoperative difficulty due to adhesions, scarring, inflammation, or bleeding. When should a surgeon continue a difficult dissection laparoscopically, convert to open, or attempt a "bail-out" maneuver? The obvious answer is that judgment should be employed. However, Strasberg has argued that a more structured, rule-based approach, similar to approaches used in the airline or nuclear power industries should be developed, to help guide surgeons faced with difficult intraoperative situations [16]. These structured approaches would involve the creation of "stopping rules," preventing the surgeon from continuing when a potentially dangerous situation is identified, before an injury has occurred. A surgeon proceeding with a dissection during a potentially dangerous situation may eventually complete a certain percentage of cases with no harm done. However, in the remaining cases, a potentially preventable vasculo-biliary injury, with devastating consequences for the patient and surgeon will have occurred, during the treatment of a relatively benign disease. It is unavoidable that certain operations will have a definite risk of serious complications, in the treatment of highly aggressive or malignant diseases (e.g., liver transplantation, Whipple, etc.). However, the risk of injuring a bile duct in order to stubbornly complete a laparoscopic cholecystectomy is not justifiable, especially when viable "bail-out" maneuvers exist. Creating exact stopping rules for cholecystectomy may not be as feasible as in other industries. Nevertheless, Strasberg has argued that the adoption of the stopping rule mind-set is more important than determining specific rules. When faced with situations such as significant bleeding, difficulty with visualization, or the inability to make progress in the course of a dissection, the surgeon should pause, review the situation at hand, seek assistance from a colleague, and consider the following alternatives: obtain additional information by performing IOC or ultrasound, proceed with conversion to an open operation (if the situation can be managed with an open approach), or proceed with a laparoscopic "bail-out" maneuver if the situation would be equally hazardous with an open approach. This last point is important, as stubbornly proceeding with an open cholecystectomy in the face of a hostile dissection may also result in significant complications. Alternatives to completion of a cholecystectomy in the case of a difficult dissection or profuse bleeding (e.g., with cirrhosis and portal hypertension), include the performance of a subtotal cholecystectomy or a tube cholecystostomy. These procedures have been shown to have acceptable outcomes and decrease the risk of vasculo-biliary injury in difficult situations.

Management of Bile Duct Injuries

Nevertheless, in spite of employing a sound technical approach with appropriate judgment, bile duct injuries occur, even among highly experienced surgeons. The complete elimination of bile duct injuries during laparoscopic cholecystectomy, despite arguments by some, will likely never occur. Thus, the appropriate management of a suspected or confirmed bile duct injury discovered intraoperatively or postoperatively will be reviewed. Although the detailed management of complicated major bile duct injuries is beyond the scope of this chapter, a surgeon performing laparoscopic cholecystectomy should be familiar with the general concepts in order to better direct the initial management and subsequent referral of these patients. Several classification systems have been described for bile duct injuries. We will use the modified Bismuth classification (A through E5) that has been described previously [15]. Briefly, type A injuries refer to bile leaks originating from the cystic duct stump or small bile ducts injured in the gallbladder bed. Type B and C injuries occur when an aberrant right hepatic duct is either occluded (type B) or transected, causing a bile leak (type C). Type D injuries involve a laceration of the common hepatic or common bile duct without ductal discontinuity. Type E injuries involve transection of the common hepatic or common bile duct, and are further classified according to the level of the injury. These injuries are classified depending on whether they occur greater than 2 cm distal to the bifurcation (E1), less than 2 cm distal to the bifurcation (E2), involve a stenosis at the bifurcation (E3), involve an occlusion of the bifurcation with non-communication between the right and left hepatic ducts (E4), or involve a combined common hepatic duct and right hepatic duct injury (E5).

It has been reported that bile duct injuries are discovered intraoperatively only approximately 32% of the time [17]. However, when there is suspicion of a major bile duct injury, the surgeon may use IOC to attempt to identify the injury, and should request assistance from a colleague. Conversion to an open operation should not be performed purely for diagnosis, but only if the surgical team is equipped to perform a definitive repair of a major bile duct injury. If the team is not sufficiently equipped to perform a definitive repair, drains should be placed laparoscopically, and arrangements made to transfer the patient to a tertiary care center with hepatobiliary surgeons for definitive management.

Type A injuries discovered intraoperatively may be treated by oversewing the leaking duct or ligating the cystic duct stump laparoscopically with a ligating loop. Type B and C injuries discovered intraoperatively usually require Roux-en-Y hepaticojejunostomy (RYHJ) to provide adequate drainage to the isolated liver segment, unless the duct is < 1 mm, in which case the small duct may be ligated. Type D injuries may be oversewn using fine absorbable suture over a T-tube if the affected circumference is less than 50% and if there is no associated thermal injury. RYHJ is indicated for more extensive type D and E injuries.

Even though some bile duct injuries are discovered intraoperatively, most are not discovered until the postoperative period. Thus, it is important to maintain a high suspicion for bile duct injuries should the patient experience significant, untoward postoperative symptoms. Patients may present with pain, sepsis, jaundice, bile fistulas, or insidiously with non-specific complaints of malaise, bloating, or constipation. Control of sepsis, drainage of fluid collections and ongoing bile leaks, and diagnosis should be the initial priorities, rather than immediate reconstruction [17]. The first-line investigation should be computed tomography (CT) to evaluate for bilomas or undrained fluid collections. After a bilious fluid collection has been drained by an interventional radiologist, the next study of choice is endoscopic retrograde cholangiopancreatography (ERCP), as it may be both diagnostic and therapeutic. Type A or D injuries may be treated endoscopically with sphincterotomy and stenting, or nasobiliary catheter placement. Type B and C injuries usually require RYHJ. Type E injuries are usually managed operatively with RYHJ reconstruction, although there have been some reports of successful management with non-operative, interventional techniques. Patients with major bile duct injuries requiring operative repair should be treated at a tertiary center by experienced hepatobiliary surgeons, as this is associated with improved long-term outcomes and reduced morbidity and mortality [18].

Preparation for the operative repair of major bile duct injuries by a hepatobiliary team usually involves a thorough assessment of the entire biliary system using a combination of CT, MRI, fistulograms, ERCP, and/or percutaneous transhepatic cholangiography (PTC) in order to account for the drainage of all hepatic segments that are to be preserved. In addition to delineating ductal injuries, imaging studies (CT or MRI angiography) are performed to evaluate for concomitant vascular injury and the need for vascular reconstruction. Preparation of the patient involves optimizing nutrition with enteral feeding, and consideration of bile refeeding to prevent fat-soluble vitamin deficiencies in patients with long-term biliary drainage [18]. The timing of definitive reconstruction varies in the literature, although in patients with uncontrolled sepsis/peritonitis, acute inflammation, thermal injury, or in the case of concomitant vascular injuries, it is generally preferable to delay reconstruction, even up to three months, until sepsis has been controlled, inflammation has subsided, and the full extent of the injury has been assessed [19].

Conclusions

In summary, laparoscopic cholecystectomy has replaced open cholecystectomy as the preferred approach to the treatment of biliary disease requiring cholecystectomy. Overall, laparoscopic cholecystectomy is a safe procedure performed with low morbidity and mortality. However, bile duct injury remains a significant risk of the operation, associated with considerable morbidity and mortality, even when managed by experienced hands. Thus, the prevention of bile duct injuries is a priority of utmost importance in the safe performance of the operation. It is imperative that general surgeons learn to recognize risk factors predisposing to bile duct injuries, employ proper techniques for the dissection and identification of the critical structures, be familiar with alternatives to completing a laparoscopic cholecystectomy in the face of a hazardous dissection, learn to recognize potential bile duct injuries, and have a pre-determined plan in place to deal with them.

Selected Readings

1. Dolan JP, Diggs BS, Sheppard BC, Hunter JG. Ten-year trend in the national volume of bile duct injuries requiring operative repair. Surg Endosc. 2005;19:967–73.

2. Dolan JP, Diggs BS, Sheppard BC, Hunter JG. The national mortality burden and significant factors associated with open and laparoscopic cholecystectomy: 1997–2006. J Gastrointest Surg. 2009;13:2292–301.

3. MacFadyen Jr BV, Vecchio R, Ricardo AE, Mathis CR. Bile duct injury after laparoscopic cholecystectomy. The United States experience. Surg Endosc. 1998;12:315–21.

4. The Southern Surgeons Club. A prospective analysis of 1518 laparoscopic cholecystectomies. N Engl J Med. 1991;324:1073–8.

5. Deziel DJ, Millikan KW, Economou SG, Doolas A, Ko ST, Airan MC. Complications of laparoscopic cholecystectomy: a national survey of 4,292 hospitals and an analysis of 77,604 cases. Am J Surg. 1993;165:9–14.

6. Targarona EM, Marco C, Balague C, Rodriguez J, Cugat E, Hoyuela C, et al. How, when, and why bile duct injury occurs. A comparison between open and laparoscopic cholecystectomy. Surg Endosc. 1998;12:322–6.

7. Russell JC, Walsh SJ, Mattie AS, Lynch JT. Bile duct injuries, 1989-1993. A statewide experience. Connecticut Laparoscopic Cholecystectomy Registry. Arch Surg. 1996;131:382–8.

8. Savader SJ, Lillemoe KD, Prescott CA, Winick AB, Venbrux AC, Lund GB, et al. Laparoscopic cholecystectomy-related bile duct injuries: a health and financial disaster. Ann Surg. 1997;225:268–73.

9. Archer SB, Brown DW, Smith CD, Branum GD, Hunter JG. Bile duct injury during laparoscopic cholecystectomy: results of a national survey. Ann Surg. 2001;234:549–58. discussion 558–549.

10. Jablonska B, Lampe P. Iatrogenic bile duct injuries: etiology, diagnosis and management. World J Gastroenterol. 2009;15:4097–104.

11. Waage A, Nilsson M. Iatrogenic bile duct injury: a population-based study of 152 776 cholecystectomies in the Swedish Inpatient Registry. Arch Surg. 2006;141:1207–13.

12. Strasberg SM. Error traps and vasculo-biliary injury in laparoscopic and open cholecystectomy. J Hepatobiliary Pancreat Surg. 2008;15:284–92.

13. Ludwig K, Bernhardt J, Steffen H, Lorenz D. Contribution of intraoperative cholangiography to incidence and outcome of common bile duct injuries during laparoscopic cholecystectomy. Surg Endosc. 2002;16:1098–104.

14. Machi J, Johnson JO, Deziel DJ, Soper NJ, Berber E, Siperstein A, et al. The routine use of laparoscopic ultrasound decreases bile duct injury: a multicenter study. Surg Endosc. 2009;23:384–8.

15. Strasberg SM, Hertl M, Soper NJ. An analysis of the problem of biliary injury during laparoscopic cholecystectomy. J Am Coll Surg. 1995;180:101–25.

16. Strasberg SM. Biliary injury in laparoscopic surgery: part 2. Changing the culture of cholecystectomy. J Am Coll Surg. 2005;201:604–11.

17. Sicklick JK, Camp MS, Lillemoe KD, Melton GB, Yeo CJ, Campbell KA, et al. Surgical management of bile duct injuries sustained during laparoscopic cholecystectomy: perioperative results in 200 patients. Ann Surg. 2005;241:786–92. discussion 793–785.

18. Connor S, Garden OJ. Bile duct injury in the era of laparoscopic cholecystectomy. Br J Surg. 2006;93:158–68.

19. Strasberg SM. Bile Duct Injury. In: Soper NJ, Swanstrom LL, Eubanks WS, editors. Mastery of endoscopic and laparoscopic surgery. Philadelphia: Lippincott Williams & Wilkins; 2009. p. 329–41.

27. Antireflux Surgery for GERD

Alexander J. Greenstein and John G. Hunter

Introduction

Gastroesophageal reflux disease (GERD) can present with a host of symptoms, the most common of which are heartburn, regurgitation, and dysphagia. In general, surgery is reserved for patients with troublesome symptoms despite adequately dosed proton pump inhibitors (PPIs) or with complications of reflux such as recurrent or refractory esophagitis, stricture, Barrett's metaplasia, and asthma. In addition, patients who are unable to tolerate medication, who are noncompliant with medication, or are unwilling to take lifelong medications are also surgical candidates.

In general, the data on antireflux surgery suggests that there is no one "best" operation for all patients, and factors such as the degree of esophageal shortening, disturbances of esophageal motility, and history of prior operations should influence the choice of operation. Nevertheless, most patients with early, uncomplicated disease can be properly treated by laparoscopic Nissen fundoplication.

Although there are important questions about antireflux surgery that have yet to be answered and long-term data is sparse, a number of series and a prospective, randomized study (up to 11 years follow-up) have revealed laparoscopic fundoplication to demonstrate comparable safety, short-term efficacy, and patient satisfaction, as well as shorter hospital stays and recuperative times than with open operation [1–4]. As with other laparoscopic surgeries, there is an associated learning curve associated with fundoplication which has been reported to be approximately 20 cases [5], but climbing the "competence" curve, as measured by operative time, complication rates and long-term outcomes, may take several hundred operations.

D.S. Tichansky, J. Morton, and D.B. Jones (eds.), *The SAGES Manual of Quality, Outcomes and Patient Safety*, DOI 10.1007/978-1-4419-7901-8_27,
© Springer Science+Business Media, LLC 2012

Complications

In most series, complications have been reported in anywhere from 3 to 10% of patients. Many of the complications are minor and are related to surgical intervention in general (urinary retention, wound infection, venous thrombosis, and ileus). Others are related specifically to the procedure or the approach (such as hollow viscus perforation, dysphagia, and pneumothorax). For the purposes of this chapter, the complications specific to this procedure will be discussed in detail and classified as either early (Table 27.1) or late (Table 27.2) complications, the latter of which can also be described as persistent side effects. The percentages in these tables were derived from a compilation of several sources [5–9].

Early Complications: Perforation

Perhaps the most feared complication of laparoscopic Nissen fundoplication is esophageal or gastric perforation. Early esophageal perforation may arise during passage of the bougie, during the

Table 27.1. Early complications.

Complication	Rate (%)
Ileus	<5
Pneumothorax	1–3
Urinary retention	<2
Urinary tract infection	1–2
Wrap herniation	<1
Perforation	<1
Hemorrhage	<1
Wound infection	<0.5
Splenectomy	<0.5
Mortality	<0.2

Table 27.2. Late complications/persistent side effects.

Complication	Rate (%)
Reflux symptoms	15
Bloating	10
Dysphagia	8

retroesophageal dissection, during greater curvature dissection with the harmonic scalpel, or during suture pull-through, while late esophageal perforation may result from inadvertent electrocautery burns during any part of the dissection. Revisional Nissen fundoplication, with intense associated perigastric fibrosis is a "set-up" for dissection related perforation.

Presentation: A leak will usually manifest itself during the first 48 h, but delayed presentations are not uncommon. Peritoneal signs will be noted if the spillage is limited to the abdomen; shortness of breath and a pleural effusion will occur if contamination extends into the chest. A well-contained perforation may present with more indolent signs such as fever, leukocytosis, malaise, hiccoughs, or left shoulder pain.

Treatment: One should consider confirmation of the site of the leak by a CT scan or contrast study with barium and/or a water-soluble contrast agent, but a high index of suspicion can justify reoperation without imaging. Optimal management consists of direct repair and drainage by thoracotomy, laparoscopy, or laparotomy if the leak is detected early. Late leaks may not be amenable to direct repair, but can usually be managed with drainage and antibiotics.

Early Complications: Pneumothorax

Both pneumothorax and pneumomediastinum have been reported. The occurrence of pneumothorax is related to breach of either pleural membrane, usually the left, during the hiatal dissection.

Presentation: Pneumothorax will present intraoperatively with a billowing out of the affected diaphragm as well as decreased unilateral breath sounds and desaturation. Tension physiology is not unusual, resulting in severe hypotension.

Treatment: If the pneumothorax is noted intraoperatively and the patient is stable, a fenestrated red rubber catheter (18 Fr) can be inserted into the pleural space. Just prior to extubation, the base of the red rubber should be removed through a port site and placed to water seal until the remaining pneumothorax has been evacuated. Once this has been accomplished, it may be drawn back from the pleural space and removed. Chest tube insertion is usually not required unless a tension pneumothorax is not rapidly alleviated by the placement of the pressure equalizing tube. As accumulated carbon dioxide rapidly dissipates following the release of the pneumoperitoneum by a combination of positive pressure ventilation and absorption, a pressure equalizing tube may not be required in all cases.

Early Complications: Hemorrhage

Hemorrhage during laparoscopic fundoplication usually originates from the short gastric vessels, a fatty liver or the spleen. Injury to the left inferior phrenic vein, an aberrant left hepatic vein, or the inferior vena cava, as well as retractor trauma to the liver may occur. Incidental splenic injury requiring splenectomy has been virtually eliminated since the advent of laparoscopic fundoplication.

Treatment: Vascular injury mandates immediate control and may require conversion to an open procedure.

Early Complications: Wrap Herniation

In a literature review that consisted of 41 papers and 10,489 procedures, early wrap herniation defined as occurring within 48 h of surgery occurred a rate of 1.3%, although other more current sources place acute wrap herniation rate at <1% [7]. This is one complication that may be more common with the laparoscopic than open approach. The explanation for this is unclear but may be related to the opening of tissue planes by the pneumoperitoneum and the reduced tendency for adhesion formation after laparoscopic compared to open surgery.

Presentation: Acute herniation of the wrap will most likely present with increased epigastric pain, tachycardia, tachypnea or retching. Gas trapping in the stomach can create an acute gastric dilation.

Treatment: The best treatment for this complication is to avoid its occurrence by routinely performing a snug crural repair and providing aggressive prophylaxis against nausea. In the event that a herniation does occur, which should be confirmed by a contrast study, immediate reoperation and reduction of the herniation with proper crural closure via pledgeted permanent sutures is mandated.

Of course, herniation of the wrap can occur slowly and thus be a late complication presenting with dysphagia or resumption of recurrence symptoms. This may be due to inadequate esophageal mobilization, an unrecognized shortened esophagus or poor closure of the crura, and will be addressed in more detail in the reoperation section.

Late Complications: Gas Bloat

Early postoperative complaints of bloating may occur in up to 30% of patients, but in less than 5% of patients do symptoms persist beyond 2 months. The pathogenesis is not well understood, and it was seen more frequently in the past when longer and tighter fundoplications were created. There are at least three reasons for bloating. First, the patient may have more difficulty belching owing to the wrap. Second, vagal trauma may contribute to delayed gastric emptying. Third, reflux patients have a tendency to swallow saliva and air to help clear the esophagus of refluxate. This habit will contribute to build-up of gastrointestinal gas.

Presentation: The patient will present with a sensation of intestinal gas and the inability to belch.

Treatment: In patients with only mild symptoms, patients should be instructed not to drink with a straw or ingest carbonated beverages and may try simethicone tablets or charcoal caplets. Metoclopramide (5–10 mg four times daily) may be helpful as a short-term treatment only – 2–3 months total – as tardive dyskinesia is associated with more chronic use. Another alternative is Erythromycin. A few patients with more serious discomfort may require nasogastric tube decompression. In patients with severe persistent symptoms, loosening a "too tight, too long" Nissen or conversion from a full to a partial fundoplication may be required. In those with documented gastroparesis, pyloroplasty can be considered.

Late Complications: Dysphagia

Despite postoperative administration of a modified dietary intake, most patients (up to 20%) initially experience some degree of dysphagia postoperatively which is usually due to either edema from intraoperative tissue dissection or hematoma of the stomach or esophageal wall. Dysphagia due to these causes should resolve after 4–8 weeks, but if dysphagia persists beyond this period, one or more of the following causes is responsible.

1. A wrap that is too tight or too long (i.e. >2.5 cm).
2. Lateral torsion of the wrap to the right due to intact short gastric vessels or a small fundus.
3. A wrap made with the body of the stomach rather than the fundus which cannot relax on arrival of the food bolus.

4.   Choice of a full wrap rather than a partial wrap in a patient with abnormal preoperative esophageal peristalsis.

Presentation: Some patients describe a "sticking" sensation in their lower or mid chest, others have persistent difficulty tolerating anything thicker than liquids.

Treatment: Patients with dysphagia that persists for more than 8 weeks or who require the resumption of antisecretory medications require evaluation of the fundoplication, typically a barium contrast study with swallow to assess the anatomic placement. Patients who have abnormally slow passage of barium through the wrap but had normal motility preoperatively should be considered for dilation. Approximately 6–12% of patients with fundoplication required dilation in various reports [10, 11]. Direct bougie dilation generally produces good results and pneumatic dilation is rarely needed. If successive dilations are ineffective, patients may require a revision (please see next section for details) or conversion to a partial fundoplication.

Failures and Reoperative Surgery

There is an incidence of approximately 15% of persistent GERD symptoms and/or physiologic evidence of continued acid exposure. All of these patients should be considered for manometry, pH studies, an esophagogram and upper endoscopy. While most of these patients can be treated with acid suppression therapy with good results, those with a sizable herniation of the wrap or persistent mechanical dysphagia are best treated with revisional surgery. In total, approximately 3–10% of patients will require revision after laparoscopic fundoplication. In a series of 241 patients who underwent revisional surgery, the indications were reflux (60%), dysphagia (55%), wrap herniation (26%), esophageal dysmotility (6%) and chest pain (6%) [12]. Unfortunately, the success rate for revisional surgery is lower than primary surgery, and about 20% of patients will continue to complain of reflux or dysphagia.

Mortality

Death is uncommon with this operation and the mortality rate for primary minimally invasive antireflux surgery has fortunately been very low (<0.2%) [7, 8]. Mortality does increase with age greater than 60 years, so GERD severity and effect on lifestyle must be considered prior to performing an antireflux procedure.

Selected Readings

1. Nilsson G, Wenner J, Larsson S, et al. Randomized clinical trial of laparoscopic versus open fundoplication for gastro-oesophageal reflux. Br J Surg. 2004;91:552–9.

2. Peters JH, Heimbucher J, Kauer WK, et al. Clinical and physiologic comparison of laparoscopic and open Nissen fundoplication. J Am Coll Surg. 1995;180:385–93.

3. Rice S, Watson DI, Lally CJ, et al. Laparoscopic anterior 180 degrees partial fundoplication: five-year results and beyond. Arch Surg. 2006;141:271–5.

4. Rattner DW, Brooks DC. Patient satisfaction following laparoscopic and open antireflux surgery. Arch Surg. 1995;130:289–93. discussion 293–4.

5. Watson DI, Baigrie RJ, Jamieson GG. A learning curve for laparoscopic fundoplication. Definable, avoidable, or a waste of time? Ann Surg. 1996;224:198–203.

6. Rantanen TK, Oksala NK, Oksala AK, et al. Complications in antireflux surgery: national-based analysis of laparoscopic and open fundoplications. Arch Surg. 2008;143:359–65. discussion 365.

7. Carlson MA, Frantzides CT. Complications and results of primary minimally invasive antireflux procedures: a review of 10,735 reported cases. J Am Coll Surg. 2001;193: 428–39.

8. Granderath FA, Kamolz T, Schweiger UM, et al. Long-term results of laparoscopic antireflux surgery. Surg Endosc. 2002;16:753–7.

9. Terry M, Smith CD, Branum GD, et al. Outcomes of laparoscopic fundoplication for gastroesophageal reflux disease and paraesophageal hernia. Surg Endosc. 2001; 15:691–9.

10. Dominitz JA, Dire CA, Billingsley KG, et al. Complications and antireflux medication use after antireflux surgery. Clin Gastroenterol Hepatol. 2006;4:299–305.

11. Malhi-Chowla N, Gorecki P, Bammer T, et al. Dilation after fundoplication: timing, frequency, indications, and outcome. Gastrointest Endosc. 2002;55:219–23.

12. Smith CD, McClusky DA, Rajad MA, et al. When fundoplication fails: redo? Ann Surg. 2005;241:861–9. discussion 869–71.

28. Complications of Bariatric Surgery

Robert B. Lim

Surgical weight loss procedures are among the most commonly performed operations in the world today. Because it is so prevalent, most general surgeons will likely have to manage bariatric patients acutely even as the surgical techniques improve and the overall complication rates decrease. Some of the reasons the outcomes from weight loss surgery (WLS) have improved are because of a better understanding of the obesity disease process, the establishment of Center of Excellence criteria, the start of minimally invasive surgical fellowships, and the use of improved equipment. Some feel that perhaps bariatric surgery probably ought to be performed only by experienced bariatric surgeons in higher volume centers with appropriate ancillary and consult expertise and in facilities where the outcomes are readily transparent. Still even in the best centers, complications will arise. As the procedure and disease are ubiquitous, it is good for all general surgeons to be familiar with these complications so that they can recognize them and initially manage them.

General Complications

DVT/PE

Pulmonary emboli (PE) are the most common cause of death after surgical weight loss procedures. Deep venous thrombi occur about 0.4–1.3% of the time and PEs occur about 0.25–3% of the time. There is great variation among practicing bariatric surgeons as to the proper prophylaxis for a venous thrombotic event. Early ambulation (a few hours after the operation) and sequential compression devices are the minimum one should use. Most start some form of anti-coagulation, like subcutaneous heparin or lovenox, preoperatively and continue it until the patient is ambulatory. Some even continue anti-coagulation for up to

D.S. Tichansky, J. Morton, and D.B. Jones (eds.), *The SAGES Manual of Quality, Outcomes and Patient Safety*, DOI 10.1007/978-1-4419-7901-8_28, © Springer Science+Business Media, LLC 2012

1 month afterward. The highest risk patients may benefit from preoperative placement of an IVC filter. Surgeons should consider consultation with a hematologist in higher risk patients to assess the risk of a thromboembolic event to aid their decisions about prophylactic measures. In all post bariatric patients who present with respiratory distress, hypoxemia or lower extremity swelling, a venous-thrombotic event should be considered in the early post operative period.

Cardiac Event

A cardiac event is the second most common cause of perioperative death, even though the overall incidence of cardiac ischemia after bariatric operations is less than 1%. Still morbidly obese patients are at an increased risk for a cardiovascular event over their lifetime when compared to normal weight individuals of the same age group. All patients with morbid obesity should be screened with an EKG preoperatively and considered for consultation with cardiology if pathology is suspected from it or from the patient's history. It should go without saying that the risk reduction from weight loss will not improve the patient's cardiac status until several months after the surgery. Therefore, WLS patients should be considered high risk for a cardiac event until their risk factors have been modified.

Pulmonary Events

Pulmonary complications are the third most common cause of mortality after bariatric surgery. The most common of these is atelectasis and its effects should not be underestimated in these patients especially if they carry a diagnosis of obstructive sleep apnea (OSA). Patients with OSA should be evaluated preoperatively for their need of positive pressure ventilation, and CPAP devices ought to be used starting the evening after surgery if they require a machine preoperatively. For those patients who do not have known OSA, then positive pressure ventilation should be considered if there is evidence of respiratory compromise from atelectasis postoperatively. The risk for injury to the gastro-jejunostomy anastomosis from positive pressure ventilation is small and it is not contraindicated in the immediate post operative period (Table 28.1).

Aspiration pneumonia can occur several months after WLS for numerous reasons that cause persistent vomiting and reflux. After Roux Y Gastric Bypass (RYGB), aspiration can result from stenosis or a

Table 28.1. Complications of bariatric surgery.

Major complications after bariatric surgery	Incidence
DVT/PE	0.4–1.3%/0.25–3%
Cardiac event (myocardial infarction)	<1
Pulmonary event	8
Malnutriton	44
Gallstones	3[a]
Psychiatric	30
Death	0.01–0.3
Complications after RYGB	
Leaks	0.7–5.1
Bleeding	0.8–4.5
Early bowel obstruction	0.2–4.5
Stenosis	9–20
Marginal ulcers	0.72–5.1
Late bowel obstructions/internal herniation	5
Weight regain	Unknown
Complications after AGB	
Acute stromal obstruction	1[b]
Gastric prolapse/band slippage	2[c]
Band erosion	1
Port flips	Unknown
Port leaks	0.4
Port infections	0.3–9
Poor weight loss/weight regain	40/25
Pouch/esophageal dilatation	Unknown
Complications after SG	
Leaks	1.4
Bleeding	0–6.4
Narrowing/stenosis	0.7
Abnormal gastric emptying	Unknown

[a]Rate decreases from 42% with the use of ursodiol for 6 months
[b]Rate decreases from 14% with the dissection of the esophageal fat pad
[c]Rate decreases from 22% with the use of the pars flaccida technique, hiatal hernia repair, and gastric imbrication

stricture. After AGB it can occur from gastric prolapsed, pouch dilatation, or simply having the band too tight.

Psychiatric

Although WLS has been shown to improve some psychiatric diseases, the incidence of psychiatric diagnoses is probably the same before and after surgery. This is because some new diagnoses manifest after significant weight loss has occurred. Certainly some people's propensity to overeat can be due to an Axis I or II disorder but most bariatric patients do not have a psychiatric illness. Preoperatively this should be determined via consultation with a mental health expert.

Postoperatively there are changes that occur with the patients that should be monitored again by behavioral health experts. The exact changes can be difficult to identify even by experts, and thus follow-up with a behavior health specialist should be part of the multidisciplinary treatment of obesity. It is important to note that the suicide rate, the incidence of alcoholism, and the rate of spousal dissatisfaction is higher in WLS patients than in those who have not undergone the procedure. Often times, though, patients just need assistance adjusting to the lifestyle changes that accompany surgical weight loss and consultation with a mental health expert can be very beneficial.

Nutritional

Malnutrition is more common after malabsorption operations such as the RYGB where it can occur in up to 44% of patients, but it can still happen to patients after an AGB and an SG. Obese patients may be malnourished prior to the operation, so they should be screened for this during their preoperative workup. Even if they are doing well postoperatively, all patients should be evaluated for malnutrition at least once per year as part of their lifelong follow-up. Many patients have not had appropriate nutritional follow up after WLS, and a full biochemical and clinical evaluation for malnutrition should be done if such patients are encountered. All WLS patients should be on lifelong supplementation. The biochemical parameters that are monitored are listed in Table 28.2, and the nutrient and vitamin deficiencies are listed in Table 28.3.

Table 28.2. Biochemical nutritional analysis.

Parameter	Lab ordered
Anemia	CBC
B12/folate	B12/folate level
Iron	Iron panel
Hypocalcemia	Calcium/vitamin D/pararthyroid hormone level
Protein	Albumin and total protein
Thiamine	Thiamine level

Table 28.3. Nutritional complications.

Deficiency	Symptoms	Incidence	Prophylaxis	Treatment
Vitamin B12/folate	Megaloblastic anemia, parathesia, peripheral neuropathy, demyelination of the corticospinal tract and dorsal columns	12–38%	350–400 mcg/d PO	2,000 mcg/m IM
Vitamin B1	Hyperemesis, Wernicke-Korsakoff syndrome, peripheral neuropathy	Unknown	0.8–1.0 mg/d	50–100 mg TID for 7–14 days
Vitamin A	Night blindness, xerophthalmia, nyctalopia, blindness	10–69	Most MVI	
Vitamin D/calcium	Myalgias, arthralgias, muscle weakness, fatigue, decreased bone mineral density, hyperparathyroidism	48–69	1.2–1.5 g/d of calcium citrate 400 IU/d ergocalciferol	
Iron	Microcytic anemia, deceased exercise tolerance, immune dysfunction, impaired thermoregulation, GI disturbances, cognitive impairment, pica	14–52	650 mg/d	IV infusion
Protein	Excessive weight loss, diarrhea, marasmus, edema, hair loss	13–18	1.2 g/kg/d	TPN
Vitamin E		4	Most MVI	
Vitamin K		68	Most MVI	
Zinc	Alopecia	Rare	MVI with zinc	

Most of the nutrients monitored are available in commercially available multivitamins, but one should not hesitate to supply other specific nutrients and vitamins if patients are lacking. Surgeons should work closely with their registered dietitians to make sure their patients are getting an adequate amount of nutrition. Any iron replacement should be accompanied with Vitamin C as it helps absorption. Thiamine deficiency should be suspected in anyone with prolonged vomiting because failure to recognize and treat this deficiency may result in an irreversible neurologic defect. If patients cannot take enough protein in orally then it can be given via total parenteral nutrition (TPN) formulas. Finally calcium, parathromone, and vitamin D levels should be monitored closely and treated aggressively with supplementation because the patient may be resorbing bone to maintain adequate serum calcium levels. Consequently they may still suffer from low bone mineral density despite having relatively normal calcium levels.

If women become pregnant after WLS then their biochemical parameters should be monitored every 2–3 months during the pregnancy. It has been recommended for pregnant women to maintain serum B12 levels greater than 600 ρg/mL and folate levels greater than 15 ng/mL after WLS, which are higher than recommended levels in nonpregnant patients.

Gallstones

Gallstone precipitation can occur after surgical weight loss in up to 38% of patients from a number of different mechanisms. The routine use of ursodiol for 6 months after WLS has been shown to decrease the incidence of gallstones down to 2% and thus is recommended. Some insurance companies will not cover the use of ursodiol after AGB surgery however.

If gallstones are present preoperatively then some may elect to remove them concomitantly if performing an RYGB or an SG. Because concomitant removal of a gall bladder with an AGB placement may put the band at an increased risk of infection, most will not perform both during the same operation. Instead they prefer a staged approach that would include removing the gall bladder first then placing a band 2–3 weeks later.

If choledocolithiasis occurs after RYGB, then performing ERCP may require either a surgically assisted transgastric approach or use of longer ballooned endoscopes that can reach the ampulla after cannulating the biliopancreatic limb. MRCP can still be used to confirm the diagnosis but an experienced endoscopist must be used to access the common bile duct. If one is not available then transfer to a facility where one is located is reasonable if the patient is stable. If they are not, then surgical common bile duct exploration may be required.

Death

The rate of mortality after WLS has decreased significantly over the past 10 years. Today patients who have had an AGB die about 0.01% of the time and the same rate is seen for SG patients. Meanwhile patients undergoing RYGB have a mortality of about 0.3%. This is down from 2% as recently as 2002. This makes WLS significantly less risky of an operation than colectomy, abdominal aortic aneurysm repair, and coronary artery bypass grafting. There are several risk factors that increase the likelihood of death after WLS, and they are male gender, age greater than 65, and surgeon's inexperience. Additionally some feel that low-volume centers, defined as less than 50 cases per year, have a higher rate of adverse complications.

Roux Y Gastric Bypass

RYGB is still considered the gold standard of WLS and over 100,000 cases are performed annually in the United States. Over the past 20 years, the overall complication and mortality rates have decreased. Today complications occur around 25% of the time but major complications occur only about 5% and the mortality again is 0.3%. Still there are many complications of which general surgeons should be aware. The first four complications should be considered as early possible complications and they usually occur within the first 30 days of an operation.

Leaks

Anastomotic leaks remain the most dreaded complication of RYGB operation. Legal statistics suggest that it is among the most litigious complications after all surgeries. There is no data that suggest a particular technique is superior to another in the prevention of leaks. Currently the leak rate in the United States remains at 1–5%. Simply having a leak does not result in legal retribution but failing to diagnose the leak in a timely manner may end up in such consequences.

The literature, though, does suggest that leaks can result from both patient and surgeon factors. Surgeons who have done fewer than 100 RYGBs have a having a higher leak rate than those who have done more than 100. So perhaps bariatric surgeons who are just starting a practice should work on lower BMI and lower risk patients until they have completed 100 cases. Also there seems to be some benefit to reducing overall complication rates if bariatric surgeons work in higher-volume centers. The Center of Excellence benchmark is for bariatric surgeons to do 50 cases per year.

There are some patient risk factors that significantly increase the chance of a leak. Males have a 33% increased risk of having a leak over females and those patients with a BMI greater than 50 kg/m^2 are 1.4 times more likely to have a leak than those who are less than 50 kg/m^2. Patients who carry a diagnosis of metabolic syndrome are also at an increased risk for leaks.

Of course leaks can still occur without these risk factors and usually there is a technical reason for it. Most leaks occur within the first 30 days after an operation. As mentioned before, no one surgical technique has been proved superior in the prevention of leaks. Additionally surgical glues like fibrin glue and stapler adjuncts such as SeamGuard® (Gore) had not proved to decrease the leak rate in prospective studies though the latter does seem to decrease postoperative bleeding.

In any anastomosis that is created, tissue ischemia is a positive predictor for leaks. This can occur on the gastric pouch side from extensive dissection of the stomach leading to devascularization of the stomach pouch. It can also occur on the roux limb side from its mobilization and division of its mesentery. When dividing the jejunum careful attention should be paid to dividing its associated mesentery perpendicularly to the intestine. If one were to divide the mesentery diagonally along the roux limb, then the tip of the limb's blood supply may be sacrificed. This can be more difficult to recognize laparoscopically (Figs. 28.1a–c and 28.2). If a retrocolic approach is used and the Peterson's defect is closed, then aggressive bites in the mesentery can lead to ischemia in the roux limb. When the gastro-jejuneal anastomosis is created, one should carefully inspect the anastomosis for signs of ischemia and surgeons should not hesitate to revise the anastomosis if they are concerned for ischemia. At the jejuno-jejunal anastomosis tissue ischemia can occur from the same mechanisms described above (Fig. 28.3).

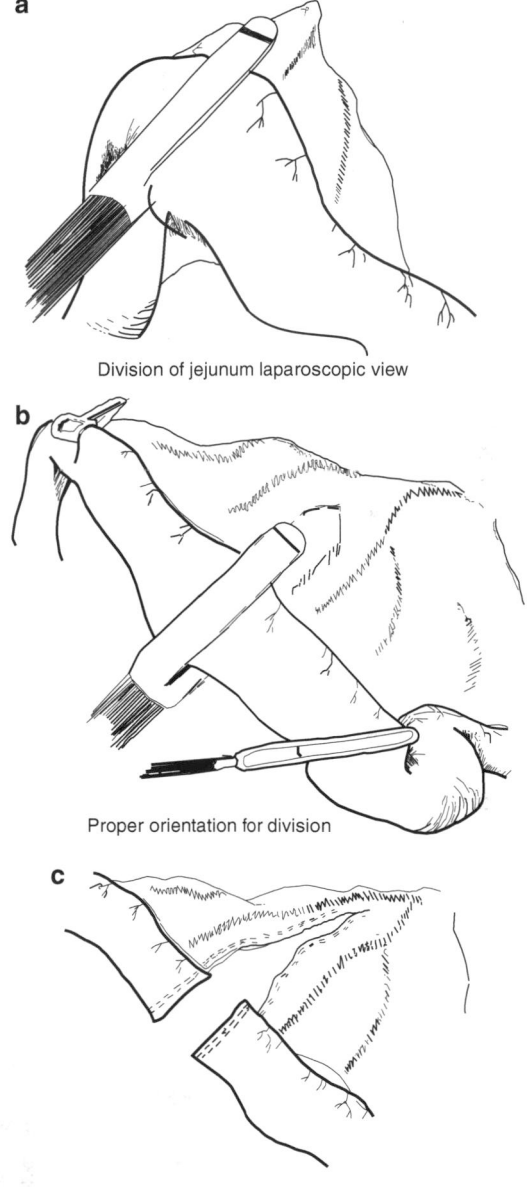

Fig. 28.1. (**a**) Division of jejunum laparoscopic view. (**b**) Proper orientation for divisionc. (**c**) Proper division of jejunum with adequate blood supply.

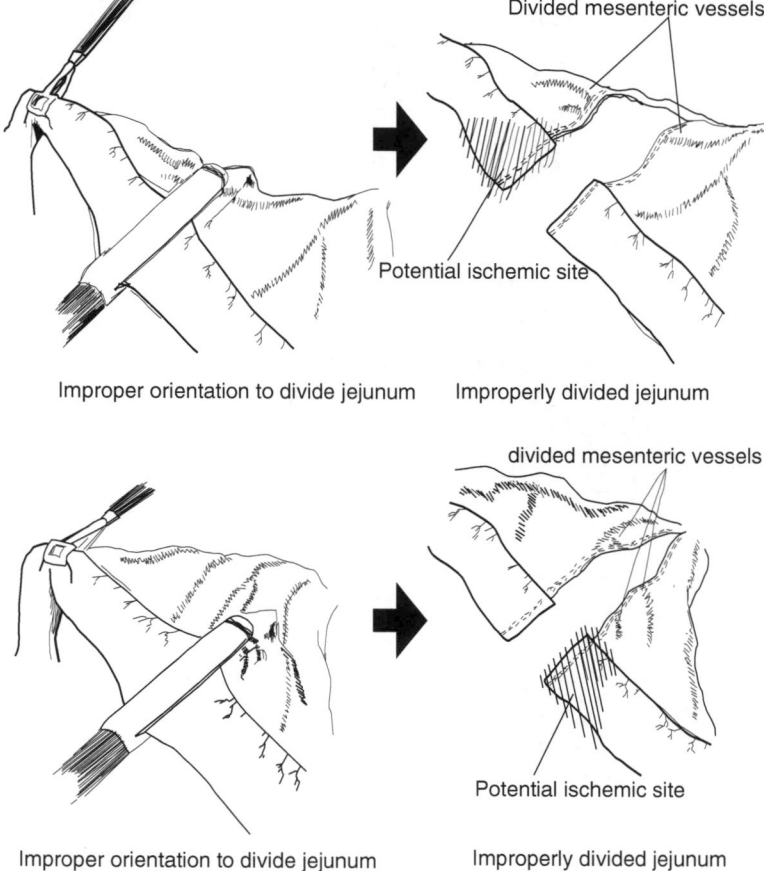

Fig. 28.2. From left to right: Improper orientation to divide jejunum, improperly divided jejunum, improper orientation to divide jejunum, improperly divided jejunum.

Tension is another variable that can negatively affect the incidence of a leak. When mobilizing the roux limb, surgeons must balance mobilization of the roux limb to avoid tension of the gastro-jejunal anastomosis with overly aggressive dissection of the mesentery that may result in ischemia. The shortest route to the gastric pouch is a retrocolic, retrogastric path, but this is technically the most challenging and a time-consuming method, and it has not been compared directly against other methods with regard to complications specifically, leak rate. The antecolic, antegastric

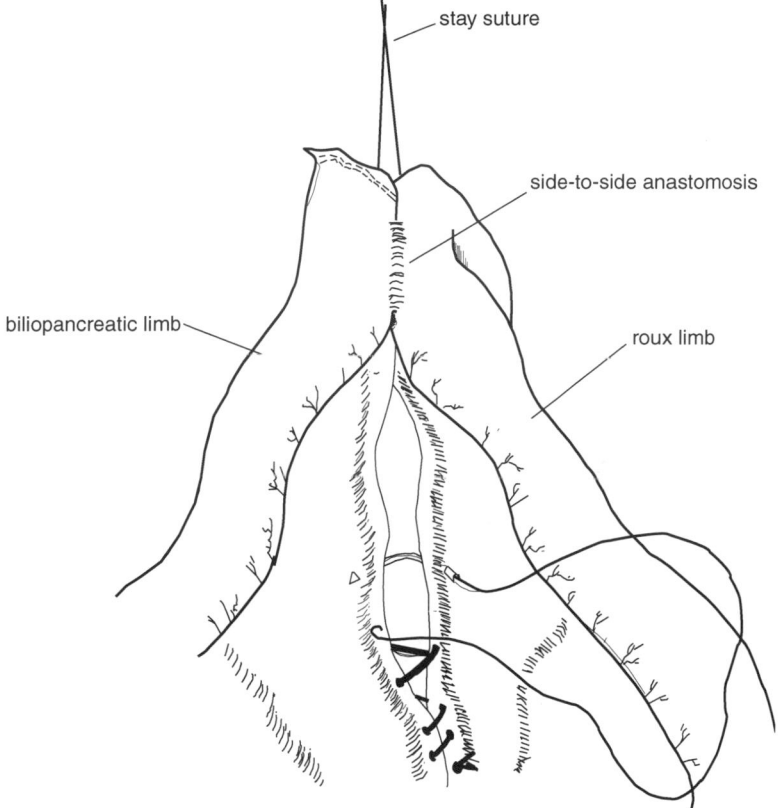

Overaggressive closure of jejunum-jejunumostomy mesenteric defect

Fig. 28.3. Overaggressive closure of the jejunum – jejunumostomy mesenteric defect.

approach is technically easier and may result in fewer internal hernias, but because it has to travel in front of the transverse colon and remnant pouch, it also represents the longest path to the gastric pouch. It, therefore, may have the most tension. Still other surgeons opt for retrocolic, antegastric, or antecolic, retrogastric approaches which may have less tension but still adds some time to the case. Again it is important to note that none of these techniques has been directly compared to one another.

Evaluation for leak should be done intraoperatively. No one method has proven superior to others. Some surgeons opt to use an endoscope and insufflate the anastomosis while it is submerged under saline. An experienced endoscopist should be used to help avoid injury to the newly created anastomosis. Others opt to inject saline, air, or methylene blue via a nasogastric (NGT) or orogastric tube (OGT). Good communication between the surgeon and person passing the NGT/OGT is imperative during this maneuver to avoid injury. The tube should be passed slowly and if resistance is encountered then the tube should be passed only after the surgeon has confirmed the resistance is not due to the tube disrupting the anastomosis or perforating the distal esophagus or gastric pouch. If methylene blue is given via an NGT or OGT, then placing a gauze pad behind the anastomosis before injection can help identify a leak. Some surgeons opt to place a drain near the gastro-jejunal anastomosis so that if a leak is found postoperatively, the drain may control it, but this is not mandatory.

If a leak occurs it can present with many different signs and symptoms. Patients may complain of abdominal pain, nausea, dyspnea, and a feeling of doom. Patients may also present with tachycardia, fevers, respiratory distress, glucose intolerance, and a leukocytosis. The most common sign of a leak is a sustained tachycardia above 120, and the most sensitive signs for a leak are a sustained tachycardia coupled with respiratory distress.

If one suspects a leak and the patient is hemodynamically unstable then surgical exploration is paramount. If a leak is found then one should widely debride the area near the leak, close the leak in two layers avoiding the use of running sutures which may loosen when the edema resolves, place multiple drains, place a nasogastric tube, and consider placement of a G-tube in the gastric remnant. The latter is to help with enteric nutrition delivery and with decompression of the intestinal tract. Since leaks increase the likelihood of other complications, patients should be placed in a monitored setting postoperatively and one should be wary of a systemic inflammatory response.

If the patient is hemodynamically stable, then workup for the patient's symptoms can occur. Specifically if the patient presents only with a sustained tachycardia, then a workup for tachycardia should be implemented. An electrocardiogram and serial cardiac enzymes should be performed to rule out a myocardial infarction. A pulmonary embolism should be ruled out with a computed tomography (CT) angiogram or traditional angiogram. Postoperative bleeding can be ruled out with serial hematocrit testing. Hypovolemia should be treated with volume resuscitation. If fever and leukocytosis are present the sources for infection should be evaluated. Other potential causes for sustained tachycardia include poor pain control, rebound tachycardia, if the patient is chronically on beta-blocker medication, and anxiety, especially if it is present preoperatively. The latter, though, should only be considered as a diagnosis of exclusion.

A leak can be diagnosed with a fluoroscopic swallow study. Here the patient should first swallow a thin contrast-like gastrograffin® to identify a large leak. If none is present then another swallow of a thicker contrast-like barium may help to identify a small leak. If the patient is to undergo a CT scan to rule out a pulmonary embolism then it is reasonable to have a CT scan of the abdomen with oral contrast to rule out the leak. One should have the patient ingest the contrast just prior to the study to evaluate for leak. It is not necessary to wait 3 h for the contrast to reach the colon before performing this exam. A CT scan has the added advantage of identifying a fluid collection that could be an abscess. The reliability of radiologic studies to detect a leak ranges from 40 to 80% meaning a negative study does not necessarily rule out a leak. Moreover, neither method is particularly adept at recognizing a leak at the jejuno-jejunostomy anastomosis.

Because of the unreliability of radiologic studies, patients, who sustain a tachycardia greater than 120 beats/min, and have no other obvious cause for their tachycardia, should be considered for urgent surgical exploration. Operation should be considered even if the patient appears good clinically and is otherwise feeling well. This is a very important concept to embrace for several reasons. One is that the longer a leak persists, the sicker the patients can become and the more difficult it may be to repair the leak. Leaks can increase the rate of all other RYGB complications. Mortality alone can increase by 35%. One of the main reasons surgeons are successfully sued after RYGB is because of failure to diagnose and treat a leak in an appropriate manner. A negative exploration is much less damaging to the patient and the physician than a leak that is allowed to persist.

If the decision to return to the operating room is made, the exploration can be done laparoscopically but this depends on the surgeon's comfort level. Sometimes small leaks can be hard to find. One should consider use of intraoperative endoscopy, insufflation, or methylene blue administered through an NGT to locate the leak. If a leak is found then the previously mentioned steps for treating a leak should be done. Use of sealants such as fibrin glue has not proven to be beneficial in this setting. If the exact leak cannot be found or if the tissue is too poor to hold a repair, then wide local debridement, placement of multiple drains, placement of a nasogastric tube, and postoperative nutrition supplementation can control the leak and eventually stop it altogether. Again the use of a G-tube in the remnant stomach to boost nutrition via enteric means can be very beneficial in this setting.

This is also a role for nonoperative management of a leak. If the patient remains hemodynamically stable and a small leak is identified radiographically but is controlled by a drain placed at the time of the initial operation, then this may be enough to prevent the sequelae of a leak. These patients should be monitored for hemodynamic instability and a worsening clinical picture that may prompt an operation. Again nutrition should be supplemented but with no G-tube, one must rely on total parenteral nutrition and the patient should be kept nothing per os (NPO). A swallow study or abdominal CT scan with oral contrast can be repeated to determine if the leak is still present. If not then the resumption of an oral diet can begin.

Bleeding

Surgical bleeding occurs up to 5% of the time after RYGB as is probably due in part to the routine use of anti-coagulation before and after the operation. Most of the bleeding occurs from staple lines, and it can occur extra- as well as intraluminally. As such patients may present with melena, hematochezia, or hematemesis. There is some data that suggest that the use of staple line adjuncts such as fibrin glue, the Duet staple, or seamguard helps reduce the incidence of bleeding but there is no data that suggest it is the standard of care. It is important to note that the stomach tissue can be thick so that use of at least a 3.5-mm size staple is probably safer. Most bleeding can be treated nonoperatively if the patient remains hemodynamically stable with the stoppage of anticoagulation, the avoidance of antiplatelet medication, correction of any coagulopathy, and transfusion of packed red blood cells. Those who do not respond to this therapy or who become stable require a surgical exploration that may also include endoscopy. In general an operation need not be delayed to localize the source of bleeding with angiography or tagged red blood cell scans.

Early Bowel Obstruction

Bowel obstructions that occur within the first 30 days after an RYGB procedure are typically the result of a technical error like failure to close a mesomesenteric defect. For those surgeons who place their patients' roux limbs retrogastrically, this can also occur at the transverse mesocolon defect and the Peterson's defect, the mesomesenteric defect between the roux limb and the transverse mesocolon. Patients with a bowel obstruction soon after an RYGB present a unique challenge because most providers would be reluctant to pass an NGT for fear of disrupting a relatively new gastro-jejunostomy anastomosis. One could consider using fluoroscopy to help facilitate this. More importantly, however, is that bowel obstructions that occur this early may be more likely to result in a small bowel resection. So if a bowel obstruction is suspected, surgeons may need to have a lower threshold for proceeding to the operating room.

Stenosis

A clinically significant stenosis can occur in up to 20% of patients and is defined as a gastro-jejuneal anastomosis that is less than 9 mm in diameter. Most patients cannot swallow solid foods at this diameter and trying to force more food down may result in swelling around the anastomosis such that even liquids cannot pass. This complication seems to occur more often with the end-to-end circular stapler technique, especially if a 21-mm stapler size is used. Weight loss does not seem to be adversely affected with use of a 25-mm stapler and the incidence of stenosis appears to be less.

The initial treatment for stenoses is endoscopic balloon dilation and fortunately this is successful in almost all patients, though they may require multiple dilations. Experienced endoscopists should do this procedure because overly aggressive dilation may result in perforation. Moreover failed dilation attempts may make it more difficult to perform subsequent procedures. Patients who present with a stenosis can be stabilized with IV fluid hydration and replacement of nutrients. Transfer to an experienced endoscopist can then be arranged. It is rare to need a surgical revision for a stenosis. Stenoses can also occur at the jejuno-jejunostomy anastomosis and these usually require surgical revision.

The following complications should be considered as long-term complications and as such they can occur at any time in the postoperative period. It is one reason why patients, who undergo surgical weight loss procedures, should be followed for the rest of their lives.

Marginal Ulcers

Marginal ulceration occurs in up to 5% of RYGBs and evidence of it can be seen within the first few weeks after an operation. Consequently some surgeons routinely place their patients on ulcer prophylaxis for 30 days after their operation. Such ulcers though can occur anytime after RYGB. The risk factors for development later on are smoking, *helicobacter pylori* infection, use of NSAID medication, and the use of permanent materials like silk when performing the anastomosis. Some surgeons recommend routine screening for *h. pylori* preoperatively so that infections can be treated prior to an operation. Others believe that even patients treated for *h. pylori* are at increased risk for marginal ulceration. Patients will typically present with epigastric pain but can also complain of melena, hematemesis, and poor PO tolerance.

Most ulcerations can be treated with a course of proton pump inhibitors and a repeat endoscopy demonstrating a healed ulcer is probably wise. Fifteen percent of ulcers are associated with a gastro-gastric fistula. Here, the stomach acid from the remnant stomach can travel to the gastric pouch and irritate the anastomosis. If a fistula is seen, then the patient should have a revision of their gastric pouch. Patients who present acutely with a perforation or peritonitis should have a revision of their pouch and their gastro-jejuneal anastomosis. Simply placing a Graham patch repair will not treat the underlying fistula.

If an ulcer is suspected in the remnant stomach or the duodenum, then identifying it would require special endoscopic techniques. These areas could be seen with a long double balloon endoscope traveling down the roux limb then retrograde up the biliopancreatic limb. Another option would be to perform a laparoscopically assisted transgastric endoscopy. If a patient presents acutely and an ulcer is found in these areas then a Graham patch can be done or if a more sinister underlying disease is suspected then a resection can be performed.

Late Bowel Obstruction/Internal Hernias

Late bowel obstructions can occur from internal herniation or from adhesive disease and ventral herniation. As such they can present like a typical small bowel obstruction with nausea, bloating, vomiting, and failure to pass flatus. These bowel obstructions can be treated with NGT decompression, IV fluid resuscitation, and NPO status. Placement of the NGT may require fluoroscopic guidance. If patients do not improve with this management or present acutely then surgical exploration should occur. One should be try to ascertain the pathway of the roux limb during the exploration, which should help them identify the potential internal hernia defects.

Patients with an internal hernia may present with chronic intermittent abdominal pain. CT scans and swallow studies may or may not identify an internal hernia. If one is seen on these films then surgical exploration should be scheduled sooner than later. If one is not seen on radiologic studies, then surgical exploration should be considered especially if no other cause of the abdominal pain can be determined after extensive workup.

Late bowel obstructions can also be caused by intussusceptions, which can travel in antegrade and retrograde fashion. They typically occur after patients have lost more than 90% of their excess weight but the exact mechanism is unknown. If the intussusception involves the jejuno-jejunostomy anastomosis then a revision of this anastomosis should be done.

Weight Regain

Significant weight regain after RYGB occurs for one of two main reasons. The first is behavioral and is due to poor diet and exercise after the surgery. Since the malabsorption effects last for about 2 years, patients who do not adjust their lifestyle permanently will be able to regain weight. The second main reason is one of several surgical etiologies. The reasons that are amenable to surgical correction are pouch dilation, too large of an initial pouch, gastro-gastric fistula, and too short of a bypass. An upper GI series can help to identify an enlarged pouch and a fistula. Revisional bariatric surgery, though, should probably only be done by experienced bariatric surgeons.

Adjustable Gastric Banding

AGB is also a very popular operation because it is easier to perform and the risk of death is significantly less than that of the RYGB at 1/1,000. The overall complication rate though can be as high as 40%. AGBs work solely by restriction but a properly adjusted band may also improve satiety.

Acute Stromal Obstruction

ASO can occur from bleeding from the proximal stomach that occurs during placement of the band. This results in the inability to swallow within the first few days after the procedure. If this occurs, patients will be unable to swallow even liquids. Dissection of the esophageal fat pad during the initial operation has been shown to decrease the incidence of this.

Band Slippage/Gastric Prolapse

Gastric prolapse occurs when the stomach migrates upward creating a large pouch. Band slippage is defined as when the band changes position such that it no longer offers restriction. If these occur, the patient will complain of a lack of restriction but may also suffer from heartburn and regurgitation. It can be demonstrated by an upper GI series that can show the band in a migrated position or a large pouch above the band. When these occur the band should be removed and a new one can be positioned appropriately. Identifying and concomitantly repairing hiatal hernias, the use of the pars flaccida technique and imbrication of the stomach over the band at the initial operation has greatly reduced the incidence of band and stomach migration.

Band Erosion

The documented rate of band erosion into the stomach is 1%, but it may be underreported. Patients can present with pain, hematemesis, and melena. They may also experience a lack of restriction. It can be diagnosed with a swallow study or upper endoscopy. It requires removal that can be done surgically, but there are increasing reports of the band being removed endoscopically.

Port Complications

(a)   *Flips.* Very simply the access port that sits beneath the skin can flip over such that it cannot be accessed. This can occur because of a poorly positioned port and the surgeon must take into consideration where the port is placed. If it is located where a skin fold occurs when the patient is in a sitting position, this may put undue pressure on the band causing it to flip. Patients should avoid dramatic movements of their abdomen and potentially traumatic injuries to their abdomen at least until the port is well incorporated because these events may cause a flip. A reoperation to correct the flip is necessary.

(b) *Leaks.* Leaks can occur at the port for one of two reasons. Only a Huber needle should be used to attempt fills and unfills of the band. If a regular needle is used to access, it will leave too wide a hole for the port to seal thus causing a leak. The second occurs if an inexperienced clinician tries to access the band and instead injures the band's tubing. For this reason, some clinicians prefer to use fluoroscopic guidance when performing a fill. A leak is suspected if there is significantly less fluid withdrawn from the band than expected. It can be proven by injecting radiopaque dye into the band under fluoroscopy that can help identify the location of the leak. Again if a leak is identified then an operation is necessary to replace the part where the leak is located.

(c) *Infection.* Infections at the level of the port are a significant complication because it may mean there is an erosion at the level of the band. If there are signs of infection over the port that has been in place for several months, then an erosion must be ruled out. If the erythema is seen within a few days after the operation, then it could be a surgical site infection instead and the patient should be admitted for intravenous antibiotics. If the infection does not clear within a short amount of time, then the entire band should probably be removed.

Gastric Pouch/Esophageal Dilatation

Gastric Pouch and Esophageal Dilatation are ill-defined entities. Patients will complain of a lack of satiety and decreased restriction due to increased reservoirs but they will also complain of regurgitation, reflux, and the feeling the food is stuck in their stomach and lower esophagus. An upper GI series can show the enlargement of the esophagus and the gastric pouch above the band. It may be confused with gastric prolapse but here the band will be in good position. It is believed that this complication occurs because of eating too much too often and this results in slow dilation over time. Patients should be reminded of proper portion sizes and proper eating and chewing habits. When these complications are seen, all the fluid from the band should be removed for a few months to give the pouch and esophagus a chance to "relax." Patients should be warned that they will likely gain weight but follow-up with a registered dietitian can blunt this. When their symptoms have resolved then the band can be slowly filled again.

Weight Regain/Inadequate Weight Loss

Similar to RYGB the most common reason people regain weight after an AGB is poor dietary and exercise habits. It is more imperative for AGB patients to comply with a good diet and exercise plan because the band only offers restriction. If patients do not limit their fat, caloric, and carbohydrate intake then their weight loss is likely to be minimal. Moreover, foods such as ice cream and desserts will not be restricted by the band and instead will slide right past it. In addition, if they do not exercise regularly, their overall weight loss is likely to be less. Every attempt should be made at proper education and reinforcement of these aspects of weight loss before revision surgery is considered. To that end, follow-up with a psychologist is also recommended to determine if the patient has an Axis I or II disorder that is preventing them from complying.

Some patients, however, will not have a psychiatric disorder that is contributing to their poor ability to comply rather they just cannot adjust to the band or are not motivated enough to use the band properly. These patients should be considered for revision surgery and most likely that will require a conversion to a Sleeve Gastrectomy or an RYGB. A surgeon who has experience with revision bariatric surgery should probably do this.

Sleeve Gastrectomy

The sleeve gastretctomy (SG) is fast becoming a very popular operation because it is significantly easier to perform than the RYGB, and it does not require as much patient compliance like the AGB. The most comprehensive data suggest that the resulting weight loss is about 50–65% after 2–5 years and the incidence of death is similar to that of the AGB at 1 in 1,000 patients. But it remains to be seen what will happen to SG patients in the long-term as the original intent of the operation was for it to be the first part of a two phased operation. Many patients are electing not to undergo the second phase because they are satisfied with the amount of weight they have lost. As of 2009, the American Society of Metabolic and Bariatric Surgeons has not advocated it as a first-line therapy for surgical weight loss though it does recognize its effectiveness.

Leaks

SGs are created by removing the greater curvature side of the stomach and subsequently creating a 150–200 cc pouch that does not readily distend. Typically the resection is done with a stapler and leaks can occur at this staple line. Staple line reinforces have not been shown to decrease the leak rate but have shown to decrease postoperative bleeding. The leak rate is around 1.4% and may be caused by the increased pressure in the stomach pouch because without the greater curve it cannot distend. Most leaks seem to occur near the angle of His where the stomach tissue is thinner. One should consider using a smaller staple height here to help prevent a leak. If one is using a staple line reinforcer, they should be cognizant of the resultant staple height with the use of this reinforcer as the later may make not allow some of the shorter staple heights to fully close the tissue.

The suspected leak can be evaluated in the same manner as suspected leaks after an RYGB. There are two ways to treat leaks: operatively and endoscopically. Some advocate stent placement endoscopically which again should be done by an experienced endoscopist. If one is not available or if the patient is unstable then surgical intervention is necessary. The leak can be identified and treated in a similar fashion to a leak after an RYGB with the exception of a G-tube placement. One should probably consider a J-tube placement for enteric feeding, though, if the extent of inflammation is great or the patient is not doing well clinically.

Bleeding

Surgical bleeding occurs mostly due to the extensive dissection of the stomach because of its rich blood supply and thicker tissue especially in the distal half of the stomach. Because of this, most bariatric surgeons will reinforce the staple line by oversewing the staple line, applying glue, or buttressing the staples. One must avoid being too aggressive with oversewing the staple line as this may result in narrowing of the stomach pouch. The incidence of bleeding is as high as 6.4%.

Narrowing/Stenosis

This phenomenon can occur if too small of a gastric pouch is made. Most bariatric surgeons advocate using at least a 36 *fr* bougie to create the pouch to avoid this but as little as 32 *fr* has been published. If the stomach is dissected free from its lesser curvature attachments, it may tend to corkscrew, which can prevent oral intake. Narrowing can also occur if oversewing of the staple line is too aggressive. The initial treatment for this is endoscopic balloon dilatation but if this fails then the SG should be considered for a revisional procedure.

Gastric Emptying Abnormalities

There is some controversy when performing an SG as to how much antrum to leave behind. If one were to leave too little then the patient would likely experience dumping and if too much is left behind then the patient may have delayed emptying and subsequent pouch dilatation. Whether the latter causes a significant clinical problem is unknown.

Most surgeons who perform an SG will leave around 5–7 cm of antrum behind and perform the gastrectomy over at least a 36 *fr* bougie. It is important to note this is neither universal nor has it been compared against other lengths and sizes in a randomized controlled study. If there is a significant clinical problem with dumping or delayed emptying then the patient should be considered for a revision surgery with possible conversion to an RYGB or a biliopancreatic diversion with a duodenal switch.

Conclusions

Bariatric surgery is very common in today's surgical world and many patients travel far from their homes to have the surgery. As a result when complications arise, they often seek relief at the nearest emergency room or care provider instead of their bariatric surgeon. Consequently most general surgeons will likely be consulted and asked to initially manage these patients. It is imperative then that general surgeons be familiar with the possible complications of all bariatric procedures. We also know now that these patients require lifelong follow-up and should be followed by a multidisciplinary team, which includes at least a bariatric surgeon, a registered dietitian, and a mental health care provider.

Selected Readings

1. Blackburn GL, Hutter MM, Harvey AM, Apovian CM, Boulton HR, Cummings S, et al. Expert panel on weight loss surgery: executive report update. Obesity. 2009;17:842–62.
2. Buchwald H, Estok R, Fahrbach K, Banel D, Sledge I. Trends in mortality in bariatric surgery: a systematic review and meta-analysis. Surgery. 2007;142:621–32.
3. Encinosa WE, Bernard DM, Du D, Steiner CA. Recent improvements in bariatric surgery outcomes. Med Care. 2009;47:531–5.
4. Longitudinal assessment of bariatric surgery (LABS) consortium, Flum DR, Belle SH, King WC, Wahed AS, Berk P, et al. Perioperative safety in the longitudinal assessment of bariatric surgery. N Engl J Med. 2009;361:445–54.
5. Jones SB, Jones DB, editors. Obesity surgery: patient safety and best practices. Woodbury, CT: Cine-Med; 2009.
6. Kelly J, Tarnoff M, Shikora S, Thayer B, Jones DB, Forse RA, et al. Best practice recommendations for surgical care in weight loss surgery. Obes Res. 2005;13:227–33.
7. Lehman Center Weight Loss Surgery Expert Panel. Expert panel on weight loss surgery. Obes Res. 2005;13:206–26.
8. Lim RB, Blackburn GL, Jones DB. Benchmarking best practices in weight loss surgery. Curr Probl Surg. 2010;47(2):69–176.
9. Moy J, Pomp A, Dakin G, Parikh M, Gagner M. Laparoscopic sleeve gastrectomy for morbid obesity. Am J Surg. 2008;196:e56–9.
10. Rosenthal R, Jones DB. Weight loss surgery: a multidisciplinary approach. Edgemont, PA: Matrix Medical Communications; 2008.

29. Complications in Colorectal Surgery

Kimberly A. Matzie and Steven D. Wexner

Introduction

All major abdominal surgeries and especially bowel resection surgeries are fraught with the same potential complications as colorectal surgeries. Common complications of abdominal operations include inadvertent enterotomy, enterocutaneous fistula, small bowel obstruction, surgical site infection, and other postoperative infections, and these are not the focus of this chapter. Complications specific to laparoscopy and endoscopy are addressed in other chapters in this manual.

This chapter focuses on several specific complications of highest concern to the colorectal surgeon: anastomotic complications, presacral bleeding, splenic injury, and ureteric injury. We do not discuss complications of anorectal surgery, or perineal or stoma complications.

Anastomotic Complications

Anastomotic complications can be the bane of a colorectal surgery practice, and they are most thoroughly discussed with the patient during the preoperative informed consent process. Part of the frustration is that even the most experienced and technically precise surgeons cannot always predict who will have an anastomotic leak. An anastomosis may appear perfect in the operating room, with excellent blood supply and no tension, and the patient could be septic from anastomotic breakdown a week later. This problem can necessitate emergency reoperation and its adverse sequelae, while more contained leaks may require drains and prolonged fecal diversion.

D.S. Tichansky, J. Morton, and D.B. Jones (eds.), *The SAGES Manual of Quality, Outcomes and Patient Safety*, DOI 10.1007/978-1-4419-7901-8_29, © Springer Science+Business Media, LLC 2012

1. Avoiding Anastomotic Complications: Both patient-related factors and technical factors may contribute to poor anastomotic healing.

    (a) *Surgeon factors*: The surgeon has control of the operative technique to ensure good blood supply of the bowel ends for the anastomosis, lack of tension, and adequate stapler function. The proximal bowel end or marginal artery should be checked for pulsatile bleeding prior to creating an anastomosis. For any colorectal anastomosis, several maneuvers are recommended to ensure the anastomosis is tension-free. These steps include division of the lateral attachments of the descending colon to medialize the colon, full mobilization of the splenic flexure with separation of the omentum from the transverse colon, and high ligation of the inferior mesenteric artery and inferior mesenteric vein. Typically good blood supply can be maintained through a preserved marginal artery even if the mesocolon is divided at its base up to the middle colic artery. If the bowel end does not demonstrate good blood flow, further colon resection must be performed until pulsatile flow is observed. Rarely, this maneuver requires resecting significantly more colon than was planned, or even performing an ileorectal anastomosis based on the ileocolic artery for blood supply.

    (b) *Patient factors*: Most patient conditions at the time of surgery are not under surgeon control, but surgeons can alter the operative approach and sometimes the timing of surgery. Malnutrition, immunosuppression, morbid obesity, local or systemic sepsis, and prior radiation are known to compromise patient healing or make abdominal and pelvic surgery more technically demanding. When operating on patients with these issues, the surgeon may choose to perform an end stoma and not a primary anastomosis at all, or may choose to create a diverting stoma to protect the anastomosis. Several months later when the patients are healthier, their intestinal continuity can be more safely restored.

2. Anastomotic Leak.

    (a) *Leak Rates*: The rate of anastomotic leak increases, even with optimal intraoperative circumstances, as the anastomosis is more distal along the bowel. Small bowel enteroenterostomies have the lowest incidence of leak, ileocolic anastomoses have reported leak rates of 1–3%, and coloanal anastomoses have reported leak rates of 10–20%. Low anterior resections are widely reported to have leak rates from 2 to 26%, as shown in Table 29.1. Ileal pouch–anal anastomosis after restorative proctocolectomy also has a high incidence of anastomotic leak. Some of the disparity in leak rates is because of widely varied definitions of anastomotic leak reported in the literature.

(b) *Risk Factors*: The only factors that have consistently borne out in nearly all studies as risk factors for anastomotic leak are a low pelvic anastomosis and male gender. When a total mesorectal excision (TME) is performed, there is potentially less bulk of tissue and poorer blood supply, creating an environment where an anastomotic dehiscence may not be contained or seal as easily as when more rectum and mesorectum remain in the pelvis. The male pelvis is typically longer and narrower than the female pelvis, making pelvic surgery technically more difficult in men. Proximal fecal diversion, most commonly with a diverting loop ileostomy, significantly decreases the clinical signs and symptoms of anastomotic leak and urgent reoperations for low anterior resection. While several authors have reported that a diverting ostomy also reduces morbidity and mortality, a recent Cochrane review did not come to that conclusion.

A myriad of retrospective studies have been written about anastomotic leak. Risk factors for leak from some of these studies include adverse intraoperative events, surgeon experience, preoperative radiation, ASA score greater than 2, obesity, smoking, use of sigmoid for the anastomosis, and use of transanal drains. Factors in some studies that protect against leak are mobilization of the splenic flexure and colonic j-pouch reconstruction. Factors that do not seem to affect anastomotic leak rate are type of anastomosis (hand-sewn vs. stapled), method of surgery (open vs. laparoscopic), bowel preparation, pelvic drain use, and tumor stage.

(c) *Leak testing*: During the operation, intraoperative leak testing is recommended to assess the anastomotic integrity. This goal can be accomplished by instilling air via a

Table 29.1. Published incidence of anastomotic leak following colorectal surgery.

Author	Year	No. of patients	No. of leaks	Percent	Comments/case mix
Vignali A, Fazio V et al. (Cleveland clinic series)	1997	1,014	29	2.9	7.7% leak <7 cm from anal verge; 1% leak more proximal
Cochrane review stapled vs. hand-sewn colorectal anastomosis (9 RCT studies)	2001	1,233 (9 studies) 825 (6 studies)	83 63	6.7 7.6	Clinical leak: 6.3% circular stapler, 7.1% hand-sewn Radiologic leak: 7.8% stapled, 7.2% hand-sewn
Colorectal cancer lap vs. open (CLASIC trial)	2005	794	48	6.0	Anastomotic dehiscence: colon cancer: 3.1%, rectal cancer: 9.2%
Colon cancer laparoscopic or open resection (COLOR trial)	2005	1,082	25	2.3	Anastomotic failure right, left, and sigmoid colectomy: open: 2.8%, laparoscopic: 1.8%
Tan WS et al. (meta-analysis LAR, non-RCT studies)	2009	10,157	1,212	11.9	Clinical leak: 13.9% without stoma, 9.3% with stoma
Cochrane review diverting ostomy LAR (6 RCT studies)	2010	648	83	12.8	Clinical leak: 19.6% without stoma, 6.3% with stoma

syringe, proctoscope, or flexible sigmoidoscope while the pelvis is filled with saline or water, or by instilling fluid such as dilute betadine in an empty pelvis. The surgeon occludes the proximal bowel and observes for air bubbles or fluid extravasation, respectively, which would indicate a leak is present. If a leak is identified, additional sutures may be applied to the unsealed area, a diverting stoma can be fashioned, and/or the anastomosis may be redone. There are some advantages to routine intraoperative endoscopic air testing rather than blind syringe air testing, specifically in addition to anastomotic air leak discovery, anastomotic bleeding, perianastomotic mucosal ischemia, and additional perianastomotic pathology can be identified and addressed. It is also recommended to examine the donuts of the circular stapler after firing, though complete donuts to not ensure a perfect anastomosis. Many groups recommend routine diverting ileostomy for any anastomosis less than 6 or 7 cm from the anal verge with TME, when there are any suboptimal patient factors, when the operation is difficult or there are any intraoperative complications. Other groups prefer more selective fecal diversion, citing the associated morbidity of stomas and stoma reversal surgery.

3. *Management of anastomotic leak*: Management of a leak depends on patient presentation. Clearly the patients with peritonitis or stool emanating through their incisions must urgently return to the operating room. Usually either a Hartmann with end stoma or a diverting stoma and drainage are needed, depending on the degree of anastomotic disruption and fecal contamination. More contained leaks may present as pyrexia, leukocytosis, diarrhea, ileus, vague pelvic pain, or generalized failure to thrive. Diagnosis can be confirmed with a CT scan with triple contrast or a water-soluble contrast enema. Clinically stable patients with localized leaks who present with the above symptoms and rectal drainage, a presacral sinus, or a presacral abscess can usually be managed with a combination of interventional radiology drains, antibiotics, local perineal procedures, and time. Anastomotic leaks may also present as enterocutaneous, colocutaneous, vaginal, or perineal fistula. Some of these patients will ultimately require temporary parenteral nutrition or fecal diversion to aid healing. When a leak is radiologically diagnosed prior to stoma closure and the

patient has no clinical signs or symptoms, then the anastomosis will often seal over time. It is recommended to repeat the water-soluble contrast enema after waiting an additional 1–3 months to assess for healing prior to stoma closure.

4. *Outcome after anastomotic leak*: Some data support that short-term mortality, long-term mortality, and local cancer recurrence are all higher for rectal cancer patients who have had an anastomotic leak and pelvic sepsis. Initial hospitalization is prolonged. In addition, a high proportion of stomas do not get reversed after patients have suffered an anastomotic leak. The long-term sequelae of a leak may include stricture or pelvic fibrosis, with subsequent poor bowel function and quality of life as a result of decreased compliance of the neorectum. This functional impairment may be similar after both clinical and subclinical (radiographic) leaks.

5. *Anastomotic Bleeding*: Many patients will have some degree of anastomotic bleeding after colorectal surgery, and it is very common for the patient's first few bowel movements to be mixed with or primarily dark blood. Even when more severe, bright bleeding occurs, as it does in up to 5% of patients, the majority of such bleeding will spontaneously stop, as illustrated in Table 29.2.

   (a) *Intraoperative management*: Intraoperatively, side-to-side anastomoses should be examined for bleeding prior to closure of the common enterotomy. Bleeding may be more frequent with the thicker linear staples, and when observed it is usually on the staple line closer to the mesentery. Bleeding sites should be controlled with interrupted sutures. Circular staple lines may be observed with a proctoscope or flexible sigmoidoscope after the anastomosis at the same time as leak testing. Sutures may be placed from the abdomen under direct vision to stop bleeding from a circular staple line. To help prevent anastomotic bleeding, the surgeon must ensure that the mesentery is not included in any of the staples lines.

   (b) *Postoperative management*: When severe bleeding is postoperatively diagnosed by multiple bright red bowel movements, a drop in hemoglobin, and/or hemodynamic instability because of hypovolemia, the patient should be transferred to a monitored setting. Intravenous fluid should be administered, serial hemoglobin and coagulation

Table 29.2. Published incidence of severe anastomotic bleeding following colorectal surgery.

Author	Year	No. of patients	No. of severe bleeding	Percent	Comments/case mix
Malik AH et al.	2008	777	6	0.8	Stapled colorectal anastomosis: 3 return to OR, 3 endoscopic
Cochrane review stapled vs. hand-sewn colorectal anastomosis	2001	662	28	4.2	5.4% Stapled; 3.1% hand-sewn (no comment on intervention)
Ishihara S et al.	2008	73	7	9.6	Bleeding identified via intraoperative colonoscopy. No postoperative bleeding events
Martinez-Serrano MA et al.	2009	1,389	7	0.5	All colorectal cases. Six managed endoscopically, 1 returned to OR

parameters monitored, and blood transfusions given if needed. Severe bleeding usually manifests within 24 h of surgery. Multiple nonoperative methods have been successful in recent years when bleeding is severe enough to require intervention. Endoscopic methods to control bleeding range from simple saline irrigation or dilute epinephrine irrigation, to adrenaline injection, cautery, and endoscopic clip application. Bleeding from proximal anastomoses that are not amenable to endoscopic control may need to be embolized or controlled with selective vasopressin via angiography in very rare instances. Conversely, very distal anastomotic bleeding may be controlled by perianal sutures or rectal packing. Bleeding will usually cease with the correction of any coagulopathy, supportive care, and time, and there are rarely any long-term sequelae for the patient. If the bleeding is such that continued transfusion is needed and/or an endoscopic view cannot be obtained, the option of last resort is to return to the operating room for re-exploration; at this point anastomotic revision will likely be required.

6. *Anastomotic Stenosis*: Anastomotic stricture commonly manifests several months after surgery, and may be clinically suspected when patients complain of obstructive symptoms including constipation, incomplete evacuation, decreased stool caliber, bloating, or pain. Stenosis is more common following colorectal, coloanal, and ileoanal anastomoses than after other colonic or small bowel resections in the absence of Crohn's disease. The incidence of infra-peritoneal anastomotic stricture is higher for stapled anastomoses than for hand-sewn anastomoses (Table 29.3). It was thought that larger circular staplers would cause less anastomosis stenosis, but this is not supported by high-quality studies. Though unpredictable, stenosis may be because of a suboptimal anastomosis with ischemia, a leak, or because of inflammation or radiation. Anastomotic stricture is usually defined in the literature as the inability to pass either a 19-mm proctoscope or 12-mm flexible scope, though it is only of clinical significance if the patient presents with obstructive symptoms. Most strictures are diagnosed during surveillance endoscopy after cancer resections, and several studies agree that the diameter of the anastomosis does not correlate with clinical symptoms of a stricture. Most of

Table 29.3. Published incidence of anastomotic stricture following colorectal surgery.

Author	Year	No. of patients	No. of strictures	Percent	Comments/case mix
Griffen FD et al. (review 10 series 1983–1990)	1990	1,483	25	1.7	Double stapled colorectal: stenosis requiring intervention
Cochrane review stapled vs. hand-sewn colorectal anastomosis (9 RCT studies)	2001	1,042 (7 studies)	50	4.3	Circular stapler: 8.0%, hand-sewn: 2.0% (no comment on intervention)
Bannura GC et al.	2004	179	8	4.4	Could not pass flexible scope. 5/8 patients needed intervention because of symptoms
Amrosetti P et al.	2008	68	12	17.6	Laparoscopic sigmoidectomy for diverticular disease

these narrowings are asymptomatic and improve with time if monitored by serial endoscopy. Many patients with distal anastomoses and proximal diversion will develop some degree of stricture while diverted. These strictures are usually soft and easily dilated with the examiner's finger. Accordingly, the surgeon should routinely examine all low anastomoses for healing and perform any dilation as necessary in clinic and in the operating room at the time of stoma reversal.

If the patient complains of symptoms that might be attributable to stenosis, the diagnosis can be made with a contrast enema or endoscopy. If an anastomotic stricture develops after a resection for malignancy, biopsies should be performed to exclude local recurrence. For symptomatic stenosis, dilation will often be successful. For coloanal or distal colorectal anastomoses, dilators of increasing sizes may be attempted. For most more proximal anastomoses, endoscopic methods of laser or argon plasma coagulation and/or hydrostatic balloon dilatation should be attempted. Outcome with these maneuvers may be more successful in patients whose resections were performed for benign conditions as opposed to malignancy. The most common complication of endoscopic dilation is restenosis. For failure of initial endoscopic measures, other more advanced techniques have been used in case series such as transanal stricturoplasty, endoscopic stricturoplasty, endoscopic resection of the stricture, or self-expanding metallic stents. Periodic biopsies should be obtained for restenosis in patients after cancer resection. Short strictures are likely more amenable to endoscopic treatment, while longer fibrotic strictures may require surgical revision. If possible upon operative re-exploration, the circular stapler anvil can be placed into the proximal lumen via an enterotomy and the circular stapler used to excise the stenosis. This type of approach will not be possible if significant pelvic scarring is present, often making these reoperations for anastomotic stricture technically demanding.

Presacral Bleeding

Pelvic bleeding most commonly occurs during proctectomy, from injury to branches of the internal iliac vessels or the presacral venous plexus. When the presacral fascia is entered, veins can be easily torn as they are anchored to the periostium of the sacrum. The surgeon must remain just posterior to the mesorectum, in the areolar tissue of the "holy plane," while dissecting the presacral space to avoid violating the presacral fascia. This should be accomplished with sharp bovie or scissor dissection and not blunt hand dissection. While massive hemorrhage is rare, it can be devastating when it occurs and significantly increase morbidity and mortality. One type of presacral bleeding can be stopped with suturing, but the torn basivertebral veins that drain the spinal column connect to the internal vertebral venous system and are extremely difficult to control.

Initially the surgeon should pack the pelvis with laparotomy sponges, inform the anesthesiologist that significant bleeding will occur, and have blood products in the operating room. Lithotomy position increases the hydrostatic pressure of the presacral plexus, so the patient's legs should be flattened and the patient taken out of Trendelenburg position. After the patient is resuscitated, the bleeding needs to be controlled. If bleeding originates from vessels of the venous plexus traveling through the sacrum at S3 to S5, attempts at suture ligation and coagulation may only make the bleeding worse. If the bleeding can be stopped with direct finger pressure, sterile thumbtacks or occluder pins can be pushed into the sacrum with the pin at a right angle to the sacrum, directly over the bleeding. If this maneuver fails, the rectus abdominus muscle may be employed in a couple different fashions; a small square of rectus muscle may be dissected and welded over the bleeding with high power coagulation, or a pedicle of rectus muscle on the inferior epigastric artery may be sutured to the sacrum to tamponade the bleeding. If all local measures fail, the pelvis should be repacked tightly with laparotomy pads, the skin closed, and the patient brought to the intensive care unit intubated. The patient should be resuscitated and with all coagulopathy corrected, and then return to the operating room 24–28 h later to remove the packs the finish the procedure.

Splenic Injury

Iatrogenic splenic injuries account for up to one-third of splenectomies, and colorectal surgeons have been responsible for one-third to one half of iatrogenic splenectomies. During colorectal surgery, the spleen is most commonly injured while the surgeon is mobilizing the splenic flexure. Because of traction on the colon and peritoneal–omental attachments, a small tear in the splenic capsule occurs either at the inferior pole or at the hilum. This is the most common mechanism of injury, and differs from an unavoidable injury when a cancer is densely adherent to the spleen or when en-bloc splenectomy is required for a splenic flexure tumor invading the spleen. To avoid splenic injury, good visualization of the splenic flexure is necessary. When mobilizing the splenic flexure, the surgeon's finger or laparoscopic instrument should stay as close to the colon as possible, releasing the peritoneal bands and the left upper quadrant omentum to stay with the spleen. For open operations, one surgeon can stand between the legs with the patient in modified lithotomy position and the other on the patient's right. Many authors believe splenic injury is less common during laparoscopic mobilization of the splenic flexure, given improved intracorporeal visualization. As shown in Table 29.4, the risk of splenic injury reported during left hemicolectomy or LAR with mobilization of the splenic flexure is 1–8%. Splenic injury is more common in patients who have had prior abdominal surgery and in obese patients. When a splenic injury occurs, blood loss, operating time, and hospital length of stay are all increased.

Initial management of a splenic injury consists of avoiding further traction and progression of the tear and improving the surgical exposure if needed. One or more of the topical hemostatic agents available should be applied and covered with laparotomy packs. The trial of hemostatic agents and packing must be given sufficient time to see if it will be successful. If the injury is near the hilum, the spleen should be mobilized and the splenic vessels controlled. Large absorbable sutures can be used with Surgicel or other hemostatic agents for tamponade, with sutures placed away from the wound to avoid further tearing. Other methods of splenorraphy have been described using absorbable mesh or omentum. Splenectomy should rarely be needed during colorectal operations, though the incidence increases once 2 attempts at conservative management have failed. Splenectomy may be necessary if there is severe injury through the hilum, the patient is hemodynamically unstable as a result of ongoing bleeding, or the patient has an underlying coagulopathy or needs medical anticoagulation postoperatively. Although the incidence of overwhelming postsplenectomy sepsis in adults is low, the mortality is high when sepsis occurs. In addition, several studies support that iatrogenic splenectomy during colorectal cancer resection results in decreased long-term patient survival.

Table 29.4. Published incidence of splenic injury during colorectal surgery.

Author	Year	No. of patients	No. of injuries	Percent	Comments/case mix
Langevin JM et al. (University Minnesota series)	1984	993	8	0.8	Total colorectal resections: 3.1% injury when splenic flexure mobilized
Marusch F et al.	2002	482	10	0.21	Low anterior resection
Malek MM et al. (Mount Sinai NY series)	2007	5,477 (open) 1,911 (lap)	13 0	0.24 0	Splenectomy only, comparison of incidence during open vs. laparoscopic colectomy
Holubar SD et al. (Mayo clinic series)	2009	13,897	59	0.42	All colectomies; 53 injuries during splenic flexure mobilization, 5 during laparoscopic surgery

Ureter Injury

Reports of ureteric injury during colorectal surgery vary between 0.2 and 5.3%, as seen in Table 29.5. Ureteric injury during colorectal surgery is the second most common type of surgery during which such injuries occur, after gynecologic surgery. Colorectal ureteric injuries account for 5–15% of all ureteral injuries by various types of surgeons. Colorectal surgeons injure the left ureter more commonly than the right. Situations which distort normal anatomic planes, such as prior abdominal surgery, radiation, malignancy, pelvic mass or adhesions, and inflammatory processes such as diverticulitis, inflammatory bowel disease, pelvic abscesses or endometriosis, increase the chance of the surgeon injuring a ureter. It is estimated that only approximately 30% of ureteral injuries are intraoperatively recognized. Immediate detection is essential to minimize patient morbidity and to optimize satisfactory healing of the ureter, with preservation of normal renal function.

1. *Anatomy*: About half of the ureter is in the abdomen and half in the pelvis. The ureter begins at the renal hilum and travels inferiorly on the anterior surface of the psoas muscle. The ureter crosses over the iliac artery bifurcation as it proceeds into the pelvis. The ureter then hugs the pelvic sidewall down toward the levator ani and enters into the posterior bladder. Blood supply to the ureter is segmental, from the renal artery, aorta, common iliac, and branches of the internal iliac artery. The blood supply to the abdominal ureter crosses from medial to lateral, while it is opposite for the pelvic ureter. Therefore, dissection of the abdominal ureter is safer laterally while dissection of the pelvic ureter is safer medially. Reoperative surgery makes the ureter more susceptible to ischemic injury during dissection.

2. *Avoiding Injury*: The best way to avoid ureteric injury is to identify the ureter, normally over the bifurcation of the common iliac artery. The ureter should be identified above the pelvic brim prior to starting a pelvic dissection. One common mistake is to confuse it with the gonadal vessels; confirmation that the suspected structure is the ureter is achieved by observing it peristalsing. Searching for a ureter during a difficult or reoperative case can require significant time and impede forward progress of the operation. Ironically, overly aggressive mobilization of the ureter to prevent injury can result in a

Table 29.5. Published incidence of ureteral injuries during colorectal surgery.

Author	Year	No. of patients	No. of injuries	Percent	Comments/case mix
Kramhoft J et al.	1975	569	9	1.6	APR & LAR, preop IVP
Anderson A and Bergdahl L	1976	111	5	4.5	APR
Leff El et al.	1982	198	4	2.0	Prophylactic ureteral stents
Hughes ESR et al.	1984	2,570	5	0.2	Colon cancer
Kyzer S and Gordon PH	1994	120	1	0.8	Prophylactic ureteral stents
Chahin F et al.	2002	66	1	1.5	All lighted stents, laparoscopic colectomy
Redan JA and McCarus SD	2009	151	0	0	All lighted stents, lap. colon, and gyn. cases

devascularization injury, which is generally not recognized until the postoperative period.

3. *Stenting*: Authors debate whether ureteric catheter placement minimizes ureter injury. There are few complications during ureteral stent placement, including inability to pass the stent, hematuria, and transient postoperative reflex anuria thought to be because of edema. While ureteral catheters do not always prevent injury, they facilitate intraoperative identification of a ureteral injury, as the stent will be visible. Some authors favor lighted stents to save time and effort in identifying the ureter. Some surgeons routinely use ureteric stents for all laparoscopic colorectal surgery, although others advocate using stents only during anticipated difficult cases. If stents are not placed at the commencement of surgery and a difficult pelvis is encountered, it only takes a few minutes during the case to readjust the drapes and pass a cystoscope and ureteric stents. If no one who performs cystoscopy is available, a small cystotomy can be made and stents intraoperatively passed by the operating surgeon. Stent placement at the beginning of the surgery requires an average of 10 min. Unfortunately, the difference in time taken to place ureteric stents compared to the time saved finding the ureters without stents has not been well documented.

4. Recognizing ureteric injury:

   (a) *Intraoperative* inspection of the ureter is essential; it has a classic peristalsis or undulating motion when carefully watched or gently manipulated with a forceps or other instrument. If there is concern about ureteric injury, the anesthesiologist should intravenously inject methylene blue or indigo carmine. The urine will turn blue or green within 10–20 min. If the dye extravasates in the operative field, then an injury is confirmed. If there is suspicion for ligation injury, intravenous pyelography may be performed in the operating room by giving 2 cc/kg of IV contrast agent and then obtaining a KUB in 10 min. This image should either demonstrate or exclude a significant injury or ligation. Every effort should be made to identify a ureteric injury at the time of initial operation, as such an identification is the single most important factor to ensure a successful outcome for the patient.

(b) Specific points during colorectal surgery when the ureter is at risk for injury:

- Ligation of the inferior mesenteric artery: The ureter must be laterally separated from the origin of the IMA, or it may be medially retracted and ligated with the artery.
- Male pelvis: In the retrovesical space, where the ureter crosses the vas deferens, the two structures may be confused and/or the ureter may be ligated or divided.
- Female pelvis: The ureter can be confused for the ovarian artery or ligated with it at the pelvic brim, and the uterine vessels and adnexa are very close to the ureter at the ovarian fossa.
- Division of the lateral stalks of the rectum: The surgeon must stay in the correct plane between the mesorectum and the pelvic sidewall, as straying too lateral risks injury to the ureter.
- Mobilizing the left or right colon, open or laparoscopically, may put the ureter at risk if the surgeon is not in the correct plane and is dissecting too far laterally and retroperitoneal.

(c) *Postoperative injury identification*: Late injury recognition may necessitate further surgical procedures and may cause loss of renal function and/or loss of the kidney.

- Several nonspecific signs and symptoms postoperatively warn the clinician that there may have been a ureteric injury, such as fever, tachycardia, oliguria or anuria, hematuria, flank or abdominal pain, ileus, and urinary fistula. Anuria should occur only if both ureters are ligated or if the patient has a single kidney, and this must be differentiated from acute tubular necrosis when the patient is anuric in the recovery room. Acute hydronephrosis will occur from a ligated or obstructed ureter, and may cause flank pain and fevers. These are both common occurrences within the first postoperative days, so diagnosis is often delayed. A transected ureter may present as a urinary fistula out of a drain, a perineal wound, the vagina, an abdominal incision, or as urinary ascites. Such injuries may not be recognized for days to weeks if the contralateral kidney and ureter are normal. If such an injury is suspected, some of the fluid should be sent to the chemistry lab for urea and creatinine measurement; urine is the only body fluid in which these values are higher than in serum.

- Radiologic Diagnosis: Intravenous pyelography may be used as the first step to identify an injury, and can diagnose the anatomic location and type of injury. It may show delayed renal function, extravasation of urine, or obstruction with hydronephrosis. CT may show intra-abdominal or retroperitoneal fluid collections or ureteric dilatation, but will show much less anatomic information. Retrograde pyelography is the most sensitive radiologic test to diagnose an injured ureter and should be performed after any positive findings on other imaging studies.

5. *Initial Management*: After postoperative diagnosis of an injury, retrograde stenting should be attempted. Some injuries may be bridged using guidewires and stents through a cystoscope, and many will heal with time. If the urologist is unable to pass a retrograde stent, then proximal decompression with a percutaneous nephrostomy tube is necessary. Then antegrade stenting can be attempted via the nephrostomy tube. If this technique is unsuccessful, surgical exploration and repair will be needed in the future.

6. *Repair of Ureteral Injuries*: Once an injury is identified, either intraoperatively or postoperatively, repair should be performed by an experienced surgeon, usually a urologist. The ureteric injury may result from ligation, crush, transection, devascularization, or thermal injury. If the injury is detected during or soon after surgery and the patient is stable, repair should immediately occur. If the patient is unstable and/or the diagnosis is significantly delayed, renal urinary drainage via percutaneous nephrostomy is recommended.

   (a) *Ligation or crush injury*: It may be sufficient to remove the suture if the ureter was ligated. A ureter crushed with a clamp may require stenting or repair. The ureter adventitia must be examined for discoloration or ischemia.

   (b) *Thermal Injury*: The injured segment should be carefully inspected. Contingent upon the length and circumference of the injury as well as the degree of thermal trauma, stenting or resection plus stenting is required.

(c) *Devascularization*: Ischemic injury to segmental blood supply occurs from overly aggressive mobilization or skeletonization of the ureter. Intraoperatively an ischemic ureter may appear dark, no longer peristalse, or a transected end will not bleed.

(d) *Primary ureter repair*: First debride ischemic or nonviable tissue, then mobilize the ureter to allow a tension-free anastomosis, and finally approximate the mucosa. Primary repair or ureteroureterostomy may be accomplished with 4–0 or 5–0 absorbable interrupted or running suture of angled spatulated ends of the ureter. This repair works best for injuries in the mid-ureter and defects less than 3 cm in length. Double J stents are used after most repairs for 4–6 weeks, and extraperitoneal drains are left in place for 48 h or until drainage is low. A primary anastomosis is the preferred method of repair when possible, if the ends are lying close enough to avoid tension and if the injury is not close to the bladder.

(e) *Advanced ureteral repairs:* If the injury is extensive, there are multiple more advanced methods of reimplanting the ureter. Extensive injury will be more common with a delayed postoperative diagnosis. Repairs include the psoas hitch, Boari flap, transureteroureteric anastomosis, and ureter replacement. The option of last resort is a nephrectomy, which should be performed only after the contralateral kidney is determined to have normal function. If a surgeon experienced in ureteral repair is not available to intraoperatively assist and an extensive injury is identified, the safest way to proceed is by placing a ureterostomy or nephrostomy tube out through the skin under direct vision, depending on the level of the injury. Never ligate the ureter without providing proximal drainage.

- *Distal injuries*: Injuries of the distal third of the ureter, less than 15 cm in length, can be repaired by reimplanting the ureter into the bladder. This reimplantation may be accomplished with just a small amount of bladder mobilization, or by using a psoas hitch or Boari flap. Most surgeons stent these repairs for 4–6 weeks. With mobilization of the lateral bladder attachments, the bladder dome may reach as high as the iliac vessels. A Boari flap is a broad-based anterior bladder flap made into a tube for ureter implantation via a spatulated end to the submucosa. The psoas hitch will not provide as much length as the Boari flap, but is technically simpler. The superior bladder is mobilized, a transverse incision is made in the anterior bladder to form a tube, the ureter is reimplanted, and the bladder is sutured to the psoas tendon. Transureteroureterostomy may be performed for lower or mid-ureteric injuries when the Boari flap is not possible, such as with a very small or fibrotic bladder. A retroperitoneal tunnel is made anterior to the great vessels, the damaged ureter is passed, and it is anastomosed at 45° end to side to the normal ureter. Many surgeons are reluctant to use this reconstruction for fear of putting the normal collecting system at risk.

- Very long injuries and proximal injuries are the most challenging to fix, and may be bridged with ileum, colon, fallopian tubes, or the appendix. Ileum is the most commonly used of these options, and may replace the entire ureter. A segment of ileum is mobilized on its blood supply and passed through the mesocolon, proximally anastomosed to the renal pelvis, and distally to the bladder.

Conclusions

The unfortunate truth is that all colorectal surgeons will likely experience some or all of these complications during their career. The incidence can be minimized using meticulous technique and including some of the principles outlined above. Avoidance of these problems is obviously better than either intraoperative recognition or postoperative reoperation and treatment. Immediate identification and repair of anastomotic leaks, anastomotic or presacral or splenic bleeding, or ureteral injuries during the operation will normally lead to an excellent patient outcome. Conversely, delayed postoperative recognition is often quite devastating with significant potentially avoidable patient morbidity.

Selected Readings

1. Bothwell W, Bleicher R, Dent T. Prophylactic ureteral catheterization in colon surgery. A five-year review. Dis Colon Rectum. 1994;37:330–4.
2. Cassar K, Munro A. Iatrogenic splenic injury. J R Coll Surg Edinb. 2002;47:731–41.
3. Hairston J, Ghoneim G. Urinary tract injuries: recognition and management. Clin Colon Rectal Surg. 2003;16:27–37.
4. Hicks T, Beck D, Opelka F, Timmcke A, editors. Complications of colon and rectal surgery. Baltimore: Williams & Wilkins; 1996.
5. Ishihara S, Watanabe T, Nagawa H. Intraoperative colonoscopy for stapled anastomosis in colorectal surgery. Surg Today. 2008;38:1063–5.
6. Li VK, Wexner SD, Pulido N, et al. Use of routine intraoperative endoscopy in elective laparoscopic colorectal surgery: can it further avoid anastomotic failure? Surg Endosc. 2009;23:2459–65.
7. Lim M, Akhtar S, Sasapu K, et al. Clinical and subclinial leaks after low colorectal anastomosis: a clinical and radiologic study. Dis Colon Rectum. 2006;49:1611–9.
8. Lustosa S, Matos D, Atallah A, Castro A. Stapled versus handsewn methods for colorectal anastomosis surgery. Cochrane Database Syst Rev. 2001;3:CD003144.
9. Malik A, East J, Buchanan G, Kennedy R. Endoscopic haemostasis of staple-line haemorrhage following colorectal resection. Colorectal Dis. 2008;10:616–8.
10. Martinez-Serrano M, Pares D, Pera M, et al. Management of lower gastrointestinal bleeding after colorectal resection and stapled anastomosis. Tech Coloproctol. 2009;13:49–53.
11. Montedori A, Cirocchi R, Farinella E, Sciannameo F, Abraha I. Covering ileo- or colostomy in anterior resection for rectal carcinoma. Cochrane Database Syst Rev. 2010;5:CD006878.
12. Remzi F, Oncel M, Fazio V. Muscle tamponade to control presacral venous bleeding. Dis Colon Rectum. 2002;45:1109–11.
13. Suchan K, Muldner A, Manegold B. Endoscopic treatment of postoperative colorectal anastomotic strictures. Surg Endosc. 2003;17:1110–3.
14. Taflampas P, Christodoulakis M, Tsiftsis D. Anastomotic leakage after low anterior resection for rectal cancer: facts, obscurity, and fiction. Surg Today. 2009;39:183–8.
15. Tan W, Tang C, Shi L, Wu K. Meta-analysis of defunctioning stomas in low anterior resection for rectal cancer. Br J Surg. 2009;96:462–72.
16. Wakeman C, Dobbs B, Frizelle F, et al. The impact of splenectomy on outcome after resection for colorectal cancer: a multicenter, nested, paired, cohort study. Dis Colon Rectum. 2008;51:213–17.

30. Solid Organ Surgery

L. Michael Brunt and Esteban Varela

Introduction

Laparoscopic solid organ surgery poses a number of unique challenges for a safe and successful outcome. These include issues of understanding the wide variety of pathologic conditions to manage, proper patient selection for operation, the potential for underlying malignancy, the need to mobilize adjacent organs, control of the organ's rich blood supply, and the need to extract specimens of varying sizes. Furthermore, solid organ surgery is less commonly performed laparoscopically compared to many other basic and advanced laparoscopic procedures, and as a result, surgeons may have relatively little experience in managing the full array of conditions which may be encountered. In this chapter, we will focus on the two most commonly performed solid organ procedures – laparoscopic adrenalectomy and splenectomy – and will review issues related to access, patient selection and preparation, and avoiding and managing complications.

Access

The location of the spleen and adrenal in the left upper quadrant and retroperitoneum, respectively, require an access approach that is typically away from the umbilicus and off the midline. Laparoscopic access to these solid organs is also facilitated by positioning in a lateral or hemi-lateral position rather than supine. For laparoscopic transabdominal lateral adrenalectomy, which is the most common approach to adrenalectomy used, the patient is in a lateral decubitus position with the affected side up.

The patient is on a bean bag mattress which is well padded and a roll is placed under the chest wall to protect the axilla. All pressure points are well padded in order to minimize the risk of a nerve compression injury

D.S. Tichansky, J. Morton, and D.B. Jones (eds.), *The SAGES Manual of Quality, Outcomes and Patient Safety*, DOI 10.1007/978-1-4419-7901-8_30, © Springer Science+Business Media, LLC 2012

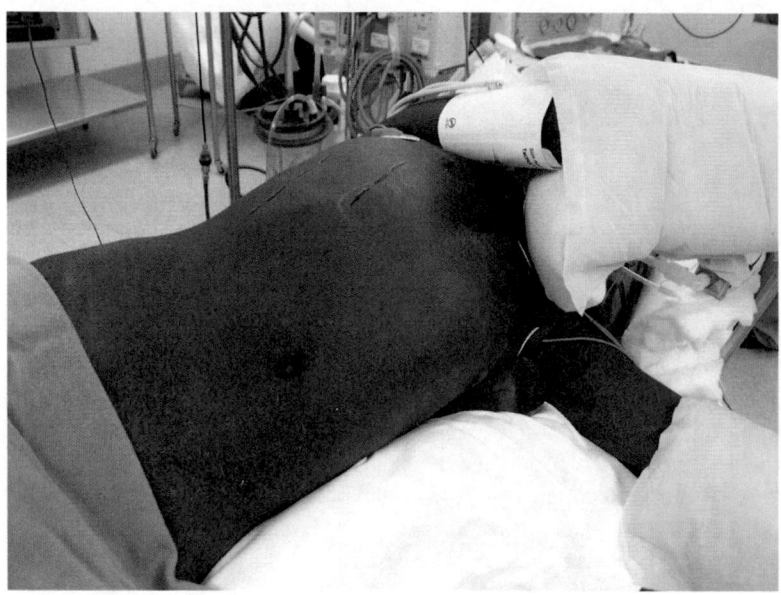

Fig. 30.1. Patient position for laparoscopic right adrenalectomy. Note how all pressure points are well padded. The anterior and posterior axillary lines are marked by the dotted lines.

or neuropraxia with the patient in this position. Important reference points are the anterior and posterior axillary lines which are marked prior to prepping and draping the patient (Fig. 30.1). Initial access can be obtained with either an open or closed approach. However, with the patient in this position, an open approach requires dissecting through multiple muscular layers and making a larger incision than is necessary with a closed approach. For adrenalectomy, the Veress needle is inserted at or just proximal to the anterior axillary line. The needle should be aspirated for blood and position confirmed with the saline drop test. After pneumoperitoneum has been established, a 5 mm port can be inserted under optical guidance. The authors caution against using a 10 mm trocar for initial access because of the additional force necessary to insert it and potentially greater consequences of an injury compared to a 5 mm port. All subsequent ports are placed under direct laparoscopic vision; if bleeding occurs at any of these sites, it should be tamponaded and will generally require no further management. Persistent bleeding at a trocar site can be controlled with a suture placed percutaneously on either side of the entry site with a suture passer which is then tied down.

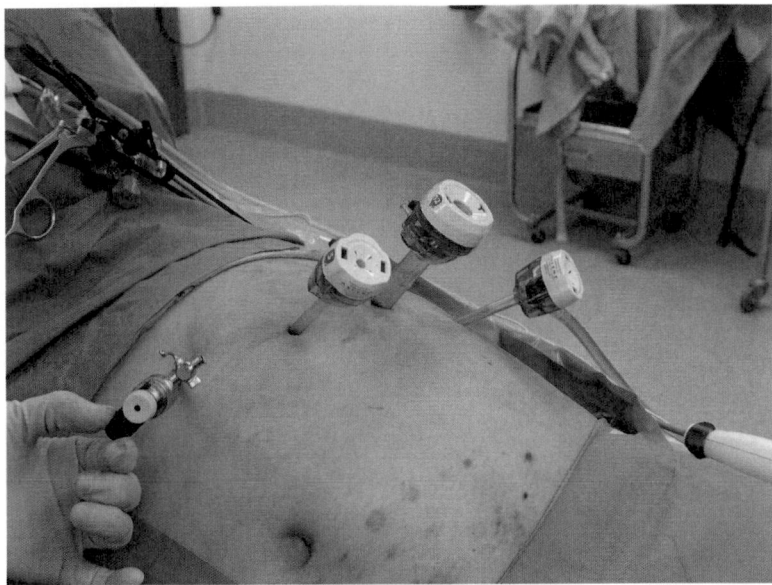

Fig. 30.2. Patient position and port placement for laparoscopic splenectomy. The ports in this case are positioned for a normal size spleen.

For laparoscopic splenectomy, a hemi-lateral position with the patient at a 30–45° angle is preferred (Fig. 30.2). The left arm is raised over the head, but a chest roll is not usually necessary since the patient is not lying on their axilla. With the patient secured to the table on a bean bag, the table can then be rolled either more laterally or medially to optimize exposure. Initial access for splenectomy varies according to patient body habitus and the size of the spleen. In patients with a normal size spleen, initial access can be obtained in a closed manner with the location of ports shifted somewhat medially compared to adrenalectomy (Fig. 30.2). In thin patients, the initial access site (and subsequent spleen extraction site) can be at the umbilicus using an open technique. An open insertion, usually umbilical, is recommended in all patients with splenomegaly to avoid injuring the spleen with the Veress needle or initial port.

Overall, major access injuries occur rarely in laparoscopic surgery and have not been reported separately for solid organ procedures. The most common access complications likely to be encountered in solid organ procedures are bleeding, usually from puncture of the liver by the Veress needle during right adrenalectomy and failure to obtain pneumoperitoneum. If blood is aspirated from the Veress needle, the needle should be removed and access attempted in another location, either closed or open. Liver bleeding will usually stop spontaneously or can be controlled with electrocautery once the laparoscopic ports are inserted. Of greater concern is bleeding in the retroperitoneum which can involve major arterial structures including the aorta; for this reason, midline closed access should not be attempted above the umbilicus. With the patient in a lateral decubitus position, the gallbladder may also be punctured during closed access on the right side, which may require cholecystectomy to avoid a postoperative bile leak. Enterotomy may also occur during access for solid organ surgery; if it involves the Veress needle or a 5 mm trocar, it may be possible to manage it by laparoscopic repair. Ten mm trocar injuries to the bowel are more likely to require resection. Recognizing that an access injury has occurred is critical to minimizing the consequences. Therefore, it is essential to inspect the initial access site in all laparoscopic solid organ cases to avoid missing such an injury.

Laparoscopic Adrenalectomy

Patient Selection and Evaluation

Proper selection and preparation of patients for adrenalectomy is one of the most important aspects of safe adrenal surgery. Therefore, it is essential for surgeons who undertake adrenalectomy to be knowledgeable about the clinical presentation and surgical indications for the various adrenal tumors. While it is beyond the scope of this chapter to review the details of the clinical presentation and biochemical evaluation of each of these tumors, the key elements of the diagnostic evaluation are given in Table 30.1 and can be reviewed in detail elsewhere [1–8]. The most common adrenal lesion encountered by clinicians today is the adrenal incidentaloma (reviewed in [9]). Since the evaluation of an adrenal incidentaloma involves both functional assessment and evaluation of a lesion's malignant potential, it provides a logical framework for evaluating all other adrenal tumors and will be considered in more detail.

The hormonal evaluation of an adrenal incidentaloma should in all cases consist of evaluation for pheochromocytoma and subclinical hypercortisolism. Only patients who are hypertensive and/or hypokalemic need to be screened for hyperaldosteronism with plasma aldosterone and renin levels. Assessment for pheochromocytoma consists of measurement of plasma-fractionated metanephrines or a 24 h urine collection for

Table 30.1. Essential diagnostic and radiographic evaluation of common adrenal tumors.

Adrenal tumor	Biochemical profile	Imaging/localization
Aldosteronoma	Elevated PAC with suppressed PRA (PAC:PRA>25–30, aldosterone >15 ng/dl and renin <0.5 ng/ml/h) 24 h urine aldosterone >12 μg/24 h	Thin section (3 mm) adrenal CT Adrenal vein sampling as indicated
Cortisol-producing adenoma	Elevated 24-h urine-free cortisol Low-dose dexamethasone test Suppressed plasma ACTH	Abdominal CT
Pheochromocytoma	Elevated plasma-fractionated metanephrines and/or urinary catecholamines and metabolites	MRI (T_2-weighted sequences showing bright appearing adrenal lesion)
Adrenal cortical carcinoma	24 h urine-free cortisol and metabolites Plasma DHEA-sulfate	CT of chest/abdomen/pelvis
Adrenal metastasis	Exclude pheo and Cushing's FNA biopsy rarely indicated	Abdominal CT, PET imaging to evaluate for extra-adrenal metastatic disease
Myelolipoma	None if radiographic appearance is unequivocal for myelolipoma	CT or MRI showing macroscopic fat

metanephrines and catecholamines. Subclinical Cushing's syndrome is most easily evaluated with an overnight dexamethasone test in which 1–2 mg of dexamethasone is given at 11 p.m. and an 8 a.m. plasma cortisol is obtained the next morning. Normal individuals should suppress cortisol levels to <1.8 μg/dl. Patients who fail to suppress should be evaluated further with a 24 h urine-free cortisol and plasma ACTH levels. An abnormality in these tests indicates some degree of autonomy in cortisol secretion. In general, patients with evidence of a hormonally active incidentaloma should undergo adrenalectomy.

The second component of the evaluation of an adrenal mass is assessment of the risk of malignancy in the lesion, which involves review of all prior imaging by the surgeon in conjunction with a radiologist. Benign lesions typically are low in attenuation (<10 Hounsfield units) on noncontrast CT, whereas malignant lesions have higher attenuation values [10]. On MRI chemical shift imaging, adrenal adenomas show loss of signal intensity on opposed phase sequences whereas malignant lesions have no loss of signal intensity. Pheochromocytomas typically appear bright on T2-weighted MRI and often are heterogeneous with areas of cystic change on CT. Adrenal myelolipomas are benign lesions comprised of fat and bone marrow elements that are distinguished radiographically by the presence of macroscopic fat. Myelolipomas are often mistaken for potentially malignant lesions by inexperienced examiners and, since they do not need to be removed, correct imaging interpretation is essential to avoid unnecessary adrenalectomy. Adrenal metastases may also present as incidentalomas, but these usually occur in the setting of known malignancy or other metastatic disease. Adrenalectomy is indicated for any solitary adrenal lesion with imaging characteristics suspicious for malignancy or lesions over 4 cm with indeterminate imaging characteristics, whether or not it is a hormonally functioning tumor.

Indications for Adrenalectomy

Most of the indications for adrenalectomy are appropriate for a laparoscopic approach. Large adrenal cortical cancers and locally invasive tumors should be approached in an open fashion. Laparoscopic adrenalectomy is more difficult in patients who are obese or those with pheochromocytomas, paragangliomas, and larger tumors (>6 cm). Patients who have had prior upper abdominal surgery on the side of the lesion, especially splenectomy or renal procedures are also more difficult. Therefore, surgeons who undertake these cases should do so only if they have the appropriate training and experience. Preoperatively, hypertension should be controlled and electrolyte abnormalities corrected. Patients with pheochromocytomas should have preoperative pharmacologic preparation with alpha adrenergic receptor blockade with phenoxybenzamine for 7–10 days in advance of surgery to avoid uncontrolled hypertensive events intraoperatively. Patients with hyerpcortisolism should be given exogenous cortisol perioperatively to avoid acute adrenal insufficiency.

Laparoscopic Approaches

The principal laparoscopic approaches to adrenalectomy are the transabdominal lateral approach and the retroperitoneal (RP) endoscopic approach. The greatest experience worldwide is with the transabdominal lateral approach but interest in the RP approach is gaining. The advantages of the former are a large working space, familiar landmarks, and more straightforward patient positioning. The latter (RP approach) provides the most direct access to the adrenals, results in short operative times (in experienced hands), and may pose less risk of bleeding. However, it can be more difficult to learn because of the lack of familiarity of most surgeons with the anatomy in the closed retroperitoneal space. The various technical aspects to these approaches to adrenalectomy are examined elsewhere [11, 12].

Adrenalectomy-Related Complications

One of the primary advantages of laparoscopic compared to open adrenalectomy has been a reduction in the incidence of postoperative complications. In a retrospective analysis from the literature, the incidence of complications was 25.2% in open adrenalectomy series but only 10.9% in laparoscopic series [13]. The lower rate of complications was primarily due to fewer wound, pulmonary, and infectious complications with the laparoscopic approach. In addition, open adrenalectomy had a significantly higher rate of associated organ injury than laparoscopic adrenalectomy (2.4 vs. 0.7%), mainly due to injuries to the spleen. In another study that analyzed adrenalectomy data from the National Surgery Quality Improvement Database from 2001 to 2004, the morbidity rate in patients undergoing open adrenalectomy was fourfold higher than in patients who had laparoscopic adrenalectomy [14]. The operative mortality associated with laparoscopic adrenalectomy is about 0.3%.

Bleeding

Bleeding is the most frequent significant complication reported with laparoscopic adrenalectomy and the most common reason for conversion to open adrenalectomy. Since even small amounts of bleeding in the retroperitoneum can obscure the operative field and dissection planes, the most effective strategy is to avoid bleeding altogether. It is important first of all to obtain good exposure in the retroperitoneum. On the right side this is done by full division of the right triangular ligament and mobilization of the right hepatic lobe medially. On the left, the splenorenal ligament should be divided up to the diaphragm and the plane between the tail of the pancreas and kidney should be separated to allow medial rotation of the tail of the pancreas and spleen together. The surgeon must use gentle retraction and should be meticulous and vigilant in hemostasis technique. A variety of methods can be used for controlling the many small vessels entering the adrenal including electrocautery or ultrasonic and bipolar coagulating devices according to surgeon preference. Clips are typically used to secure the adrenal vein although with the retroperitoneal approach, the vein may be sealed with a bipolar coagulator.

Potential sources of major bleeding during adrenalectomy are the inferior vena cava (IVC), renal veins, renal arterial branches, and adjacent organs (liver, pancreas, spleen, kidney). Special care must be taken with the adrenal vein on the right side which is short and empties directly into the IVC. Excessive traction on the adrenal gland/tumor and right adrenal vein can result in a tear of the vein into the vena cava which can be difficult to control. One must also be cognizant of the location of the IVC relative to the dissection plane and instrument positions at all times to avoid injuring it; similarly, once clips have been applied to the adrenal vein, one should be careful to avoid catching them with an instrument or suction device and potentially dislodging them. If bleeding occurs, it can usually be managed by tamponade of the bleeding site with an atraumatic instrument as most minor bleeding will cease with this maneuver alone. If this fails, use of thermal energy or clips may be used as appropriate as long as this does not risk violation of the tumor capsule. Major bleeding that is not controllable laparoscopically should be managed by prompt conversion to open operation.

High-Grade Complications/Adjacent Organ Injury

One of the primary benefits of a laparoscopic approach to adrenalectomy has been a lower incidence of injury to adjacent organs. The most common solid organ injured during laparoscopic adrenalectomy is the liver which may be punctured during initial access or lacerated by the retraction device. Most liver lacerations of this nature are superficial and will stop with time and pressure and/or cauterization. The risk of liver laceration may be reduced by thorough mobilization of the right triangular ligament and medial rotation of the right hepatic lobe. Splenic capsular tears may also occur and usually stop with conservative measures since incidental splenectomy has been described rarely. Other injuries that may occur include renal vessel injury, especially superior pole renal artery branches, and injuries to the ureter, pancreas and colon.

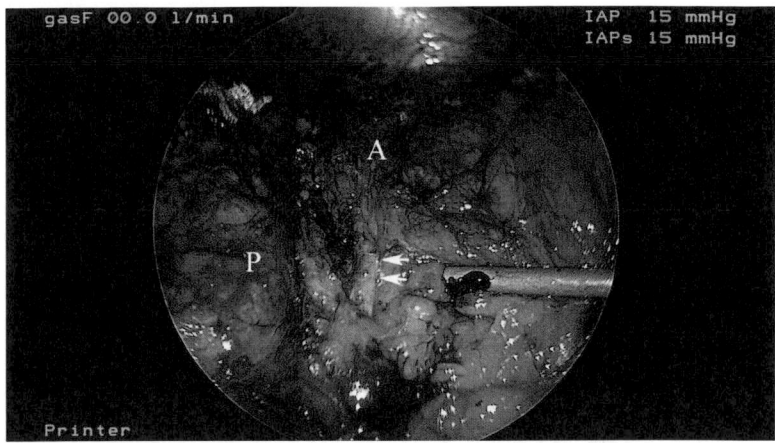

Fig. 30.3. Relationships of tail of pancreas, kidney, and adrenal during laparoscopic left adrenalectomy, transabdominal flank approach (P – pancreas, A – adrenal, *arrows* point to adrenal vein).

Despite the lower overall complication risk, a number of major, high-grade complications involving injury to adjacent organs have been described, and others undoubtedly occur that are never reported. Tessier et al. [15] reported six cases referred to multiple tertiary centers in which major organ injury occurred. These included a case of complete transection of the porta hepatis and another that involved ligation of the right hepatic artery during right adrenalectomy for pheochromocytoma, both of which required treatment by liver transplantation; ligation of the left ureter which led to hydronephrosis and loss of renal function; and a case of renal artery injury that led to nephrectomy. Cases in which the tail of the pancreas has been mistaken for the adrenal and inappropriately resected have also occurred. This may occur because the pancreatic tail is very close to the adrenal and is usually encountered before the adrenal gland is seen with the lateral flank approach. The key to avoiding this complication is threefold: (1) understanding the anatomic relationship of the pancreatic tail to the kidney and adrenal (Fig. 30.3); (2) always making a positive identification of both adrenal and pancreas; and (3) identifying the splenic artery and vein which should be coursing with the tail of the pancreas back toward the splenic hilum. An excessive number of or unusually positioned vessels encountered during the dissection should also raise this possibility to the surgeon. If there is any suspicion that the pancreatic parenchyma has been violated, a closed suction drain should be placed and tested for amylase after the patient has resumed a regular diet.

Tumor Recurrence

For patients with malignant or potentially malignant adrenal tumors, the most important outcome measure is the oncologic result, regardless of the technique used for adrenalectomy. Adrenal malignancies may be more difficult to remove laparoscopically for a number of reasons including larger tumor size and extension of tumor outside the adrenal capsule. In general, conversion rates to open adrenalectomy have been higher for malignant tumors than for benign adrenal lesions (reviewed in [16]) Overall, local tumor recurrence after laparoscopic resection of adrenal metastases have been low. However, in one series local or regional tumor recurrence developed in three of five patients with suspected or unsuspected adrenal cortical carcinomas removed laparoscopically [17] and there have been other anecdotal reports of recurrences of primary adrenal cancers after laparoscopic resection as well. More concerning is the observation from MD Anderson regarding the pattern of local recurrence after resection of adrenal cortical cancer: in their review, peritoneal carcinomatosis developed in five of six patients (83%) after laparoscopic resection compared to only 8% of patients with local recurrences after open adrenalectomy [18].

Finally, local recurrence of apparently benign adrenal lesions has also been reported. Li et al. [19] reported three cases of recurrent pheochromocytomatosis that occurred after laparoscopic adrenalectomy. In each of these patients, multiple small tumor nodules were found in the adrenalectomy bed at open reoperation. The mechanism of recurrence in these cases was felt to be tumor fragmentation and/or excessive tumor manipulation during the laparoscopic dissection. These findings emphasize the importance of experience in dealing with these more difficult tumors and suggest that until data prove the oncologic safety of laparoscopic resection of large adrenal cortical cancers, these rare tumors should be approached in an open fashion.

Other Complications

Other major complications such as deep vein thrombosis and pulmonary embolism occur rarely following adrenalectomy with a reported incidence of 0.8 and 0.5%, respectively. Pneumatic compression stockings should be used perioperatively to minimize the risk of venous thromboembolism and consideration should be given to subcutaneous heparin prophylaxis as well in higher risk patients such as the morbidly obese. Trocar site hernias are infrequent as well, provided that the fascia is closed at all port sites that are 10 mm or larger.

Postoperative Complications

Acute adrenal insufficiency may occur following adrenalectomy for Cushing's syndrome or after bilateral adrenalectomy and can result in refractory hypotension. To prevent this complication, at-risk patients should receive glucocorticoid replacement postoperatively. Patients with Cushing's syndrome may take 6–12 months or longer to recover adequate function of the pituitary–adrenal axis in order to be weaned off replacement. In addition, patients who undergo bilateral adrenalectomy should be given both glucocorticoid and mineralocorticoid replacement lifelong. After resection of pheochromocytoma, patients may experience a period of hypotension from the alpha blockade which usually resolves within 24 h. Transient pressor support with intensive care monitoring may be indicated for patients who fail to respond to crystalloid or colloid administration. Pheochromocytoma patients may also experience rebound hyperinsulinemia from catecholamine-induced suppression of insulin secretion by the tumor and, therefore, are at risk for hypoglycemia in the early postoperative period.

Laparoscopic Splenectomy

Patient Selection and Preoperative Preparation

As it is the case in laparoscopic adrenalectomy, proper selection and preparation of patients for splenectomy is one of the most important aspects of safe spleen surgery. Laparoscopy has also become the standard approach for spleen removal. The most common indications for laparoscopic splenectomy are hematologic and neoplastic pathology that may increase the risk for perioperative morbidity such as bleeding and infection [20]. This morbidity is related to significant length of stay and overall hospital costs. Most of the complications encountered after or during laparoscopic splenectomy are technical in nature. Therefore, patient selection and preoperative preparation is of essence for a safe laparoscopic splenectomy. Not uncommonly, patients requiring a splenectomy present with hematologic disorders such as anemia, thrombocytopenia and coagulopathy that must be investigated and optimized prior to surgery.

Targarona et al. identified predictors for complications after laparoscopic splenectomy. These included patient's age, spleen weight, malignancy, and learning curve [21]. Common reasons for conversion to an open splenectomy approach included: bleeding, spleen size, and intra-abdominal adhesions. Overall, the morbidity for laparoscopic splenectomy can be as high as 20%. Although operative times are longer for laparoscopic vs. open splenectomy, in general, laparoscopic splenectomy has been associated with a significant reduction in morbidity, with fewer pulmonary, wound, and infectious complications [22, 23].

Indications for Splenectomy

The most common indications for laparoscopic splenectomy are listed in Table 30.2. These included most commonly hematologic (red and white cell, platelet disorders) followed by neoplastic and other conditions.

Table 30.2. Potential indications for splenectomy.

Red blood cell disorders
Autoimmune hemolytic anemia
Spherocytosis
Elliptocytosis

White cell disorders
Hodgkin's lymphoma
Non-Hodgkin's lymphoma
Myeloproliferative disorders (myelofibrosis)
Chronic lymphocytic leukemia
Chronic myeloid leukemia
Hairy cell leukemia

Platelet disorders
Idiopathic thrombocytopenic purpura (ITP)
HIV related ITP
Evans syndrome
Thrombotic thrombocytopenic purpura

Others
Splenic trauma
Splenic abscess/infarct
Cysts
Angiomatosis
Splenic tumors
Hypersplenism (portal hypertension)

Splenectomy-Related Complications

Bleeding

Bleeding is the most common technical complication during and after open and laparoscopic splenectomy. Bleeding may account for up to one-third of all complicated cases. It is also related to a high number of conversions from laparoscopic to an open technique. However, the use of vessel-sealing energy devices has shown to decrease both intraoperative bleeding and operative time during laparoscopic splenectomy [24, 25].

Adjacent Organ Injury

Injuries to adjacent organs happen uncommonly and may involve the pancreas, colon, stomach, and diaphragm. The great majority are related to the use of energy devices, vigorous tissue traction, and dissection. The judicious use of these energy devices and prompt injury recognition or conversion to an open technique may avoid significant morbidity including gastric, colonic, or pancreatic leaks that may ultimately require a reoperation and prolonged hospital stay. Particularly important is the vicinity of the tail of the pancreas to the splenic hilum. If transection of the pancreatic tail is indicated, this may be safely accomplished by the use of mechanical stapling devices with buttressing. Data have suggested that the use of stapling buttressing materials during pancreas stapling and transection may decrease the incidence of pancreatic leaks which may occur in 26% of pancreatic resections without buttressing [26].

Thromboembolic (Splenic/Portal Vein Thrombosis)

Portal vein thrombosis is a relatively common complication of splenectomy (which may occur up to 8% of cases), particularly in patients with splenomegaly. Presenting symptoms may include anorexia, abdominal pain, fever, and both elevated leukocyte and platelet counts. A high index of suspicion, early diagnosis by contrast-enhanced computed tomography, and prompt anticoagulation are key to a successful outcome [27, 28].

Post-Splenectomy Sepsis

The spleen plays a major role in the body's immunity as it is part of the reticulo-endothelial system. Therefore, asplenia and the subsequent absence of splenic macrophages increase the susceptibility to bacterial infections. Post-splenectomy sepsis or overwhelming post-splenectomy infections is a rare but potentially fatal infectious complication. Infection is most commonly caused by encapsulated organisms such as the *Streptococcus pneumonia*. The risk of post-splenectomy sepsis has been estimated at under 0.5% per year with a 5% lifetime risk [29]. However, these incidence figures are largely based on studies reported prior of the routine use of vaccine prophylaxis. The groups at greatest risk are children with thalassemia and sickle cell anemia and is greatest during the first 2–3 years after splenectomy. The administration of preoperative vaccines such as the pneumococcal vaccine polyvalent, hemophilus influenza type b (Hib) and meningococcal vaccines directed to encapsulated organisms, and patient education regarding the need for antibiotics in the event of an upper respiratory infection or sore throat are the safest strategies to prevent sepsis after spleen removal.

Selected Readings

1. Stowasser M. Update in primary aldosteronism. J Clin Endocrinol Metab. 2009; 94:3623–30.
2. Funder JW, Carey RM, Fardella C, et al. Case detection, diagnosis, and treatment of patients with primary aldosteronism: An Endocrine Society Clinical Practice Guideline. J Clin Endocrinol Metab. 2008;93:3266–81.
3. Findling JW, Raff H. Diagnosis and differential diagnosis of Cushing's syndrome. Endocrinol Metab Clin N Am. 2001;20:729.
4. Tomiato A, Merante-Boschin I, Opocher G, Pelizo MR, Schiavo F, Ballota E. Surgical versus conservative management for subclinical Cushing syndrome in adrenal incidentalomas: a prospective randomized study. Ann Surg. 2009;249:388–91.
5. Reisch N, Peczkowska M, Januszewicz A, Neumann HP. Pheochromocytoma: presentation, diagnosis and treatment. J Hypertens. 2006;24:2331–9.
6. Guerrero MA, Schreinemakers JMJ, Vriens MR, Suh I, Hwang J, Shen WT, et al. Clinical spectrum of pheochromocytoma. J Am Coll Surg. 2009;209:727–32.
7. Allolio B, Fassnacht M. Adrenocortical carcinoma: clinical update. J Clin Endocrinol Metab. 2006;91:2027.
8. Brunt LM. Gastrointestinal tract and abdomen. Disorders of the adrenal glands. In: Ashley SW, editor. ACS Surgery (online). Philadelphia: Decker Intellectual Properties; 2010. DOI: 10.2310/7800.S05C38.

9. Brunt LM, Moley JF. Adrenal incidentaloma. In: Cameron JL, editor. Cameron's current surgical therapy. 9th ed. Philadelphia: Mosby Elsevier; 2008. p. 597–602.

10. Yip L, Tublin ME, Falcone JA, Nordman CR, Stang MT, Ogilvie JB, et al. The adrenal mass: correlation of histopathology with imaging. Ann Surg Oncol. 2010;17:846–52.

11. Tessier D, Brunt LM. Laparoscopic adrenalectomy. In: Soper NJ, Swanstrom LL, Eubanks WS, editors. Mastery of Endoscopic and Laparoscopic Surgery. 3rd ed. Philadelphia: Lippincott, Williams & Wilkins; 2009. p. 410–20.

12. Walz MK, Alesina PF, Wenger FA, et al. Posterior retroperitoneoscopic adrenalectomy-results of 560 procedures in 520 patients. Surgery. 2006;140:943.

13. Brunt LM. The positive impact of laparoscopic adrenalectomy on complications of adrenal surgery. Surg Endosc. 2001;16:252–7.

14. Turrentine FE, Henderson EG, Khuri SF, et al. Adrenalectomy in veterans affairs and selected university medical centers: results of the patient safety in surgery study. J Am Coll Surg. 2007;204:1273–83.

15. Tessier DJ, Iglesias R, Chapman WC, Kercher KW, Matthews BD, Gorden L, et al. Previously unreported high grade complications of adrenalectomy. Surg Endosc. 2009;23:97–102.

16. Brunt LM. Minimal access adrenal surgery. Surg Endosc. 2006;20:351–61.

17. Kebebew E, Siperstein AE, Clark OH, et al. Results of laparoscopic adrenalectomy for suspected and unsuspected malignant adrenal neoplasms. Arch Surg. 2002; 137:948.

18. Gonzalez RJ, Shapiro S, Sarlis N, Vassilopoulos-Sellin R, Perrier ND, Evans DB, et al. Laparoscopic resection of adrenal cortical carcinoma: a cautionary note. Surgery. 2005;138:1078–86.

19. Li ML, Fitzgerald PA, Price DC, et al. Iatrogenic pheochromocytomatosis: a previously unreported result of laparoscopic adrenalectomy. Surgery. 2001;130:1072–7.

20. Tessier DJ, Pierce RA, Brunt LM, et al. Laparoscopic splenectomy for splenic masses. Surg Endosc. 2008;22:2062–6.

21. Targarona EM, Espert JJ, Bombuy E, et al. Complications of laparoscopic splenectomy. Arch Surg. 2000;135:1137–40.

22. Brunt LM, Langer JC, Quasebarth MA, Whitman ED. Comparative analysis of laparoscopic versus open splenectomy. Am J Surg. 1996;172:596–9. discussion 9–601.

23. Winslow ER, Brunt LM. Perioperative outcomes of laparoscopic versus open splenectomy: a meta-analysis with an emphasis on complications. Surgery. 2003;134:647–53. discussion 54–5.

24. Barbaros U, Dinccag A, Deveci U, et al. Use of electrothermal vessel sealing with LigaSure device during laparoscopic splenectomy. Acta Chir Belg. 2007;107:162–5.

25. Misawa T, Yoshida K, Iida T, et al. Minimizing intraoperative bleeding using a vessel-sealing system and splenic hilum hanging maneuver in laparoscopic splenectomy. J Hepatobiliary Pancreat Surg. 2009;16:786–91.

26. Yamamoto M, Hayashi MS, Nguyen NT, Nguyen TD, McCloud S, Imagawa DK. Use of Seamguard to prevent pancreatic leak following distal pancreatectomy. Arch Surg. 2009;144:894–9.

27. Winslow ER, Brunt LM, Drebin JA, Soper NJ, Klingensmith ME. Portal vein thrombosis after splenectomy: a case series. Am J Surg. 2002;184:631–6.
28. Winslow ER, Klingensmith ME, Brunt LM. Problem of portal venous thrombosis after splenectomy. Ann Surg. 2005;242:745. author reply –6.
29. Davidson RN, Wall RA. Prevention and management of infections in patients without a spleen. Clin Microbiol Infect. 2001;7:657–60.

31. Minimally Invasive Esophagectomy: Complications and Management

Francis Rosato, Nathaniel Evans, and Ernest Rosato

Introduction

Over the past 10 years, minimally invasive esophagectomy has become an accepted approach to the management of esophageal and gastroesophageal benign and malignant neoplasms. There are many interpretations of the minimally invasive esophagectomy. Currently, the most frequently performed surgeries include combined thoracoscopic esophageal mobilization and laparoscopic gastric mobilization with creation of a cervical esophagogastrostomy anastomosis ("3-hole" esophagectomy); laparoscopic Ivor-Lewis technique, utilizing a laparoscopic mobilization of the stomach followed by a thoracoscopic intrathoracic esophagogastrostomy anastomosis; laparoscopic transhiatal esophagectomy, utilizing a laparoscopic mobilization of the stomach and a trans-abdominal laparoscopic mediastinal esophageal dissection, combined with a cervical esophageal blunt dissection and creation of an esophagogastrostomy anastomosis in the neck. All of these procedures are based upon previously described open surgery techniques; however, there are unique challenges faced during the laparoscopic mobilization and resection phases, which can affect patient outcome. Last, the postop management of these patients has evolved in a way that has reduced length of stay and accelerated return of GI function. Much of this is the result of the minimally invasive nature of the surgery, combined with better postoperative intensive care, and adherence to predetermined postoperative pathways which speed patient recovery, reduce length of stay, and accelerate return to normal activity. The following illustrates the common perioperative complications following esophagectomy, and the current options for their management.

D.S. Tichansky, J. Morton, and D.B. Jones (eds.), *The SAGES Manual of Quality, Outcomes and Patient Safety*, DOI 10.1007/978-1-4419-7901-8_31, © Springer Science+Business Media, LLC 2012

Preoperative Preparation

1. All patients are staged with a high definition, multislice CAT scan of the chest, abdomen, and pelvis. It is particularly important to note any vascular anomalies in the celiac axis and/or superior mesenteric artery blood supply to the stomach, duodenum, and proximal small bowel. Strictures of the celiac axis may predispose to anomalous blood supply to the gastric conduit. The stomach conduit is most frequently supplied by the right gastroepiploic artery, which is a branch of the gastroduodenal arcade. The right gastric artery supplies the lesser curve of the stomach and is often left intact as additional blood flow to the gastric conduit. Accessory and replaced left hepatic arterial branches which arise from the left gastric trunk occur in 20–25% of patients. These vascular anomalies can be managed intraoperatively by simple ligation and division with an expected transient elevation of liver enzymes. Aberrant replacement of the entire hepatic arterial inflow from the left gastric trunk is a rare anatomic variant present in approximately 1% of patients. This is best appreciated preoperatively and managed by selective dissection and preservation, or vascular bypass.

2. In cases of malignancy, patients are staged with a PET scan to rule out unexpected distant disease which may impact the operative plans.

3. Pulmonary function testing is performed in all of the patients in whom thoracoscopy is to be performed. This includes a baseline arterial blood gas, spirometry, room air saturation, and calculated diffusion capacity.

4. Patients with significant cardiac risk factors undergo preop cardiac evaluation as dictated by the American College of Cardiology/American Heart Association 2007 guidelines for perioperative cardiovascular evaluation and care for noncardiac surgery.

5. *Bowel preparation.* Because of the possibility of extension of tumors into the cardia and fundus of the stomach, which may necessitate colon interposition as an alternative replacement, we routinely bowel prep our patients with mechanical bowel preps. We have stopped utilizing antibiotic prep given the increased risk for *C. difficile* infection.

6. All patients undergo routine preadmission testing to include liver function testing, coagulation studies, CBC, and electrolytes and nutritional parameters.

7. Patients are admitted the same day as surgery.
8. If the patient has received induction chemotherapy and/or radiation therapy, we try to perform the esophagectomy approximately 6 weeks postcompletion of the radiation therapy to avoid excessive radiation-induced fibrosis of the esophagus.
9. Routine staging laparoscopy is not performed as a separate procedure for esophageal carcinomas. Selective performance of separate staging laparoscopy for tumors involving the cardia of the stomach or where there is a high suspicion of metastatic disease is performed at the surgeon's discretion. Performance of left gastric artery ligation is not carried out on a routine basis as part of the preconditioning, although there are reports which support this as a technique to improve blood supply to the planned resultant arterial arcades (right gastric and right gastroepiploic), and in an attempt to enhance collateralization in the gastric fundus.

General Considerations

1. Patient should be positioned on the bed with either beanbag or gel roll support during the thoracoscopic mobilization. Left lateral decubitus position with adequate support of the upper extremities and placement of an axillary roll to prevent axillary neuropraxia is the standard position for thoracoscopic mobilization.
2. Insufflation of CO_2 especially during the abdominal portions of the surgery can result in dissection of carbon dioxide into the mediastinum and subcutaneous spaces, which results in increasing CO_2 absorption in the blood stream and resultant acidosis. During the thoracoscopy portion, we attempt to hyperventilate the remaining lung and continuously monitor end-tidal CO_2. If the patient's acid base balance becomes problematic then addition of bicarbonate and/or temporary re-insufflation of the collapsed right lung is utilized to return the pH to normalcy. During the abdominal portions, we try not to open the hiatus of the abdomen until the end of the epigastric mobilization to prevent loss of CO_2 into the mediastinum and thus minimize both loss of CO_2 and insufflation pressure, and decrease secondary absorption of CO_2.
3. *Temperature management.* Expanding carbon dioxide utilized as the insufflation agent is a cause of hypothermia during

prolonged surgical procedures. The average operative time for a laparoscopic/thoracoscopic esophagectomy is approximately 5–7 h and during that time significant heat loss can occur. We, therefore, recommend the use of heated CO_2 tubing to raise the temperature of the insufflation gas to that of body temperature. Liberal use of heating blankets and insulating padding help minimize temperature loss as well.

4. *Fluid management.* While these cases tend to be long, the actual fluid losses during the laparoscopic surgical procedure are minimal due to the positive pressure from the CO_2 and the lack of an open incision. However, there can be a systemic inflammatory response especially following collapse and re-insufflation of the right lung, which precipitates hypotension during the surgery. We have pursued a course of fluid restriction in an attempt to prevent postoperative volume overload. The use of hypertonic saline, temporary vasopressors, and anti-inflammatory agents have been helpful in avoiding fluid overload both intra- and postoperatively. We work closely with the anesthesiology team to avoid excessive fluid administration.

5. *Airway management.* Patients are initially intubated with a single lumen tube during which time preoperative bronchoscopy and upper endoscopy are performed as final staging for the tumor. Conversion to a double lumen tube or a bronchial blocker setup is then carried out by the anesthesiologist with bronchoscopy guidance. This is always performed in consort with the surgeon to ensure that after positioning adequate lung desufflation will be achieved without airway compromise. At the completion of the thoracic portion of the surgery, the double lumen tube is changed to a single lumen and this is maintained postoperatively until the patient has awoken satisfactorily for extubation. We strive for early extubation in the OR/ICU as part of the critical pathway for early recovery.

Surgical Technique for "3-hole" MIE

Thoracoscopic Portion

The patient is placed in the left lateral decubitus position. The right chest is prepped. The following ports are typically placed: (1) at the anterior axillary line in the 8th intercostal space (10 mm port); (2) at the posterior axillary line in the 7th intercostal space (10 mm); (3) below the tip of the scapula (5 mm); (4) 4th intercostal space in the anterior axillary line (10 mm); and (5) between the 1st and the 4th ports for suction (5 mm). An Endo Stitch is placed at the tendinous portion of the right diaphragm. This is brought through the skin using a Carter-Thompson device and maintained on tension to retract the diaphragm. The dissection starts anteriorly at the pericardium. The harmonic scalpel is used to incise the pleura and separate the periesophageal fat from the pericardium. The subcarinal lymph node package is then completely removed, separating it carefully from the left and right main stem bronchi. The azygous vein is divided with an Endo GIA using a vascular load. Nodal tissue around the esophagus is dissected and brought with the specimen. The esophagus is then carefully separated from the trachea and the dissection then proceeds cephalad to the thoracic inlet. The pleura, posteriorly, is then incised anterior to the thoracic duct. The esophagus and periesophageal tissue are dissected away from the aorta; aortoesophageal branches are clipped and divided. An intercostal block with Marcaine is performed at the level of ribs 6, 7, 8, and 9, and a single chest tube is inserted.

Laparoscopy

The patient is then repositioned in the relaxed lithotomy position. A trans-umbilical approach is used for insertion of the 12-mm camera port. The remaining 5-mm ports are placed in the right lateral subcostal position and the left subcostal position. A mid-axillary 12-mm port is inserted in the right subcostal position. Using these ports, the greater curvature of the stomach is mobilized, with fastidious preservation of the gastroepiploic arcade. The short gastric vessels are divided and the fundus is mobilized. The greater omentum is divided along the gastro-epiploic arcade and the stomach is completely mobilized down to the origin of the right gastroepiploic arterial system. The lesser curve is then mobilized and the right diaphragmatic crus identified. The phreno-esophageal ligament is incised and the retrocardia space is established. The right crus is opened by incising it with the Harmonic scalpel to allow for easy placement of the conduit. At this point, the left gastric artery is divided with the endovascular GIA stapler, and the nodal tissue is swept up with the specimen. Next, the 12-mm port site is enlarged to an approximately 5-cm incision and a Lap Disk wound protector is inserted.

Neck Incision and Completion

The left neck is approached through an oblique incision paralleling the anterior border of the sternocleidomastoid. The platysma and strap muscles are divided as is the inferior thyroid artery. The left recurrent largyngeal nerve is identified and preserved throughout its course. It is important to avoid excessive retraction to prevent stretch injury to the nerve. The esophagus is then encircled and transected with a GIA-75 linear cutting stapler. The distal end of the divided esophagus is attached to a chest tube as a mediastinal placeholder and delivered with the stomach through the wound protector in the right upper quadrant small incision. The stomach is tubularized extracorporeally with a GIA-75 stapler and the suture line is oversewn with a running 3-0 PDS suture. A pyloromyotomy is also performed through this incision. The proximal tip of the stomach tube is then attached to the mediastinal chest tube placeholder and the stomach, in proper orientation, is delivered back up into the left neck, where a side-to-side esophagogastrostomy anastomosis is performed with an Endo GIA stapler. The nasogastric tube is positioned through this anastomosis. The anastomosis is then completed with a TA-60 stapler or handsewn. A tacking suture is then placed from the staple line to the prevertebral fascia to keep this anastomosis in the neck region. Alternatively, the stomach can be tubularized laparoscopically with several applications of an endo GIA stapler and an intracorporeal pyloroplasty or pyloromyotomy performed. The resected specimen is attached to the newly created gastric tube and delivered through the neck incision in proper orientation. At this point, a #14 French red rubber catheter is placed laparoscopically as a feeding jejunostomy tube.

Synopsis of Surgical Technique for Ivor-Lewis MIE

The operation is begun with the patient in relaxed lithotomy position and the laparoscopic portion is performed as above. At the completion, the conduit is placed back into the abdominal cavity in the correct orientation so that it can be delivered into the chest for the next portion. The patient is then placed in the left lateral decubitus position and VATS ports are placed as above. The dissection proceeds as previously described except for that done towards the thoracic inlet. Once the esophagus is dissected circumferentially to the level of the azygous vein, it is sharply divided at this level and removed through a slightly enlarged posterior surgeon's port (#2, above).

At this point, a 29 EEA anvil is placed inside the esophagus. An EndoStitch is used to create a pursestring to secure the anvil in the esophageal lumen. The conduit is grasped and opened so that the EEA shaft can be placed into it. The spike from the EEA is brought out from the side of the conduit and docked into the anvil. The EEA is then fired and removed. At this point, an Endo GIA blue load is used to amputate that tip of the stomach and remove it from the chest. Another EndoStitch is used to tack the stomach to the diaphragmatic crura. The intercostal nerve block and chest tube placement proceed as described earlier.

Postoperative Complications

Historically, transhiatal, transthoracic, and three-hole esophagectomy have been characterized by high mortality and a surgical morbidity that approaches 50%. This is, in part, due to the magnitude of the surgery and the comorbidities inherent in the patient population. Minimally invasive esophagectomy has not shown a significant reduction in overall morbidity and mortality in most series. Several series have shown, however, decreased percentages of serious complications as graded by the Clavien Scale and significant reductions in pulmonary complications. Minimally invasive esophagectomy has been associated with equivalent tumor resection, operative time, and lymph node harvest. The most common complications following minimally invasive esophagectomy parallel those seen in open esophagectomy.

1. The most common pulmonary complication following esophagectomy remains pneumonia. Approximately, 25% of patients will experience some type of lung consolidation requiring antibiotics and aggressive pulmonary toilet. Aspiration pneumonia especially in the early postoperative period is particularly problematic. Esophagectomy patients have lost their lower esophageal sphincter and may also have vocal cord paresis predisposing them to aspiration during swallowing. Maintenance of aspiration precautions in the early postoperative period is critical to avoid aspiration and the associated chemical pneumonitis, which can predispose to adult respiratory distress syndrome. Patients are closely monitored during their postop recovery in an ICU setting with pulse oximetry and daily chest X-ray. Patients who develop vocal cord paresis receive speech pathology evaluations with videofluoroscopy to evaluate their swallowing function and rule out silent aspiration. Routine

postop pulmonary toilet including incentive spirometry, nasotracheal suctioning, and bronchoscopy for those patients who suffer from lobar collapse are mandatory to prevent pneumonia. A laparoscopic approach usually allows for early mobilization of the patients due to decreased pain and smaller incisions.

2. *ARDS or adult respiratory distress syndrome.* The adult respiratory distress syndrome can be seen as sequelae of aspiration pneumonia, postlung re-expansion, postradiation, or associated with systemic sepsis. This occurs in approximately 5% of patients during their postoperative stay. Neoadjuvant radiation therapy can predispose to an ARDS picture secondary to lymphatic obstruction from radiation therapy. We strive to perform esophageal resections within 6 weeks of the completion of radiation therapy to ensure that this lymphatic obstruction is minimized. ARDS is managed with a standard postoperative ventilator protocol weaning oxygen and positive end expiratory pressure rapidly in an attempt to minimize barotrauma as well as oxygen toxicity. Recurrent laryngeal nerve palsy is present approximately in 10–15% of patients following cervical dissection for a cervical esophagogastrostomy anastomosis. As noted earlier, laryngeal nerve palsy can predispose to aspiration, which can produce respiratory failure and prolong both the ICU and hospital course. All patients in whom there is a suspicion of laryngeal nerve injury during the dissection are extubated over a bronchoscope to allow for evaluation of the vocal cords at the time of extubation. Patients who have paresis are evaluated by ENT and early medialization of the cords is performed to minimize vocal abnormalities. Last, these patients receive speech pathology evaluation to rule out silent aspiration prior to being advanced to a house diet.

3. *Pleural effusions.* The frequency of pleural effusion is directly related to the approach to the esophageal tumor. Pleural effusions in the right chest are uncommon given the drains placed during transthoracic procedures; however, contralateral pleural effusions can develop. Proper fluid management, diuretics, and pleural drainage control this in symptomatic patients. Pleural effusion in transhiatal esophagectomy remains a common finding postoperatively and is managed in a similar fashion. Prophylactic placement of bilateral chest tubes is often

advocated to prevent complications related to lung parenchymal compression from postoperative effusions.

4. *Esophageal stricture.* Esophageal stricture occurs in approximately 5% of intrathoracic esophagogastrostomy anastomosis and approximately 20% of cervical esophageal anastomosis. This is thought to be a function of tension and ischemia at the anastomotic line. While many surgeons prefer a hand-sewn anastomosis, the development of endoscopic stapling devices has allowed for the performance of large esophagogastric anastomosis in a side-to-side fashion. This has reduced the stricture rate in the modern era. The use of end-to-end stapling devices and the performance of anastomosis in the well-vascularized body region of the gastric conduit has also minimized stricture in the transthoracic approach.

5. *Gastric conduit ischemia.* The stomach is a richly vascularized tissue for the creation of a conduit to replace the resected esophagus. Inflow is preserved through the right gastroepiploic and often the right gastric arteries. As noted in the preoperative preparation section, high-definition CT angiography allows the surgeon to review the blood supply to the planned stomach conduit and identify any areas of vascular irregularity, which may produce ischemia in the postoperative period. The routine use of gastric conduit preconditioning either by laparoscopic division of the left gastric inflow or preoperative embolization is not routinely performed in most centers, but may be a way to enhance blood supply to the conduit prior to surgery in those patients who have marginal inflow. Anastomotic leak occurs in approximately 9% of all esophagectomies. Historically, the leak rate in the thoracic anastomotic region has been less than that seen in the cervical esophagogastrostomy. Most cervical esophagogastric leaks can be managed with simple open drainage of the wound at the bedside. Approximately, 1% of the patients will require return to the operating room for revision and/or washout of the neck anastomosis. Intrathoracic anastomoses that leak are associated with a high mortality. Early return to the operating room with thoracoscopic washout of the right pleural space and repair of the anastomotic leak with an intercostal muscle pedicle flap or pericardial fat pad covering, combined with wide drainage of the region, has reduced the mortality associated with an intrathoracic leak to less than 5% in most series. Recent small series have described

the use of covered esophageal wall stents to bridge the anastomotic leak in stable patients and facilitate control and healing of the esophago-pleural fistula.

6. *Chylothorax*. Chylothorax is a relatively rare, but devastating complication following esophagectomy. It can be due to large tumors, which involve the GE junction and necessitate resection of the thoracic duct as it travels through the aortic hiatus. The thoracic duct crosses the midline from right to left at approximately the second to third thoracic vertebrae which can predispose the duct to inadvertent injury during blunt dissection and even open transthoracic procedures. Last, dissection in the left neck can sometimes disrupt the thoracic duct as it drains into the left subclavian-innominate venous system leading to postoperative chyle leak. Diagnosis is confirmed by the presence of chylomicrons and/or lipid in the effluent from the drains. Chyle leak in the neck and abdomen is usually handled by the drains in these areas and will usually close with conservative measures consisting of TPN and/or elemental diets. Thoracic duct injury in the chest, which is under negative pressure can lead to a chylothorax. Detection of thoracic duct injuries in the early postoperative period mandates return to the operating room for thoracoscopic examination and suture ligation of the injured duct. The use of high fat or cream jejunostomy tube feeding to identify the site of leak is quite helpful intraoperatively. In those patients in whom return to the operating room is not possible due to clinical decline or intrathoracic adhesions, the performance of a lymphangiogram followed by trans-abdominal percutaneous embolization of the thoracic duct by interventional radiology can speed the closure of the chyle leak. Successful management of a chylothorax requires adequate pleural drainage to prevent pulmonary compromise, nutrition support in the form of TPN or elemental diets, and early closure or embolization of the leak to minimize long-term debilitation.

7. Cardiovascular events remain quite frequent in the minimally invasive esophagectomy patient. The most common postop cardiovascular complication is the development of an atrial arrhythmia, which occurs in approximately 35–40% of patients. Myocardial infarction is a function of the patient's preoperative cardiac risk index and remains relatively low in well-prepared

patients. Management of atrial arrhythmias includes rate control, volume monitoring, electrolyte management, and anticoagulation as needed if early conversion cannot be achieved. Management of myocardial infarctions includes supportive care and early coronary artery catheterization for those patients who have acute occlusions of a major coronary artery branch.

8. *Wound infection.* Wound infection is a minor complication affecting approximately 2% of patients in most series. The most common site for a wound infection remains the neck incision in those patients who have a cervical esophagogastrostomy anastamosis secondary to soilage at the time of the anastomosis. Neck wound infection can also be an early indicator of an anastomotic leak. Management of wound infections require opening of the wound to establish good drainage, and the use of antibiotics in those patients who develop deep space infections or cellulitis.

9. *Conduit fistulas.* Conduit fistulas can be secondary to an esophagogastric anastomotic disruption or a staple line disruption in the gastric conduit. Early suture line disruption usually presents with acute clinical decompensation and requires return to the operating room for repair and drainage. Late postoperative fistulas into the mediastinum or pleural spaces may be asymptomatic, especially if they spontaneously drain back into the esophageal conduit. Those that result in abscess formation may require percutaneous or thoracoscopic drainage as dictated by the location and symptom complex.

Summary

Minimally invasive esophagectomy offers advantages in terms of shorter length of stay, decreased blood loss, and greater patient's satisfaction. Serious morbidity may be reduced but mortality remains similar to open esophageal surgery. Further advances in technology and postop management will certainly improve the outcome in this high-risk patient population (Tables 31.1 and 31.2).

Table 31.1. Summary MIE complications.

Complication	Percent (%)
Mortality	(6.8)
Atrial arrythmias	(41)
Myocardial infarction	(0)
Pneumonia	(25)
Effusion	(2)
ARDS	(4)
Conduit necrosis	(2)
Anastomotic leak	(9)
Anastomotic stricture	(6)
Recurrrent laryngeal Nerve injury	(14)
Chylothorax	(1)
Wound infection	(4)

Table 31.2. Comparison of complications: MIE vs. open surgery.

	Minimally invasive ($n = 65$)	Open ($n = 53$)	p-value
Mortality	5 (7.7%)	4 (7.5%)	1.0
Overall complications	31 (48%)	32 (60%)	0.1
Major complications (grades 3–5)	13 (20%)	23 (41%)	0.008
Minor complications (grades 1–2)	18 (28%)	12 (23%)	0.5
Respiratory failure/ARDS	5 (7.7%)	12 (21%)	0.03
Pneumonia	5 (7.7%)	10 (18%)	0.11
Anastomotic leak	9 (14%)	6 (11%)	1.0
DVT/PE	1 (1.5%)	6 (11%)	0.04

DVT deep venous thrombosis, *PE* pulmonary embolism, *ARDS* adult respiratory distress syndrome
Source: "Oncologic Efficacy is Not Compromised, and May be Improved with Minimally Invasive Esophagectomy"

Selected Readings

1. Luketich JD, Alvelo-Rivera M, Buenaventura PO, et al. Minimally invasive esophagectomy: outcomes in 222 patients. ANN Surg. 2003;238:486–94. discussion 494–5.

2. Pham TH, Terry KA, Dolan JP, et al. Comparison of perioperative outcomes after combined thoracoscopic-laparoscopic esophagectomy and open Ivor-Lewis esophagectomy. Am J Surg. 2010;199:594–8.

3. Sgourakis G, Gockel I, Radtke A, et al. Minimally invasive versus open esophagectomy: meta-analysis of outcomes. DIG DIS SCI DOI 10.1007/s10620-010-1153-1.

4. Berger AC, Bloomenthal A, Weksler B, et al. Oncologic efficacy is not compromised, and may be improved with minimally invasive esophagectomy. JACS (in press).

32. Video-Assisted Thoracic Surgery: Complications and Management

Michael R. St. Jean

History of VATS: Since the first use of a thoracoscope by Hans Jacobaeus in the treatment of pleural adhesive disease as a result of artificial pneumothorax therapy for tuberculosis in 1910, the desire to access the hemithorax with minimal tissue damage and discomfort remained relatively unattainable until the advent of the laparoscopic revolution some 80 years later. The instrumentation and application of techniques utilized during the more common laparoscopic cholecystectomies and fundoplications saw renewed interest in a minimally invasive approach to thoracic diseases and conditions. However, there were aspects of thoracic surgery that posed initial hurdles for this burgeoning technology. The relative rigid confines of the hemithorax as opposed to the more expansible abdominal wall of laparoscopy required an adaptive approach to tackling thoracoscopic procedures. The development of specialized angular instruments, low-pressure CO_2 insufflation techniques and coordinated single lung ventilation paved the way for a greater variety of procedures which were once limited to thoracotomy to be amenable to this video-assisted technology. Nearly two decades after the explosion of laparoscopic techniques into the surgical armamentarium, there remains but a select few procedures which have not made the transformation to minimally invasive surgery.

The benefits to a thoracoscopic surgical approach to the chest are well documented and supported by similar findings with laparoscopic surgery that have been long standing [1, 2]. They are all interrelated to reduced postoperative pain, reduced immunologic compromise, a reduction in intravenous and intrathecal or epidural anesthetic which results in a more rapid return to normal activities, reduced hospital days and reduction in overall cost [3, 4]. Unfortunately, as all surgical procedures, there are associated complications, although relatively risk-reduced compared with open thoracotomy or median sternotomy; these are what we will focus on along with strategies for avoidance and management.

D.S. Tichansky, J. Morton, and D.B. Jones (eds.), *The SAGES Manual*
of Quality, Outcomes and Patient Safety, DOI 10.1007/978-1-4419-7901-8_32,
© Springer Science+Business Media, LLC 2012

Complications: Although major complications associated with video-assisted thoracoscopic surgery are rare, the most frequent complications can be categorized into persistent air leak; postoperative infection/empyema; hemorrhage; intercostal neuralgias and injury to intrathoracic or intraabdominal structures [5]. The majority of these may be minimized with an attentive, situational as well as anatomical awareness, throughout surgical dissection. Furthermore, several may be related with the simple hasty introduction to the thoracic cavity. Undisciplined dissection through the intercostals muscle layers without clear identification of tissue planes could easily result in a triad of intercostal nerve injury producing prolonged postoperative neuropathy, adjacent arterial injury producing hemorrhage control issues, as well as inadvertent visceral pleural disruption leading to persistent air leak. Predictive factors for complication risk may correlate with a cautious patient selection with regard to age, extent of planned surgery, as well as preoperative immune status [6–8]. I shall attempt to outline a strategy for prevention as well as management of the most frequent thoracoscopic complications. Emerging technologies may present opportunities for reduction or even elimination of various operative risks that will alter future management algorithms.

Persistent Air Leak

The definition of what constitutes a persistent air leak after thoracic surgery varies in as much distinction as the myriad of techniques used to treat this often recalcitrant condition. Most thoracoscopic as well as thoracic surgeons would agree that the presence of an air leak beyond 5–7 days postprocedure would qualify. The true incidence of this complication after purely thoracoscopic procedures remains low, with studies indicating a range of 1–13% [3, 6, 7]. This correlates with the proposed intent of this minimally invasive technique to minimize the degree of tissue trauma to the friable visceral pleural surface while still achieving the goal of the operation. Persistent air leak is often the result of unrecognized visceral pleural disruption related to inadequate parenchyma closure after pulmonary wedge resection or overly aggressive lysis of intrapleural adhesions. The culprit may in fact reside in the all too often hands of marginal visualization of the operative field. Insuring the appropriate placement of stapling devices on normal lung parenchyma with adequate visualization of lung surface to avoid bullae or division across fibrotic alveolar tissue precludes potential for problematic air leaks [9]. Patience in the ability to maximize the panoramic view of the thoracic cavity is paramount to surgical success with minimal adverse events. The precise coordination of surgical, anesthesia and nursing personnel will allow for the surgeon's videoscopic reference to the operative field to be optimized. The combination of proper patient positioning, single lung ventilation augmented with low flow CO_2 insufflations as needed, along with appropriate trocar location, provides the thoracoscopic surgeon with the optimum hemithorax panorama. Proper patient positioning should allow the ready application of two to three trocar insertions through the thoracic cage with adequate triangulation to avoid unnecessary and troublesome "sword fighting." Potential alternate trocar sites may be identified prior to incision in support of target lesions in the posterior mediastinum or apical regions. With the patient properly positioned, the extent of maneuverability in the thoracic cavity will be limited without single lung ventilation. Coordination with the anesthesia staff is critical to insure proper patient ventilation while maintaining an adequate degree of intrathoracic mobility. Haste is the enemy at this point. Adequate decompression of the nonventilated lung may require several minutes. An appropriately deflated lung allows for a comprehensive inspection as well as palpation of the surface for irregularities or target lesions. If this view is still insufficient to proceed with the required dissection, then the addition of low flow CO_2 insufflations may allow for additional decompression of the lung, as well as expansion of the ipsilateral hemidiaphragm augmenting visualization of the entire hemithorax. Preoperative radiologic reviews, as well as the presence of imaging studies in the operating room, allows the precise placement of instrumentation to minimize trocar incisions while optimizing access to the planned anatomical area of operation. They also offer the opportunity to identify potential aberrant structures which could pose potential roadblocks or hazards during dissection.

These techniques allow for the manipulation of lung parenchyma to be incorporated into stapling devices with decreased bulk and reduced shearing forces on the divided tissues. More precise dissection can be achieved with minimized disruption of alveolar surface. Additionally, the increased space within the hemithorax allows for greater standoff between any visceral–parietal pleural adhesions to be divided closer to the thoracic cage, thereby reducing the risk of visceral pleural violation. In recent years, the armamentarium of the surgeon for dealing with this issue has expanded significantly. The addition of buttressing strips to stapling devices has resulted in reports of increased control of air leaks with reduction in duration postoperatively [10]. These bovine pericardium Peri-strips Dry (Biovascular/Synovis Surgical Innovations, St. Paul, MN) strips act to increase fibrosis along the staple line. Alternatively, Seamguard Bioabsorbable (WL Gore & Associates, Flagstaff, AZ) provides a scaffolding for the deposition of Type I collagen by incorporating a biocompatible copolymer of a polyglycolic acid–trimethylene carbonate and is advertised to decrease air leaks as well as staple line bleeding. Their use during stapled division of incomplete fissures or nonanatomic wedge resections has shown to statistically decrease duration of postoperative air leaks. Consequently, incorporation of these buttressing devices has been shown to reduce the duration of air leak as well as subsequent chest tube drainage time. The additions of the buttressing materials as collagen extracellular matrix allows for increased fibrosis, resulting in greater tolerance to bursting strength. Their utilization in gastrointestinal procedures with reductions in staple line leakage during bariatric procedures spawned further applications to thoracic and lung volume reduction procedures [10, 11]. Another implement is the addition of a topical tissue adhesive. The use of agents such as Tisseel (Baxter International, Inc., Deerfield, IL) or other fibrin glue adhesive mixture combinations to cover areas of staple lines or visceral pleural disruptions have gained popularity. The use of various application techniques with fibrinogen in combination with thrombin and vicryl mesh as a substrate on areas of alveolar air leakage in porcine models has shown promise [12]. The exact timing and combination of sealants to provide optimum tissue level repair in human patients remains under dispute pending further clinical investigation.

It must be stressed that the implementation of these techniques or materials serves only as a companion to meticulous surgical dissection including instrument awareness. The inability to focus on the area of surgical dissection while maintaining spatial awareness of both hands' instruments invariably leads to inadvertent tissue insult. Areas of dissections should be manipulated gently, if not minimally, with atraumatic instruments or the use of the surgeon's fingers through trocar access sites. At the conclusion of the dissection, gradual ventilation of the ipsilateral lung through coordination with the anesthesia team combined with gentle saline irrigation may allow for identification of minor visceral disruptions and potential sites for air leak. The use of staple buttressing materials or tissue adhesives over traumatized lung parenchyma surfaces may be applied based upon our above review and surgeon preference. If there is no evidence of visceral pleural insult, or the dissection did not involve the lung parenchyma, then tube thoracostomy may be avoided in select cases with suctioning of pleural space by silicone catheter timed with a maximal inspiratory delivery. However, the majority of cases will require the utilization of at least one tube thoracostomy. In cases with minimal bleeding and limited dissection, the use of smaller 24–32fr tubes is usually sufficient. Proper tube placement may be equally important to the prevention or potential management of a persistent air leak. Therefore, delegating this minor task to the least experienced member of the surgical team should be avoided and attention paid to proper positioning. Apical placement of the tube tip is important for adequate relief of potential pneumothorax but so is avoidance of locating fenestrations over areas of identified air leak or visceral pleural injury. This could result in an inordinately prolonged air leak or formation of a bronchopleural fistula in rare cases. Ideally, the chest tubes will be removed by standard criteria: drainage is less than 200 ml/24 h; no evidence of air leak and a properly expanded lung field revealed by chest radiograph. If an air leak persists for greater than 5 days, rarely is repeat surgical intervention warranted unless the original procedure indication was recurrent pneumothorax. First, insure that the tube thoracostomy system is intact, including the drainage device, and that the tube has not migrated. Second, attempt a minor manipulation of the chest tube to dislodge any potential adhesions over parenchyma air leaks and observe for decrease in flow over the next 24 h. Third, if the leak is associated with a persistent pneumothorax, consider computerized tomography or fluoroscopic guided placement of an additional thoracic catheter. The optimum use of water seal suction in preference to wall suction, even in circumstances of small residual pneumothorax, has gained clinical favor to mitigate prolongation of alveolar-air leakage [13]. For recalcitrant air leaks, the literature has recently demonstrated the use of image guided delivery of tissue adhesives to be an effective option [14]. In the face of persistent air leak, chemical pleurodesis represents a low probability of success. The use of a talc slurry or vaporized talc is the recommended derivative. The use of Doxycycline as a chemical pleurodesis agent is fraught with painful side effects often warranting significant narcotic premedication or dosing that may impair respiratory therapy.

Infection and Empyema

Unless dealing with a preexisting pulmonary infectious process, the majority of VATS procedures would be categorized as clean surgical cases and as such have a relatively low incidence of postoperative infectious complications when adhering to prophylactic antibiotic regimens. Rovera et al. demonstrated an overall surgical site infection rate of 1.7% in a series of 346 consecutive patients undergoing various thoracoscopic procedures [15]. Antibiotic prophylaxis compliance was above 90% in the study population. The only predictor of increased incidence of surgical site infection was a FEV1 of <70% of predicted ($p < 0.05$). The incidence of pneumonia was 3% in the VATS procedure group. This data correlates well with more recent studies by Solaini and Winter, demonstrating similar rates with positive predictors related to patient age, surgical extent and patient preoperative immune status [6, 8].

The use of preoperative prophylactic antibiotic dosing, as well as a practice of early physiotherapy and ambulation postoperatively, along with adequate pain control, were hallmarks to both of the above studies. Adherence to patient selection criteria to optimize preoperative physiologic conditioning may be warranted in selected patients. Minimally invasive principles which advocate smaller as well as fewer incisions provide an appreciable decrease in surgical site volume to act as nidus for postoperative infections. Similarly, the adaptation of tissue handling oncologic principles to the thoracoscopic arena from lessons learned in laparoscopic colorectal cancer resections have witnessed greater utilization of endoscopically designed specimen retrieval devices. The end result is a reduction in the exposure of potential respiratory tract pathogens to port sites while maintaining positive control of the oncologic specimen.

Since the incidence of postoperative surgical infections after VATS is relatively low, the occurrence of post-VATS empyema is rare. However, the use of this modality in the treatment for reclamation of the pleural space with concurrent evacuation of infectious fluid collections as a primary therapy for empyema management is gaining acceptance. Early intervention with disruption of all pleural adhesions, elimination of potentially infected inflammatory tissue and reestablishment of normal inspiratory volume mechanics is routinely performed thoracoscopically. Rarely the need for a minithoracotomy to free a trapped segment or loculation is augmented through an appropriate extension of a port site. Standard removal criteria for postoperative tube drainage should be adhered to and catheters extracted at the earliest opportunity.

Hemorrhage

In researching this chapter, the most common cause or reason offered for conversion of thoracoscopic procedures to thoracotomy regardless of size was hemorrhage followed by a close second of what is termed thoracoscopic failure to complete the procedure [16]. The conversion of a purely VATS procedure to a small anterior lateral thoracotomy or minithoracotomy extension of port site should not in my opinion be considered a technical failure. Rather a demonstration of sound surgical judgment. Hemorrhage from VATS procedures is a rare occurrence with only slightly higher rates reported in thoracoscopic lung lobectomies or formal resections [3]. The exponential improvement in intracorporeal suturing techniques, along with the above-mentioned staple line buttressing materials and extensive array of ligaclip application devices, provides the modern surgeon with a myriad of tools to adequately control all but the most voluminous of operative bleeding sites. Special circumstances do exist with regard to VATS that may augment the surgeon's efforts for hemostasis. An experienced surgical team with the appropriate applicable dedicated instruments should be available for all thoracoscopic cases. A variety of angulated thoracoscopes will allow for proper visualization of bleeding sites in the posterior apex or along the margins of the diaphragm and thoracic wall. Now it is not the time to discover that your VATS lobectomy set is in fact a laparoscopic cholecystectomy tray with a 0° endoscope.

For minor surface hemorrhages, application on dry sponge and gentle pressure or possible topical application of fibrin or thrombin soaked products may suffice. The use of human fibrinogen concentrates such as Tisseel (Fibrin Sealant, Baxter International Inc., Deerfield, IL) as adjuncts to sealing superficial bleeding sites is a prime example. With larger bleeding sites, maintaining proper visualization and rapid control are paramount to preventing accumulating blood from absorbing available light in the chest cavity. Angulated atraumatic clamps are specifically designed for the limited mobility of the chest wall and can be introduced through port sites in the chest wall to obtain hemostatic control or traction to deliver the area of concern into proper view for repair. Similarly, these clamps can provide a means to apply direct sponge stick pressure on otherwise inaccessible areas, thereby allowing time for added exposure or instrumentation as necessary. In the case of inadvertent injury to the central hilum, great vessels or pericardium, only the most skilled of thoracoscopic surgeons may be comfortable approaching such an injury without at least a minithoracotomy for added dexterity, tactile feedback and improved visualization of the area. More commonly, the bleeding sites to be encountered will consist of a persistent intercostal vessel bleed related to a laceration or an apical staple line bleed. The latter can usually be managed with an additional vascular staple load or figure of eight suture ligation. Ask one of your trauma colleagues about bleeding intercostals and invariably they will relate a tale of protracted chest tube bleeding resulting in eventual thoracotomy only to discover the source an intercostal injury adjacent to fracture or penetrating wound. Since the arterial flow through the vessel is sourced through the internal mammary anteriorly as well as the aorta from the posterior, there often exists two hemorrhage sites. These tend to retract within the intercostals musculature, further frustrating control attempts. If the bleeding is originating from a trocar site, then application of digital pressure may allow the placement of ligaclips from an alternate port. Alternatively, the use of a Foley catheter with a 30-cc balloon filled with saline and retracted against the chest wall may control small venous bleeding or temporarily allow control for suture ligature. The use of an open technique for entry into the chest cavity while placing trocars should minimize such injuries by allowing direct visualization of the superior rib surface to concentrate on separation of the muscle fibers from this surface of the interface. Additionally, the utilization of bladeless endoscope viewing trocars such as Endopath Xcel (Ethicon Endo-Surgery, Inc., Cincinnati, OH) optical tips allow layer by layer tissue examination through the videoscope separating the tissues while allowing the surgeon to orient entry to the chest cavity safely.

Intercostal Nerve Injury and Neuralgia

Historically, the standard posterior lateral thoracotomy incision garners the dubious distinction of the most painful surgical incision. Following in the wake of the laparoscopic evolution and expansion, the implementation of advanced thoracoscopic techniques have significantly expanded the scope of eligible procedures to this approach. Accordingly, as referenced previously, the same advantages of decreased pain, hospital length of stay and return to normal activities propelled VATS beyond the traditional thoracotomy. The standard approach for the majority of VATS procedures entails an initial array of three trocar sites 5–12 mm in size. Initial port placement is usually centered in the mid axillary line at the seventh or eighth intercostals space. Additional trocars are inserted under direct visualization through the videoscope at the initial entry site. Allowing the incision site and subsequent chest cavity entry to be centered over the intercostal space affords the surgeon with circumferential mobility of the instruments while minimizing torque or leveraging on the superior nerve bundle. Specific trocar designs have developed to reduce the incidence of intercostals nerve trauma. Oblong ports such as the Snowden-Pencer Thora-port (Cardinal Health, Dublin, OH) are designed to allow simultaneous use of multiple instruments while minimizing forces against the rib surfaces through orientation parallel to the rib curvature. Alternatively, the use of ports or trocars themselves may be obviated for introduction of an instrument or stapling device that may capable of functioning without the added diameter trocar impinging on surrounding structures. Angulated atraumatic tissue graspers or sponge clamps are usually reusable and offer a more ergonomic alternative to longer disposable instruments devised for the larger abdominal cavity. The implantations of these techniques are goal oriented to minimize potential nerve injury as well as possible inadvertent rib fractures that will contribute to the patient's postoperative pain and recovery. Prophylactic injection of trocar sites with paracostal infiltration of a long acting local anesthetic such as Bupivacaine may offer the patient several hours of analgesia. Care must be taken to avoid inadvertent vascular injury or injection to the corresponding arteries and veins.

Postoperatively, if the patient should manifest signs and symptoms of neuropathic chronic pain corresponding to a trocar or port site then prompt enlistment of a Pain Management specialist may offer the patient an algorithmic approach to resolution and or treatment. Radiofrequency as well as cryoablation therapies for such neuropathic symptoms may provide prompt relief rather than repeated oral narcotic analgesic dosing fraught with risk. Recent literature suggests that the incidence of true intercostals neuralgia may be masked by visceral pain pathways. Meegers et al. in a review of a group of patients who underwent thoracic surgery including VATS as well as thoracotomy found that less of the chronic pain sufferers demonstrated a clear neuropathic etiology. Although the prevalence of chronic pain patients was higher in the VATS cohort (47 vs. 40%), this was not a significant predictor of chronic pain. Younger age, radiotherapy exposure, performance of pleurectomy and more extensive surgery were all statistically significant predictors of postoperative chronic pain [17].

Discussion and Future Directions

The evolution of thoracoscopic surgery over the past two decades has seen the implementation of the minimally invasive techniques to the most complex of thoracic surgeries from esophagectomies to pneumonec-tomies. Despite the additional complexity of these procedures, the benefits of thoracoscopy continue to propel this modality into further subspecialty areas. Orthopedic, neurosurgical and vascular surgeons are utilizing the capabilities of HD (high definition) video clarity, minimized incisions and reduced analgesic requirements to added patient benefit. More recently, the method of single incision laparoscopic surgery (SILS) may precede adaptation to the thoracic surgery arena. Minimally invasive valve replacement is already becoming standard in the cardiovascular specialty. The use of single thoracic trocars as access to simple thoracoscopic procedures will continue to broaden the candidate pool for which numerous modalities may be employed. Thoracentesis may be replaced by thoracoscopic directed pleural biopsy at the bedside. Transesophageal access to the mediastianal and pleural cavities for biopsy of hilar lymphadenopathy or other pathology has developed as an extension of Natural Orifice Translumenal Surgery (NOTES). The development of Full HD video camera/scope combinations allows greater panoramic range while emulating three-dimensional views to enhance surgical accuracy of dissection (Karl Storz, Tuttlingen, Germany). All of these advances serve to augment the surgeon's capabilities in delivery of the optimum care with minimal morbidity. The applicable patient population for thoracoscopic surgery like the specialty continues to evolve as referenced in this review. From pediatric to geriatric, the age boundaries remain fluid. Despite the expansion of scope for which VATS may be applied, it is the surgeon's duty to remain focused on the optimal patient safety and minimal procedural morbidity. The careful use of patient selection, meticulous video guided dissection with judicious attention to oncologic principles will serve the novice thoracoscopic surgeon well.

Selected Readings

1. Kaiser LR. Video-assisted thoracic surgery. Current state of the art. Ann Surg. 1994;220:720–34.
2. Landreneau RJ et al. Postoperative pain-related morbidity: video-assisted surgery versus thoracotomy. Ann Thorac Surg. 1993;56:1285–9.
3. Villamizar NR et al. Thoracoscopic lobectomy is associated with lower morbidity compared with thoracotomy. J Thorac Cardiovasc Surg. 2009;138(2):419–25.
4. Schuchert MJ et al. Anatomic segmentectomy for stage I non-small-cell lung cancer: comparison of video-assisted thoracic surgery versus open approach. J Thorac Cardiovasc Surg. 2009;138(6):1318–25.
5. Imperatori A et al. Peri-operative complications of video-assisted thoracoscopic survey (VATS). Int J Surg. 2008;6 Suppl 1:78–81.

6. Solaini L et al. Video-assisted thoracic surgery (VATS) of the lung: analysis of intraoperative and postoperative complications over 15 years and review of the literature. Surg Endosc. 2008;22(2):298–310.

7. Mun M et al. Video-assisted thoracic surgery for clinical stage I lung cancer in octogenarians. Ann Thorac Surg. 2008;85(2):406–11.

8. Winter H et al. Predictors of general complications after video-assisted thoracoscopic surgical procedures. Surg Endosc. 2008;22(3):640–5.

9. Haraguchi S et al. Postoperative recurrences of pneumothorax in video-assisted thoracoscopic surgery for primary spontaneous pneumothorax in young patients. J Nippon Med Sch. 2008;75(2):91–5.

10. Stammberger U et al. Buttressing the staple line in lung volume reduction surgery: a randomized three center study. Ann Thorac Surg. 2000;70(6):1820–5.

11. Mery CM et al. Profiling surgical staplers: effect of staple height, buttress and overlap on staple line failure. Surg Obes Relat Dis. 2008;4(3):416–22.

12. Itano H et al. The optimal technique for combined application of fibrin sealant and bioabsorbable felt against alveolar leakage. Eur J Cardiothorac Surg. 2008;33(3):457–60.

13. Cerfolio RJ. Recent advances in the treatment of air leaks. Curr Opin Pulm Med. 2005;11(4):319–23.

14. Carillo EH et al. Thoracoscopic application of a topical sealant for the management of persistent post traumatic pneumothorax. J Trauma. 2006;60(1):111.

15. Rovera F et al. Infections in 346 consecutive video-assisted thoracoscopic procedures. Surg Infect. 2003;4(1):45–51.

16. Koren JP et al. Major thoracic surgery in octogenarians: the video-assisted thoracic surgery (VATS) approach. Surg Endosc. 2003;17(4):632–5.

17. Steegers MA et al. Only half of the chronic pain after thoracic surgery shows neuropathic component. J Pain. 2008;9(10):955–61.

33. Robotic Surgical Outcomes and Safety

Bryan J. Sandler and Santiago Horgan

Minimally invasive surgery has ushered in many new advances within the field of surgery since its introduction two and a half decades ago. This evolution has dramatically improved hospital length of stay, improved postoperative pain, cosmesis, overall physiologic insult of surgery, and shortened time to return of physical activity when compared with conventional open surgical procedures. Improved imaging, instrumentation, and skills training within this field even led to the development of surgical robotics, microsurgery, and extension into surgical endoscopy via natural orifice surgery.

The driving forces behind these advances are multi-factorial, including patient, physician, and industry concerns, and have altered surgical training significantly. Laparoscopic skill acquisition has become a focus of surgical education and training as more focus on minimally invasive techniques has become commonplace. As this process has evolved, the reliance upon standard laparoscopic instrumentation has demonstrated limitations and led to the development of new surgical tools such as ultrasonic shears and coagulators, suture devices, and endoscopic stapling devices. Despite these advances, the limitations of depth perception, rigid instrumentation, limited ability to work within anatomically confined space, reliance upon trained operative assistants, and increasingly complex ergonomics remain significant challenges.

Technological advancement in the field of surgical robotics has attempted to address several of these limitations. While a number of robotic surgery devices have been developed, such as the Automated Endoscopic System for Optimal Positioning (AESOP; Computer Motion, Santa Barbara, CA), the Zeus Surgical System (Computer Motion), and the da Vinci Surgical System (Intuitive Surgical, Sunnyvale, CA), the da Vinci Surgical System (dVSS) is currently the only U.S. Food and Drug

D.S. Tichansky, J. Morton, and D.B. Jones (eds.), *The SAGES Manual of Quality, Outcomes and Patient Safety*, DOI 10.1007/978-1-4419-7901-8_33, © Springer Science+Business Media, LLC 2012

Administration approved telerobotic surgical system available in the market. This system has current applications within a wide variety of surgical fields, including general, urology, gynecology, hepatobiliary, colorectal, otolaryngology, and cardiothoracic surgery.

Computer-Assisted Surgical System

The dVSS, as previously stated, is the only FDA approved commercially available robotic surgical system currently available. The term "robotic" system is a bit misleading, when applied to the dVSS, as this implies a level of "intelligence" that is independent of the operating surgeon. This system lacks adaptability that is often necessary in a surgical situation, and instead relies upon the interpretation of the operator to adequately assess and respond to changes in the surgical field. Telepresence in surgery is the remote operation of a robot to perform a surgical procedure. Within this context, the dVSS is more accurately described as a computed-assisted telemanipulator, where the surgeon sits at a remote console and controls the surgical instrumentation that is in direct contact with the patient.

The da Vinci Surgical System consists of three components: a surgeon control console, a tower with video and insufflation electronics, and a patient-side chassis with three or four arms on which the operative instruments and videoscope are mounted. The surgeon console is an ergonomically designed interface with the hands and feet in a comfortable position located below the eyes, which peer down into the operative field image. The surgeon's hands control the end-effector instruments, which are interchanged on the patient-cart side by the operative assistant, and an image of these instruments are projected in the operative field within the surgical console. The camera position is manipulated through the hand controls when a foot-pedal is depressed on the surgeon console. Magnification is possible, an important feature, as the loss of haptic feedback must be countered by accurate interpretation of visual cues. The visual magnification is matched by hand-motion scaling, allowing increased surgical precision and fine or very fine motor control by scaling down the surgeon's hand motion to match the scale of the camera image.

Safety Advantages and Disadvantages

The robotic platform has several computer-aided advantages over traditional laparoscopic surgical approaches. These improvements help address several patient and procedural-related challenges posed with advanced laparoscopy.

Imaging

Improved imaging and visualization with a high-resolution, three-dimensional reproduction of the operative field through the utilization of a dual-lens, multi-chip digital camera is superior to that seen with standard laparoscopic imaging. The adjustable magnification and direct surgeon control of the camera eliminates the need for a trained surgical assistant often required in the operative field with laparoscopy. Assistant fatigue or distraction, the result of an independent operative assistant who is responsible for adequate imaging of the surgical field, is eliminated, as the primary surgeon controls the focal point of the endoscopic image.

Motion

Improved motion characteristics are a benefit of using the dVSS due to several computer-enhanced functions of the surgical tools. The movement of the surgical instrumentation is more representative of a surgeon's natural wrist movement because of tremor filtration, motion scaling, and advanced instrument articulation seen with the dVSS. Each instrument has 7° of motion freedom, which results in improved operative dexterity and the ability to operate within anatomically challenging spaces when compared with traditional laparoscopy. This allows for technically challenging tasks such as suturing, delicate dissection, and even choreographed and coordinated manipulation of a moving target, such as stable visualization, resection, and suturing of a beating heart within the closed chest cavity. Additionally, the dVSS console is designed to improve surgeon ergonomics and help address fatigue often encountered with advanced laparoscopic surgical procedures.

Cost and Storage

While there are significant advantages to using the dVSS when compared with traditional laparoscopy, there are several limitations to this system. These surgical systems are quite costly, with an estimated cost of approximately $1.75 million US dollars for the da Vinci S-system in 2009. The instrument has a large surgical footprint, requiring significant space to store. This often requires a specially designed operative suite, with additional space to accommodate the surgeon's console, the patient-side cart, and the video tower. Remote surgeon-console use has been described outside of the USA but is currently not approved by the FDA.

Limited Patient Positioning and Access

In addition to the large surgical footprint of the dVSS, the functional impact to the surgical field is a substantial concern that must be anticipated. When the dVSS is "docked" to a patient for an operative procedure, the patient positioning is relatively fixed so as to avoid inadvertent injury during instrument manipulation. This fixed patient position also makes changing the operative field of focus difficult and inefficient when compared with traditional laparoscopy. The patient-side cart also restricts access to the patient, limiting anesthesia and nursing contact with the patient during the procedure (Fig. 33.1). This may pose a significant problem when intra-operative problems, such as pneumothorax or hypotension, require swift access to the thoracic cavity, for instance during robotic foregut procedures. The limited access also makes intra-operative endoscopy challenging, as access to either the mouth or the perineum is often difficult with the patient-side cart in place.

Operative Assistant Dependence

As the surgeon sits at a console that is remote from the sterile operative field, there are consequences of this arrangement that require team preparation and a well-trained surgical assistant within the operative field. Some loss of direct surgeon access to the operative field is also a

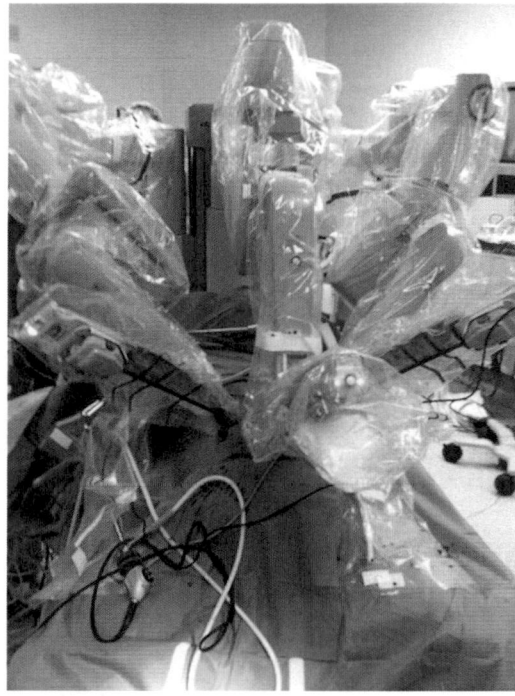

Fig. 33.1. An example of limited access in intra-operative endoscopy.

limitation when intra-operative bleeding is encountered as the lack of a surgeon-controlled suction/irrigation device mandates dependence upon the operative assistant. This dependence is amplified as the surgeon relies upon the assistant for suctioning, while often also waiting for the assistant for instrument exchange or clip applier introduction. The loss of tactile feedback can result in tissue injury as well as suture fracture, which require significant surgeon training and experience to avoid. Lastly, with the focused magnification and fixed arm positions, shifting surgical focus into a new area or even moving to a new quadrant within the abdomen requires removal of all instruments and camera so repositioning can occur without patient injury, again a coordinated function of the surgical team and on-field operative assistant.

Minimally Invasive Robotic Mentoring

The dVSS has several features that allow for supervision and proctoring during complex surgical procedures. The most simple is the touch-screen feature, allowing drawing between the on-field screen and the surgeon-console, a feature that helps with intra-operative novice surgeon training and demonstration. The addition of computer-aided skills simulation programs for the da Vinci Si System also allows for safe learning environments for novice robotic surgeons without the added pressure and time constraint of intra-operative teaching. Lastly, the addition of the da Vinci Si System Dual Console (Fig. 33.2) provides real-time proctoring through the same three-dimensional surgical view and telemanipulation shared between the primary and mentor surgeon during a surgical procedure. These features each contribute significantly to the safe training and improved skills acquisition of novice robotic surgeons while maintaining patient-safety.

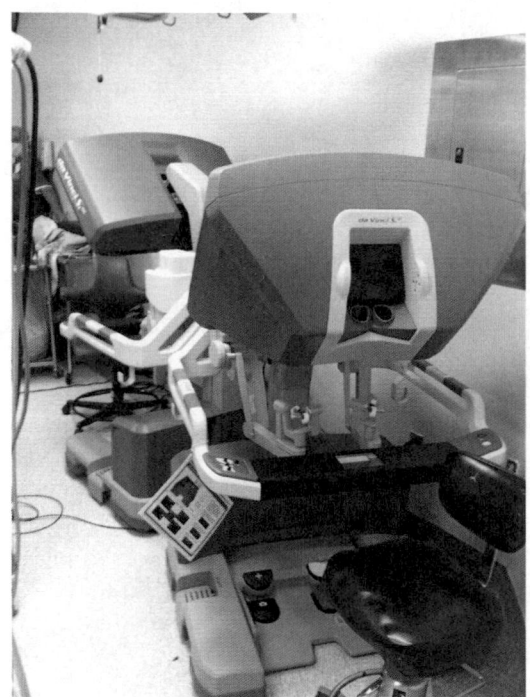

Fig. 33.2. The da Vinci Si System Dual Console.

Robotic Surgical Outcomes

General Surgery

Current applications of the dVSS within general surgery include many adaptations from advanced laparoscopic techniques. Foregut surgical procedures, such as fundoplication, esophageal surgery, as well as gastric bypass, and many colorectal and even liver resections or transplantation procedures have been described.

Fundoplication

Several randomized and nonrandomized trials have examined the use of the dVSS for robotic-assisted fundoplication and compared this with conventional laparoscopic surgery. Morino et al. showed equivalent clinical results between robotic-assisted fundoplication and conventional laparoscopic fundoplication in a series of 50 randomized patients. Significant differences were seen in operative times and total hospital costs, while short-term reflux measures, including Demeester scores, pH values, and incidence of dysphagia were equivalent. As more instrumentation becomes available and with increased use of the fourth-arm on the dVSS, less dependence upon a surgical assistant is necessary. The addition of the robotic ultrasonic dissector has provided greater independence for the primary surgeon. Despite these advances, robotic fundoplication, whether done as a Nissen, a Dor, or another type, all seem to take significantly longer with use of the robot and also comes with added cost to the surgical procedure, without measurable improvements in anti-reflux surgical outcomes.

Achalasia Surgery

Heller myotomy has been performed using the dVSS for the past 10 years. Like other robotic-assisted surgical procedures, Horgan et al. demonstrated that there appears to be a steep learning curve associated with this procedure. Use of the dVSS is associated with a lower esophageal perforation rate, when compared with a conventional laparoscopic Heller myotomy. Reasons for this include better visualization with the three-dimensional view provided by the dVSS, allowing for greater surgical precision, along with tremor elimination and greater freedom of motion, provided by the wristed instruments of the dVSS. Quality of life after Heller myotomy also appears to be consistently improved following robotic Heller myotomy, an additional benefit over conventional laparoscopic myotomy. Overall, Heller myotomy performed using the dVSS appears to be associated with a lower esophageal perforation rate and a better quality of life following surgery, a finding that appears to be consistent in the literature.

Esophageal Surgery

Use of the dVSS for esophageal resection has been retrospectively compared with both open and laparoscopic esophageal resection and appear to have similar overall oncologic outcomes. The introduction of the robot for this surgical application is certainly in its infancy, with very small numbers found in trials comparing these methods. Despite the small volume of published data on this use, a recent meta-analysis by Clark et al. shows improved ICU length of stay, estimated blood loss, and lymph node retrieval after robotic-assisted esophageal resection with a similar hospital length of stay when compared with laparoscopic resection. Most interesting in this paper is the similar overall operative time between robotic-assisted resection versus conventional laparoscopic resection, a parameter that may improve with additional robotic experience. Overall, the use of the dVSS seems to be associated with equivalent oncologic outcomes at this time, but with the spread of its use for this application, increasing familiarity with the device, and better technology, patient outcomes may improve significantly when used for esophageal resection.

Gastric Bypass

Roux-en-Y gastric bypass is a technically demanding laparoscopic operation that requires extensive bowel manipulation and ability to perform technically challenging intra-corporeal bowel anastomoses. While many surgeons prefer a laparoscopic approach for this operation with its reduced patient morbidity in this high-risk population, several have described the use of the dVSS for multiple steps of this procedure. Some of the limitations of conventional laparoscopy encountered include limited visualization given the thick abdominal wall or hepatomegaly, loss of adequate dexterity with standard laparoscopic instruments, and increased surgeon fatigue during these technically challenging procedures. Most commonly, the gastro-jejunal anastomosis is constructed with the use of the dVSS, which allows for better visualization of this critical anastomosis in an obese patient. This is often a hybrid-type operation, with the first portion performed laparoscopically, creating the Roux-en-Y limb. Many then use the dVSS for the second stage of the operation, completing the jejuno-jejunostomy and performing the gastro-jejunostomy as well. Snyder et al. described this technique and showed lower gastrointestinal leak rate for their robotic-assisted RYGB technique compared with their traditional laparoscopic RYGB. Ayloo et al. demonstrated, in their single-surgeon series, that there is a learning curve when establishing a robotic-assisted RYGB program, which was approximately 30 cases, after which their operative times were significantly shorter when using the dVSS for the gastro-jejunal anastomosis. Overall, robotic-assisted RYGB appears to be safe and effective, and in some series, is associated with a lower gastrointestinal leak rate, than that seen with traditional laparoscopic RYGB.

Colorectal Surgery

Use of the dVSS has been described for several disease processes involving the colon and rectum, both benign and malignant. Resection of the right, left, and sigmoid colon resection have been described in the literature for benign and malignant colorectal diseases. Anterior rectal resections, with complete mesorectal resections have also been attempted with the dVSS for the treatment of rectal cancer. Maseo et al. performed a meta-analysis of several published series examining the efficacy of the dVSS in several abdominal operations, including colorectal resections. A similar length of stay, complication number, estimated blood loss was found between robotic-assisted colorectal resection and conventional laparoscopic resection, although total operative time and total operative costs were found to be higher in the dVSS colorectal resection studies.

Solid Organ Surgery

Minimally invasive solid-organ surgery is an expanding field of interest, but has been slow to evolve, when compared with other abdominal procedures, given the relative lower incidence of solid organ pathologies. Robotic-assisted adrenal, spleen, pancreatic, and renal resections have been described in the literature with similar outcomes as those seen with conventional laparoscopic resection, but often with a trend toward higher procedural costs and longer operative length.

One emerging application for dVSS in solid organ surgery is that of living donor nephrectomy for renal transplantation. Avoidance of target organ injury, with adequate vascular and ureteral resection margins is critical in this group of patients undergoing elective donor nephrectomy. The superior visualization provided by the dVSS, along with the improved instrument dexterity allows for this operation to be completed safely, with similar estimated blood loss, operative time, length of stay, and warm ischemia time as seen with conventional laparoscopic donor nephrectomy.

Head and Neck Surgery

Minimally invasive approaches to cervical disease have been developed, reducing the size of neck incisions and providing remote access to the thyroid gland through a gasless axillary approach. Several extra-cervical approaches have been developed that may eliminate the neck incision entirely. These techniques are challenging and technically very difficult to complete. As a result, the dVSS has been applied to this technique, allowing better visualization in three dimensions, better range of motion of instrument tips, and the other benefits of robotic-assisted minimally invasive surgical techniques. The largest series of minimally invasive thyroid surgical techniques comes from Kang et al. in Korea, where a gasless, transaxillary robotic-assisted thyroid surgery has been proven safe and feasible. This is a gasless technique, performed through an axillary incision, which reproduces a view similar to that seen with an open surgical approach to the thyroid. Several other approaches have been described: transcervical, anterior chest wall, breast, and axillary approaches. Each allows remote access to the thyroid or parathyroid glands in the neck through a sub-platysmal plane. Oncologic outcomes have not yet been established, however central lymph node dissection has been described through this remote access technique. As with most new techniques, operative times are significantly longer with the robotic-assisted remote approach to the neck, but the technique shows promise.

Conclusions

Robotic surgical applications will continue to grow as the technology improves. The addition of haptics as well as greater primary surgeon independence through the addition of other instrumentation will allow for more comfort and easier transition from open surgical techniques into a robotic approach. The motion and visual aspects of the current system are impressive, but as technology advances, the size, ease of use, and overall footprint will continue to improve. This will allow the technology to become adapted by a wider range of surgeons and allow its spread to other fields, including crossover into endoscopy and, eventually, into natural orifice surgery. Device size and function will eventually become so small and easy to use that endoluminal and transluminal applications will allow for the use of surgical robotics in a bedside setting under minimal sedation. The image quality will continue to grow through camera and monitor improvement and the three-dimensional integration become so imperceptible that surgeons will feel that true virtual reality surgery will be possible. The addition of CT- or ultrasound-based patient data integration into an image may allow for virtual vision of deep tissue structures in three dimensions, helping to avoid critical structures, not visible on the surface of the operative field. Computer technology will continue to evolve and allow greater development of the robotic telepresence in surgery, allowing significant expansion of our current surgical capabilities.

Selected Readings

1. Ayloo SM, Addeo P, Buchs NC, Shah G, Giulianotti PC. Robot-assisted versus laparoscopic Roux-en-Y gastric bypass: is there a difference in outcomes? World J Surg. 2011;35(3):637–42.
2. Clark J, Sodergren MH, Purkayastha S, Mayer EK, James D, Athanasiou T, Yang GZ, Darzi A. The role of robotic assisted laparoscopy for oesophagogastric oncological resection; an appraisal of the literature. Dis Esophagus. 2011;24(4):240–50.
3. Horgan S, Galvani C, Gorodner MV, Omelanczuck P, Elli F, Moser F, et al. Robotic-assisted Heller myotomy versus laparoscopic Heller myotomy for the treatment of esophageal achalasia: multicenter study. J Gastrointest Surg. 2005;9(8):1020–9.
4. Huffmanm LC, Pandalai PK, Boulton BJ, James L, Starnes SL, Reed MF, et al. Robotic Heller myotomy: a safe operation with higher postoperative quality-of-life indices. Surgery. 2007;142(4):613–8.

5. Kang SW, Jeong JJ, Yun JS, Sung TY, Lee SC, Lee YS, Nam KH, Chang HS, Chung WY, Park CS. Robot-assisted endoscopic surgery for thyroid cancer: experience with the first 100 patients. Surg Endosc. 2009;23(11):399–406. Epub 2009 Mar 5.

6. Maeso S, Reza M, Mayol JA, Blasco JA, Guerra M, Andradas E, et al. Efficacy of the Da Vinci surgical system in abdominal surgery compared with that of laparoscopy: a systematic review and meta-analysis. Ann Surg. 2010;252(2):254–62.

7. Morino TM, Pellegrino L, Giaccone C, Garrone C, Rebecchi F. Randomized clinical trial of robot-assisted versus laparoscopic Nissen fundoplication. Br J Surg. 2006;93(5): 553–8.

8. Snyder BE, Wilson T, Leong BY, Klein C, Wilson EB. Robotic-assisted Roux-en-Y Gastric bypass: minimizing morbidity and mortality. Obes Surg. 2010;20(3):265–70. Epub 2009 Nov 3.

34. Complications in Single-Incision Laparoscopic Surgery

Homero Rivas

Introduction

Laparoscopic surgery, and other minimally invasive techniques, continues to revolutionize how surgery is being performed, particularly compared to the historically crude practices prior to twentieth century surgery. What is even more exciting is that laparoscopic innovations are evolving the mindset of most of today's surgeons so they are pursuing additional minimal access surgical approaches, with their ideally quicker healing times and better outcomes, to accomplish what has for years been performed with conventional surgery. In addition, minimal access surgery itself has spun off other new and potentially improved techniques, including: Natural Orifice Translumenal Endoscopic Surgery (NOTES™), Single-Incision Laparoscopic Surgery, etc. [1–8]. Unlike basic laparoscopy, these latter techniques are quite sophisticated and exhilarating attempts to create a new scarless or nearly scarless paradigm of surgery.

In surgery or medicine, as in any other industry, any new technology will always present new and different implications and applications among users and end-receptors (in this case surgeons and patients) ranging from helpful to disruptive. There is a certain level of adjustment, in terms of training, due to the advent of single-incision laparoscopic surgery. Even though this concept is very similar to earlier laparoscopy, in reality it demands a new set of skills and knowledge which not all laparoscopists may have attained. There is a learning curve, but its potential benefits have attracted a great deal of deserved interest.

D.S. Tichansky, J. Morton, and D.B. Jones (eds.), *The SAGES Manual of Quality, Outcomes and Patient Safety*, DOI 10.1007/978-1-4419-7901-8_34, © Springer Science+Business Media, LLC 2012

Technical Aspects

To better understand the issues influencing the adoption of single-port laparoscopic surgery it is helpful to briefly describe the surgical techniques involved. As we have noted before, since the inception of laparoscopy surgeons have made continual efforts in further reducing the number of ports required for any given surgery. Reports of single-incision laparoscopy go back to the mid-1990s [9, 10]; however this technique was not widely adopted at that time due to numerous reasons, especially technical difficulties and a reactionary inertia among many surgeons at the time. During the last few years, however, since the inception of NOTES™ [1], there has been a strong resurgence of interest in single-incision laparoscopy and hybrid approaches. Overall, the concept behind the single-port technique is the creation of a single skin incision in the abdomen, and then either a single incision in the fascia (with the use of a multi-channel port device) or the alternative of making multiple different fascial incisions for the placement of several different ports all through the same single skin incision. The proposed main benefits of either of these single-incision laparoscopic techniques is to provide positive cosmetic results, with virtually no scar, and also potentially less wound-related complications from multiple operative sites which will ultimately lead to better patient outcomes [2–8].

Factors Affecting Outcomes and Predicting Potential Complications

In general, patient outcomes and safety from any given surgical procedure may be affected by three different, but equally important, factors: the patients' health (or disease); surgeons (expertise, training and his/her surgical team); and technology used [11]. All are interrelated and dependent on each other, but we will try to single out some very important considerations.

First, not every patient or disease may be conducive for a minimal access surgical approach, much less for single-incision laparoscopy. Sound patient selection is, without a doubt, one of the most important determinants of success in any surgery or medical treatment, not just with this technique. This is true with any technological or technique innovation, both in diagnosis and therapeutic medicine. Presently, there is still a lack of widespread and commonplace experience with single-incision laparoscopy, yet it is a reasonable conjecture that simple patients with simple pathologies are the most adequate candidates for this approach. Therefore, one might think that patients who are morbidly obese, those with multiple previous abdominal procedures (especially umbilical or ventral hernia repairs with mesh), very tall patients, or patients with multiple co-morbidities, may be avoided (at least at an early point of a surgeon's single-port use experience) as common patients with whom to use this technique. As we gained more experience, more complex and sicker patients may be safely amenable to this technique [3–7]. Realistically these more serious patients are those who may ultimately benefit the most from single-port surgery, but until there is a critical mass of surgeons and experience this important clinical group should continue to be treated with conventional laparoscopic and at times open surgical techniques.

With this in mind, it may not be ideal for all surgeons to incorporate the single-port technique into their surgical arsenal just yet. This technique does demand a special set of skills which are highly sophisticated when compared to basic laparoscopy. Many surgeons may decide that it is simply not worth the effort (at least presently) for them to dedicate the time, patience and hard work to learn and attain competency with the needed new skill-set. Surgeons with no extensive knowledge, training or experience with this technique, including thorough familiarity of the instrumentation needed, will likely fail and potentially may harm even with the most ideal and suitable patient [12].

As a still evolving technique, most of the technology which has been used for the single-port approach has not actually been specifically designed for this laparoscopic technique. In general, multiple instrumentation from conventional laparoscopy and flexible endoscopy has been utilized to perform single-incision laparoscopy [2]. This situation represents a great void in the growing laparoscopy marketplace, and there has been an almost immediate response from the medical device industry, as well as globally from innovative scientists and surgeons, looking to fill this gap. Clearly, any technological innovation will have an inherited barrier to adoption with its inherent demands of a new learning process in how it is to be used and mastered. Most of the technological advances in single-incision laparoscopy are still not obvious or very intuitive, adding complexity to the overall process. This engineering challenge itself may represent a potential source of utilization complications if the appropriate techniques are not mastered prior to their use; therefore, it is very important to understand any technological limitations that may lead to unforeseen complications without the proper prior training, whatever the new port device manufactures or designers may claim.

Complications Arising from Single-Incision Laparoscopy

Generally speaking, all complications inherent to laparoscopy will also be potential issues in single-incision laparoscopic surgery [2–8, 13–18]. Until large clinical trials are available to show otherwise, many surgeons and patients may suspect that complications would be more common with the new, and somewhat complex, single-port approach. Presently, most clinical series have not revealed a higher complication rate, or more severe types of complications, after single-incision laparoscopy. In fact, the available research has shown similar outcomes with single-incision laparoscopy as compared to traditional laparoscopy, with the addition of some of its proposed and unique advantages such as improved cosmesis from virtually no visible scars [2–10].

Yet there may be a subset of potential complications, which may prove to be as common or more common with the single-port technique as compared to other techniques. Of particular interest is that electrical injuries could be, at least in theory, more prone to occur. These may take place as a result of the closed proximity of laparoscopic instruments, with near or complete contact, to each other [13–17]. Even fully insulated instruments could potentially develop coupled-capacitance when using monopolar energy; or even direct-coupling if there would be a disruption or break in the instruments' insulation. Due to this potential risk, however unlikely, it is still much more attractive to use advanced forms of energy, such as bipolar sealant instruments, ultrasonic energy, etc. Whenever monopolar energy is chosen, it should be cautiously used and it would be of paramount importance that it be, if possible, both potentially disposable yet still of a very high quality of instrumentation [13–15].

One of the biggest challenges when performing single-incision laparoscopy is to obtain adequate exposure and visualization of the target treatment area, while still maintaining optimal ergonomics. This challenge may tempt some surgeons to sacrifice visualization to be able to perform a given procedure. This is a serious mistake. Compromising proper visual exposure will inevitably increase the risk of potential complications. A good rule to follow is that no surgical spectator, viewing the images on a monitor screen, should be able to distinguish between a surgery which is done by conventional laparoscopy versus a single-incision one. Both should give the same exposure regardless of the number of incisions in the abdomen [2–4, 8]. With this rule in mind there is admittedly a very prevalent and inherent challenge to single-incision laparoscopy in attaining proper retraction of tissues and organs. Numerous efforts are being implemented to solve this issue: from primitive ways using needle and sutures to retract, to much more sophisticated endo-grabbing or magnetic systems [2, 19]. Each one of these platforms may have inherent complications related to their use (mainly potential tissue trauma) that may be dependent to the expertise of their respective use.

As stated before, endoscopic complications are the same as in conventional laparoscopy, however the main difference is that intra-operative complications may be much more difficult to manage if one must stick to this single-incision laparoscopic technique. A very low threshold should be customary when considering adding additional ports and/or finalizing a case with conventional laparoscopy, or even, if needed, converting to an open approach [2–8]. Bleeding, in particular, is much more challenging to control with present single-port technology, especially with a limited number of hands and with less-than-optimal ergonomics. Bleeding can also easily compromise adequate visualization of critical anatomical structures, and therefore it becomes even more important to place additional trocars sooner rather than later. Failure to complete a surgery via single-incision laparoscopy may not be a problem in itself, but failure to recognize the necessity of conversion to traditional laparoscopy or even open surgery could be a serious one. Despite the advantages and benefits of single-incision laparoscopy, a cautious and conservative approach, as with any surgical approach, should be the paradigm.

One concern many surgeons express about single-port technique is the possibility of a higher incidence of incisional umbilical hernias. The rationale behind this worry is that single-incision laparoscopy requires a bigger fascial incision, of 2–2.5 cm, to accommodate a multi-channel port device. Of even more concern is the scenario when multiple fascial incisions are used in close proximity to each other. This could potentially render a very weak fascia with multiple openings which may subsequently be prone to development of hernia. Presently these are only pragmatic speculations, and it will be only after long-term prospective evaluation of clinical series when either of these situations could be proven to be true or not. As of this writing there is no clinical evidence of increased hernia rates [3–8]. Also, in the case of many surgical procedures where a specimen needs to be extracted from the abdomen, this situation proves invalid, as even with conventional laparoscopy a bigger fascial incision would be needed for organ extraction.

Perhaps the historical adoption of laparoscopic cholecystectomy 25 years ago is not the ideal model of how to roll-out the continued adoption of single-incision laparoscopy [18, 20]. Most surgeons would remember the days when laparoscopy was first widely adopted and how injuries of the biliary tree were experienced more often than conventional surgery. Even when a cholecystectomy can be simple in nature, it can represent a formidably complex problem when complications cascade from a biliary duct injury [18, 20]. With the further development of economies of scale and scope of these conventional laparoscopic techniques, injuries such as these are now not much more common than with open surgery, as long as some principles of exposure and technique are followed. The same standards and pattern should apply to single-incision laparoscopy, even though right now any evidence showing this trend is very limited – so far there is no documented increase in bile duct injuries with this single-incision technique [3–8]. Recent studies have demonstrated that the critical view of the structures of the Hepato-cystic triangle (triangle of Calot) can be adequately attained, to reproduce a safe single-incision laparoscopic cholecystectomy [3, 4, 8]. One must emphasize the paramount importance of responsible training and adoption of this technique to avoid the catastrophic mistakes of fast adoption with laparoscopic cholecystectomy over two decades ago.

Lastly, it should be noted that unlike the potential complications of conventional laparoscopic surgery, single-incision laparoscopy is unlikely ever to experience situations such as, bleeding from epigastric or iliac vessels, urinary bladder injuries, etc., which may be an intrinsic result of placing different trocars away from the midline or in the pelvis. These types of injuries only present themselves in single-port laparoscopy if one creates a point-of-entry at a place different than the umbilicus, or if the target operative site is the actual site of injury (i.e. inguinal hernia, hysterectomy, etc).

Final Remarks

With any technological or medical technique innovation, there are challenges that must be faced in matching a strong interest in the advance with its responsible and transparent adoption. We as pioneers and early adopters have a responsibility to prospectively gather clinical data to establish adequate evidence-based medicine to substantiate the adoption or rejection that single-port laparoscopy may have. Animal and dry models should be used as much as possible to gain expertise in this technique before even considering implementing it clinically. Also, patients must always clearly understand the intrinsic differences and challenges of this technique as compared to conventional laparoscopy, before ever agreeing to undergo a single-incision laparoscopic procedure. In general, single-incision laparoscopic surgery appears safe, reproducible, and with complications very similar to those of conventional laparoscopy. Sound selection of patients and proper training in this technique and of its required technology are critical for its safe and successful adoption. In addition, this technique promises additional, potential benefits such as better cosmesis, less pain, less related wound complications, etc., over conventional endoscopic techniques.

Selected Readings

1. Rattner D. ASGE/SAGES Working Group. ASGE/SAGES Working Group on Natural Orifice Translumenal Endoscopic Surgery. October 2005. Surg Endosc. 2006;20(2): 329–33.
2. Gill IS, Advincula AP, Aron M, Caddedu J, Canes D, Curcillo 2nd PG, et al. Consensus statement of the consortium for laparoendoscopic single-site surgery. Surg Endosc. 2010;24(4):762–8.
3. Rivas H, Varela E, Scott D. Single-incision laparoscopic cholecystectomy: initial evaluation of a large series of patients. Surg Endosc. 2010;24(6):1403–12.
4. Curcillo 2nd PG, Wu AS, Podolsky ER, Graybeal C, Katkhouda N, Saenz A, et al. Single-port-access (SPA) cholecystectomy: a multi-institutional report of the first 297 cases. Surg Endosc. 2010;24(8):1854–60.
5. Lee PC, Lo C, Lai PS, Chang JJ, Huang SJ, Lin MT, et al. Randomized clinical trial of single-incision laparoscopic cholecystectomy versus minilaparoscopic cholecystectomy. Br J Surg. 2010;97(7):1007–12.
6. Ahmed K, Wang TT, Patel VM, Nagpal K, Clark J, Ali M, Deeba S, Ashrafian H, Darzi A, Athanasiou T, Paraskeva P. The role of single-incision laparoscopic surgery in abdominal and pelvic surgery: a systematic review. Surg Endosc. 2010 Jul 10. [Epub ahead of print].
7. Antoniou SA, Pointner R, Granderath FA. Single-incision laparoscopic cholecystectomy: a systematic review. Surg Endosc. 2010 Jul 7. [Epub ahead of print].
8. Rawlings A, Hodgett SE, Matthews BD, Strasberg SM, Quasebarth M, Brunt LM. Single-incision laparoscopic cholecystectomy: initial experience with critical view of safety dissection and routine intraoperative cholangiography. J Am Coll Surg. 2010; 211(1):1–7.

9. Navarra G, Pozza E, Occhionorelli S, Carcoforo P, Donini I. One-wound laparoscopic cholecystectomy. Br J Surg. 1997;84(5):695.

10. Dávila F, Weber A, Dávila U, Lemus J, López J, Reyes G, Domínguez V. Laparoscopic cholecystectomy with only one port (with no trace): a new technique. Society of Gastrointestinal Endoscopic Surgeons, 1999 Annual Congress, San Antonio, TX.

11. Murphy MM, Ng SC, Simons JP, Csikesz NG, Shah SA, Tseng JF. Predictors of major complications after laparoscopic cholecystectomy: surgeon, hospital, or patient? J Am Coll Surg. 2010;211(1):73–80.

12. Santos BF, Enter D, Soper NJ, Hungness ES. Single-incision laparoscopic surgery (SILS) versus standard laparoscopic surgery: a comparison of performance using a surgical simulator. Surg Endosc. 2010 Jun 29. [Epub ahead of print].

13. Montero PN, Robinson TN, Weaver JS, Stiegmann GV. Insulation failure in laparoscopic instruments. Surg Endosc. 2010;24(2):462–5.

14. Wu MP, Ou CS, Chen SL, Yen EY, Rowbotham R. Complications and recommended practices for electrosurgery in laparoscopy. Am J Surg. 2000;179(1):67–73. Review.

15. Nduka CC, Super PA, Monson JR, Darzi AW. Cause and prevention of electrosurgical injuries in laparoscopy. J Am Coll Surg. 1994;179(2):161–70. Review.

16. Callery MP, Strasberg SM, Soper NJ. Complications of laparoscopic general surgery. Gastrointest Endosc Clin N Am. 1996;6(2):423–44. Review.

17. Crist DW, Gadacz TR. Complications of laparoscopic surgery. Surg Clin North Am. 1993;73(2):265–89. Review.

18. Wu YV, Linehan DC. Bile duct injuries in the era of laparoscopic cholecystectomies. Surg Clin North Am. 2010;90(4):787–802.

19. Dominguez G, Durand L, De Rosa J, Dacnguise E, Arozamena C, Ferraina PA. Retraction and triangulation with neodymium magnetic forceps for single-port laparoscopic cholecystectomy. Surg Endosc. 2009 Jul;23(7):1660–6. Epub 2009 May 5.

20. Soper NJ. Laparoscopic cholecystectomy. Curr Probl Surg. 1991;28(9):581–655.

35. NOTES: Common Complications and Management

Denise W. Gee and David W. Rattner

Natural orifice translumenal endoscopic surgery (NOTES) may have potential advantages when compared with traditional transabdominal or transthoracic surgical approaches. These include better cosmesis, fewer incisional hernias, decreased postoperative pain, and quicker return to full function. Human NOTES procedures performed worldwide thus far seem to confirm these benefits. Nevertheless, caution is warranted especially since NOTES access to the abdominal or thoracic cavity involves traversing organs such as the esophagus, stomach, bladder, vagina, or rectum. Safe access is imperative when performing NOTES procedures. In fact, the SAGES/ASGE White Paper on NOTES identified safe access to the peritoneal cavity as one of the fundamental barriers that needed to be overcome in order for NOTES to be ready for human clinical use [1].

Currently, the most commonly performed human NOTES procedures, appendectomy and cholecystectomy, utilize transgastric and transvaginal approaches. If access to the peritoneal or thoracic cavity is obtained blindly, potential damage to surrounding structures may occur. This issue was brought to light in a recent animal study examining the high rate of injuries caused by NOTES gastrotomy creation [2]. NOTES gastrotomy-related complications occurred in 13.2% of animals with a 7.9% major complication rate (splenic laceration, mesenteric tear, and fatal diaphragmatic injury) and 5.3% minor complication rate (abdominal wall injuries and minor gastrotomy site bleeding). Laparoscopic guidance resulted in fewer injuries (5.5% vs. 15.5%) but this did not reach statistical significance. The authors, therefore, concluded that gastric punctures should be made either with laparoscopic visualization or other techniques with noncutting devices. In human studies thus far, puncture through the stomach or vagina is regularly monitored using a laparoscope or second endoscope [3]. This avoids the risk of damaging surrounding organs.

D.S. Tichansky, J. Morton, and D.B. Jones (eds.), *The SAGES Manual of Quality, Outcomes and Patient Safety*, DOI 10.1007/978-1-4419-7901-8_35,
© Springer Science+Business Media, LLC 2012

In an early report of human NOTES cholecystectomy, five patients underwent transgastric hybrid cholecystectomy. The postoperative course was uneventful in all patients and no complications occurred. Postoperative pain was minimal, with three patients requiring no analgesia after surgery [4]. Another retrospective case–control study compared transvaginal and laparoscopic cholecystectomy. The authors found that women in the transvaginal group reported significantly less postoperative pain, less nausea or vomiting, and lower analgesic consumption. The recovery room stay was shorter and the rate of general and surgical complications was lower [5]. Although there was much initial concern about dyspareunia or other gynecological problems after transvaginal access, this has generally not been a major patient complaint.

In a recent prospective multicenter NOTES trial [6], 362 patients underwent transvaginal or transgastric NOTES procedures. Intraoperative complications occurred in 5.8% of patients (Table 35.1) and postoperative complications (Table 35.2) occurred in 3.04% of patients. Management of each of these complications is detailed in Tables 35.1 and 35.2. Five patients required reoperation due to peritonitis, esophageal perforation, or biliary fistula. No deaths occurred. Most other complications were successfully managed similar to a laparoscopic or open operation. Nearly 25% of patients undergoing NOTES cholecystectomy and appendectomy required no postoperative analgesia. Transgastric surgery appeared to have a higher complication rate than transvaginal surgery highlighting the fact that transvaginal approaches may be a safer route especially given the ability to directly visualize access and closure routes with less potential for complications such as fistula and peritonitis.

The largest patient series to date consists of 551 patients in the German Registry for Natural Orifice Translumenal Surgery [7]. All of the patients in the registry were female and nearly all procedures were performed transvaginally (in two cases no access route was specified). A hybrid approach with tranvaginal access and one or more additional abdominal ports was used in 99.3% of the patients. In this series, 85.3% of the procedures were cholecystectomies. Other procedures included appendectomies (7.3%), gastric surgery including bariatrics (1.2%), and colon surgery (2.5%). Interestingly, complications occurred only in patients undergoing cholecystectomies (intraoperative 1.3% and postoperative 1.8%). Details are shown in Table 35.3. Bladder injuries occurred in four patients but were repaired with sutures or managed conservatively with an indwelling catheter. Postoperative complications included bleeding in three patients and vaginal or urinary tract infection

Table 35.1. Intraoperative complications of NOTES procedures, IMTN study.

Type of complication	Number	Original procedure	Evolution	Grade[a]
Cystic artery bleeding	5	TV cholecystectomy	Intraoperative laparoscopic or endoscopic treatment	I
Appendix vessels bleeding	4	3 TV appendectomies; 1 TG appendectomy	Intraoperative laparoscopic or endoscopic treatment	I
Gastric access bleeding (epiploic vessels)	1	TV cholecystectomy	Conversion to open surgery, suturing	IIIb
Gastric wall perforation (inflammatory adhesions)	1	TV cholecystectomy	Laparoscopic suturing	IIIb
Bowel serosal laceration	1	TV cholecystectomy	Intraoperative suturing	IIIb
Esophageal perforation and mediastinitis	1	TG cholecystectomy	Conservative, TPN, conversion to laparoscopy, dismissed after 16 days	IVa
Abdominal wall injury	1	TG appendectomy	Conversion to laparoscopic surgery	IIIb
Vaginal laceration	3	TV cholecystectomy	Conservative	I
Intra-abdominal hypertension	2	1 TV cholecystectomy; 1 TV cancer staging	Desufflation and fluid therapy	I
Total	21 (5.8%)			

Note: *NOTES* natural orifice translumenal endoscopic surgery, *TV* transvaginal, *TG* transgastric

[a]Grade classification of surgical complications according to Dindo et al. Zorron R, Palanivelu C, Galvao Neto MP, Ramos A, Salinas G, Burghardt J, et al. International multicenter trial on clinical natural orifice surgery—NOTES IMTN study: preliminary results of 362 patients. Surg Innov. 2010 Jun;17(2):142–58

Table 35.2. Postoperative complications of NOTES procedures, IMTN study.

Type of complication	Number	Original procedure	Evolution	Grade[a]
Umbilical port infection	5	TG cholecystectomy	Conservative	II
Peritonitis	1	TG cholecystectomy	Streptococcus faecalis, laparoscopic reoperation, drainage, antibiotics, good PO course	IIIb
Biliary leak	2	TV cholecystectomy using laparoscopic clips or suture	1 nasobiliary drainage, 1 laparoscopic reoperation and drainage	IIIa, IIIb
Prolonged ileus	1	TG appendectomy	Conservative	I
Esophageal hematoma	1	TG cholecystectomy	Conservative	II
Dyspareunia	1	TV cholecystectomy	Conservative	I
Vaginal granuloma	1	1 TV cholecystectomy; 1 TV rectosigmoidectomy	Conservative	I
Urinary tract infection	2	1 TV cholecystectomy; 1 TV rectosigmoidectomy	Antibiotic therapy	II
Subcutaneous and mediatinal emphysema	1	1 TV neprectomy	Conservative	IVa
Total	11 (3.04%)			

Note: *NOTES* natural orifice translumenal endoscopic surgery, *TV* transvaginal, *TG* transgastric

[a]Grade classification of surgical complications according to Dindo et al. Zorron R, Palanivelu C, Galvao Neto MP, Ramos A, Salinas G, Burghardt J, et al. International multicenter trial on clinical natural orifice surgery–NOTES IMTN study: preliminary results of 362 patients. Surg Innov. 2010 Jun;17(2):142–58

Table 35.3. Details of intraoperative and postoperative complications.

Age	BMI	Length of operation (min)	Details of complication and action taken (if specified)	Length of hospital stay (d)
Intraoperative				
39	21.3	211	Rectum injury	8
59	28.9	68	Serosa injury of the rectum	9
47	27.6	43	Adhesions, small bowel injury, conversion to open surgery	9
61	32.1	55	Bladder injury (adhesions after hysterectomy)	6
67	30.1	55	Bladder injury, cystoscopy, indwelling catheter for 3d	6
68	31.1	150	Bladder injury, laparoscopic suture (two additional trocards), cystoscopy	12
29	34.3	63	Bladder injury, indwelling catheter	10
Postoperative				
59	28.9	68	Postoperative bleeding	9
57	23.5	50	Vaginal bleeding	3
26	26.2	60	Vaginal bleeding	3
39	n/a	40	Abscess in the pouch of Douglas 3 weeks after surgery, laparoscopic drainage, further course without problems	10 (2 hospital stays)
50	28.6	76	Emesis	8
21	28.7	46	Urinary tract infection	4
60	30.0	80	Would infection	4
38	19.2	36	Vaginal mycosis	2
80	n/a	n/a	Bacterial vaginitis	
74	26.0	56	Abdominal pain, laparoscopy without pathological findings	

Note: All reported complications occurred in cholecystectomies. Seventeen complications occurred in 16 patients as 1 patient had an intraoperative complication (serose injury of the rectum) and a postoperative complication (postoperative bleeding)

Lehmann KS, Ritz JP, Wibmer A, Gellert K, Zornig C, Burghardt J, et al. The German registry for natural orifice translumenal endoscopic surgery: report of the first 551 patients. Ann Surg. 2010 Aug;252(2):263–70 in three patients. One patient was readmitted because of an abscess in the pouch of Douglas that was treated laparoscopically.

In this registry, 20 operations were converted to laparoscopy and 7 to open surgery. Subgroup analysis of this series revealed that patients with a BMI ≥ 25 kg/m^2 had a higher probability of conversion and the duration of their operations was longer. Older patients also had a higher conversion rate with patients ≥65 years being more than three times more likely to have a conversion compared with patients <65 years. Finally, it was found that while institutional case volume did not influence the probability of conversions or complications, there was an effect on length of operations and number of trocars used.

Based on the findings of these two large trials, the transvaginal access route, though only applicable to half of the population, may be safer than the transgastric route. Many of the complications of the early human NOTES experience could be due to the learning curve of the operating surgeons and should decrease over time. The key to performing NOTES procedures is to ensure that the same safe surgical principles are maintained despite a new approach. Methods of managing NOTES complications include low threshold to convert to laparoscopic or open technique. As with any invasive procedure, patients should be closely monitored so that complications can be detected as early as possible and remedied appropriately.

Although the complication rate has been low, complications such as infection and bleeding have been seen in human NOTES studies to date. Human trials investigating transgastric instrumentation of the peritoneal cavity have shown contamination of the peritoneal cavity, but the contamination was found to be clinically insignificant [8–10]. Gastric lavage with antibiotic or betadine solution along with preoperative intravenous antibiotic administration may decrease the incidence of infection. In the human studies described above, severe bleeding resulted in conversion to laparoscopic or open procedures. Although bleeding can often be addressed with conventional endoscopic methods of injection, thermal, or mechanical therapy, current studies have focused on improving methods of hemostasis. Fritscher-Ravens et al. conducted a randomized controlled study comparing different methods of obtaining endoscopic hemostasis following artificially induced hemorrhage in the peritoneal cavity [11]. The study assessed several methods of hemostasis including an endoscopic suturing device, prototype monopolar electrocautery forceps, and forced argon plasma coagulation (FAPC). In the end, FAPC was found to have significantly faster times in controlling bleeding and in achieving complete cessation of blood loss when compared with the other methods.

If this is to be used intraperitoneally, it is essential to prevent high intraperitoneal pressures from developing. A recent study comparing the use of prototype flexible bipolar forceps (FBF) with conventional laparoscopic bipolar forceps (LBF) showed that transgastric FBF was as effective as LBF in achieving hemostasis in a porcine model [12]. These studies are promising since they demonstrate the ability to manage difficult complications even in the NOTES setting. It will be important to extend these studies to look at hemostatic methods in the thorax since vessels within the chest, including intercostal arteries and veins, can be difficult to access due to surrounding bony structures (i.e., ribs, vertebral bodies).

Recently, NOTES transanal endoscopic rectosigmoid resection was performed in a 76-year-old female with T2N2 rectal cancer treated with preoperative chemoradiation [13]. Complete mesorectal excision was performed and the patient's postoperative course was uneventful. The final pathology revealed pT1N0 with 23 negative lymph nodes and negative margins. Similar NOTES colorectal procedures have been performed on other patients in Spain with equally successful results. Patient pain can be controlled with oral analgesics and there has been no evidence of postoperative complications such as leak or fistula formation. More NOTES colorectal work is being performed around the world.

Another increasingly studied access route is transesophageal NOTES for procedures in the mediastinum and thorax. Security of the esophagotomy closure is paramount yet the ideal method of closure has yet to be identified. Sumiyama et al. [14] and Gee et al. [15] have performed survival NOTES studies in swine by creating an esophageal submucosal tunnel. The mucosal flap valve offsets the entry and exit sites in the esophageal wall and upon withdrawal of the endoscope, no additional closure device is required. These studies have demonstrated good clinical outcome with no evidence of large abscess or mediastinitis. Another group has experimented with endoscopic suturing devices for the closure of transesophageal entry sites [16]. While the endoscopic sutures successfully closed the mucosal defects in the esophagus, there were remaining defects in the esophageal muscular wall on necropsy. More recently, a group reported the first use of resorbable sutures at transgastric NOTES access sites, which could have applicability to esophageal sites as well [17]. It is unclear whether the use of endoscopic sutures or the submucosal tunneling technique will be superior in allowing proper healing of the transesophageal exit conduit without infectious complications. Animal trials comparing the outcomes of these different techniques have not yet been published.

Placement of an esophageal stent may produce even better outcomes than endoscopic suturing or tunneling techniques. In humans, observational studies have looked at the utility of esophageal stent placement following esophageal perforations. In a recently published survival animal series, safe esophageal closure was demonstrated with a prototype retrievable, antimigration stent [18]. Access to the mediastinum and thorax was obtained with the submucosal tunneling technique and a stent was placed at the completion of the procedure. All swine thrived clinically, except for a brief period of mild lethargy in one animal who improved with short-term antibiotic therapy. The submucosal tunnels were completely healed and no esophageal bleeding or stricture formation was observed [18]. Esophageal stent placement successfully diverted intraluminal contents from the tunnel thus preventing contamination of the mediastinum and thorax and allowed animals to resume their oral intake in the immediate postoperative period. The authors concluded that the submucosal tunneling technique combined with esophageal stent placement is a safe and effective method of esophageal closure in thoracic NOTES procedures. Though observational evidence for stents seems promising, randomized trials remain to be performed to better assess their utility in treating iatrogenic esophageal perforations.

The ease of esophageal submucosal tunnel creation naturally led many groups to study the feasibility of transesophageal and transcervical endoscopic Heller myotomy in animal and cadaver models [19–22]. These studies demonstrated relative ease of myotomy, both posteriorly and anteriorly, with minimal surrounding trauma and ability to extend the myotomy onto the stomach. The self-approximating mucosal flap was either left alone to serve as closure [21], or clips were used [20]. More recently, this procedure was performed in 17 humans with no serious complications [19]. During follow-up, additional treatment or medication was necessary in only one patient who developed reflux esophagitis which was well controlled later with proton pump inhibitors.

Esophageal closure technique, the risk of esophageal leak, and infections including mediastinitis, pneumonia, and bacteremia are major concerns when attempting to access the thoracic cavity via a transesophageal route [23]. Large studies investigating infectious complications have not been reported and are challenging to complete due to limitations of the animal model. The trials summarized in Table 35.4 suggest infectious complications could be low. Pneumothorax or hemothorax is another potential adverse event in transesophageal NOTES procedures. These complications have also been observed in swine NOTES thoracic studies. Conventional interventions such as needle decompression or chest tubes can be performed, though there was never a need for chest tube placement in the animal studies reviewed in Table 35.4 [23].

Table 35.4. Closure techniques and associated complications in swine transesophageal NOTES studies.

Study	Esophageal closure strategy	Early complications	Late complications	Morbidity (n)	Mortality (n%), (n)
Fritscher-Ravens et al. [16]	Prototype T-tag device (n=6), EndoClip (n=3)	Pericardial hematoma (acute animal)	None	1	None
Sumiyama et al. [14].	SEMF	Pleural injury resulting in death	None	None	25%, (n=1)
Gee et al. [15]	m-SEMF+EndoClip (n=2), m-SEMF only (n=2)	None	Subclinical esophageal abscess	1	None
Sumiyama et al. [25]	SEMF+EndoClip	Descending aorta injury	Esophageal mucosal ulceration at SEMF site	1	20%, (n=1)
Willingham et al. [26]	m-SEMF+EndoClip	Pneumothorax requiring angiocatheter decompression	N/A	1	None

SEMF submucosal endoscopy with mucosal flap safety valve, *m-SEMF* modified SEMF, *EndoClip* metal clip applied to esophageal mucosa, *N/A* not applicable

Turner BG, Gee DW. Natural orifice transesophageal thoracoscopic surgery: A review of the current state. World J Gastrointest Endosc. 2010 Jan 16;2(1):3–9

In a systematic review of thoracic NOTES procedures, mortality was found to be 5% and morbidity 19%, when combining all published studies of thoracic-related studies using a NOTES technique [24]. The review included two studies where thoracic procedures were accomplished with a transvesicular, transdiaphragmatic, or transgastric approach, while the remaining five studies were transesophageal. The morbidity and mortality in the combined studies represent one of the major challenges in creating a new, minimally invasive technique and underscores the technological improvements necessary before transesophageal NOTES can be used for intrathoracic or trans-mediastinal procedures in humans.

For the time being, a hybrid approach using laparoscopic guidance in NOTES procedures allows safe access to the abdominal and thoracic cavities and is a safe bridge to pure NOTES procedures in humans. Device development remains imperative as these technological advances will help minimize risk of postoperative leaks and aid in the management of procedure complications. New instruments may also help decrease procedure times. Currently, transvaginal approaches have been the most widely utilized and seem to be the safest but will only be available to female patients. Therefore, ongoing work with gender-independent access routes is essential. At this point in time NOTES procedures are a promising alternative to traditional approaches. Complications that occur during NOTES procedures to date have not been unique and can be managed in much the same manner as if they had occurred during a laparoscopic or open procedure.

Selected Readings

1. Rattner D, Kalloo A. ASGE/SAGES Working Group on Natural Orifice Translumenal Endoscopic Surgery. October 2005. Surg Endosc. 2006;20(2):329–33.
2. Sohn DK, Turner BG, Gee DW, Willingham FF, Sylla P, Cizginer S, et al. Reducing the unexpectedly high rate of injuries caused by NOTES gastrotomy creation. Surg Endosc. 2010;24(2):277–82.
3. de Sousa LH, de Sousa JA, de Sousa Filho LH, de Sousa MM, de Sousa VM, de Sousa AP, et al. Totally NOTES (T-NOTES) transvaginal cholecystectomy using two endoscopes: preliminary report. Surg Endosc. 2009;23(11):2550–5.
4. Dallemagne B, Perretta S, Allemann P, Asakuma M, Marescaux J. Transgastric hybrid cholecystectomy. Br J Surg. 2009;96(10):1162–6.
5. Hensel M, Schernikau U, Schmidt A, Arlt G. Comparison between transvaginal and laparoscopic cholecystectomy: a retrospective case–control study. Zentralbl Chir. 2010 May.

6. Zorron R, Palanivelu C, Galvao Neto MP, Ramos A, Salinas G, Burghardt J, et al. International multicenter trial on clinical natural orifice surgery: NOTES IMTN study: preliminary results of 362 patients. Surg Innov. 2010;17(2):142–58.

7. Lehmann KS, Ritz JP, Wibmer A, Gellert K, Zornig C, Burghardt J, et al. The German registry for natural orifice translumenal endoscopic surgery: report of the first 551 patients. Ann Surg. 2010;252(2):263–70.

8. Hazey JW, Narula VK, Renton DB, Reavis KM, Paul CM, Hinshaw KE, et al. Natural-orifice transgastric endoscopic peritoneoscopy in humans: initial clinical trial. Surg Endosc. 2008;22(1):16–20.

9. Narula VK, Happel LC, Volt K, Bergman S, Roland JC, Dettorre R, et al. Transgastric endoscopic peritoneoscopy does not require decontamination of the stomach in humans. Surg Endosc. 2009;23(6):1331–6.

10. Narula VK, Hazey JW, Renton DB, Reavis KM, Paul CM, Hinshaw KE, et al. Transgastric instrumentation and bacterial contamination of the peritoneal cavity. Surg Endosc. 2008;22(3):605–11.

11. Fritscher-Ravens A, Ghanbari A, Holland C, Olagbeye F, Hardeler KG, Seehusen F, et al. Beyond NOTES: randomized controlled study of different methods of flexible endoscopic hemostasis of artificially induced hemorrhage, via NOTES access to the peritoneal cavity. Endoscopy. 2009;41(1):29–35.

12. Park PO, Long GL, Bergstrom M, Cunningham C, Vakharia OJ, Bakos GJ, et al. A randomized comparison of a new flexible bipolar hemostasis forceps designed principally for NOTES versus a conventional surgical laparoscopic bipolar forceps for intra-abdominal vessel sealing in a porcine model. Gastrointest Endosc. 2010;71(4): 835–41.

13. Sylla P, Rattner DW, Delgado S, Lacy AM. NOTES transanal rectal cancer resection using transanal endoscopic microsurgery and laparoscopic assistance. Surg Endosc. 2010;24(5):1205–10.

14. Sumiyama K, Gostout CJ, Rajan E, Bakken TA, Knipschield MA. Transesophageal mediastinoscopy by submucosal endoscopy with mucosal flap safety valve technique. Gastrointest Endosc. 2007;65(4):679–83.

15. Gee DW, Willingham FF, Lauwers GY, Brugge WR, Rattner DW. Natural orifice transesophageal mediastinoscopy and thoracoscopy: a survival series in swine. Surg Endosc. 2008;22(10):2117–22.

16. Fritscher-Ravens A, Patel K, Ghanbari A, Kahle E, von Herbay A, Fritscher T, et al. Natural orifice transluminal endoscopic surgery (NOTES) in the mediastinum: long-term survival animal experiments in transesophageal access, including minor surgical procedures. Endoscopy. 2007;39(10):870–5.

17. von Renteln D, Eickhoff A, Kaehler G, Riecken B, Caca K. Endoscopic closure of the natural orifice transluminal endoscopic surgery (NOTES) access site to the peritoneal cavity by means of transmural resorbable sutures: an animal survival study. Endoscopy. 2009;41(2):154–9.

18. Turner BG, Cizginer S, Kim MC, Mino-Kenudson M, Ducharme RW, Surti VC, et al. Stent placement provides safe esophageal closure in thoracic NOTES(TM) procedures. Surg Endosc. 2011;25(3):913–8.

19. Inoue H, Minami H, Kobayashi Y, Sato Y, Kaga M, Suzuki M, et al. Peroral endoscopic myotomy (POEM) for esophageal achalasia. Endoscopy. 2010;42(4):265–71.

20. Perretta S, Dallemagne B, Allemann P, Marescaux J. Multimedia manuscript. Heller myotomy and intraluminal fundoplication: a NOTES technique. Surg Endosc. 2010;24(11):2903.

21. Pauli EM, Mathew A, Haluck RS, Ionescu AM, Moyer MT, Shope TR, et al. Technique for transesophageal endoscopic cardiomyotomy (Heller myotomy): video presentation at the Society of American Gastrointestinal and Endoscopic Surgeons (SAGES) 2008, Philadelphia, PA. Surg Endosc. 2008;22(10):2279–80.

22. Spaun GO, Dunst CM, Arnold BN, Martinec DV, Cassera MA, Swanstrom LL. Transcervical Heller myotomy using flexible endoscopy. J Gastrointest Surg. 2010;14(12):1902–9.

23. Turner BG, Gee DW. Natural orifice transesophageal thoracoscopic surgery: A review of the current state. World J Gastrointest Endosc. 2010;2(1):3–9.

24. Clark J, Sodergren M, Correia-Pinto J, Zacharakis E, Teare J, Yang GZ, et al. Natural orifice translumenal thoracoscopic surgery: does the slow progress and the associated risks affect feasibility and potential clinical applications? Surg Innov. 2009;16(1): 9–15.

25. Sumiyama K, Gostout CJ, Rajan E, Bakken TA, Knipschield MA, Chung S, et al. Pilot study of transesophageal endoscopic epicardial coagulation by submucosal endoscopy with the mucosal flap safety valve technique (with videos). Gastrointest Endosc. 2008;67(3):497–501.

26. Willingham FF, Gee DW, Lauwers GY, Brugge WR, Rattner DW. Natural orifice transesophageal mediastinoscopy and thoracoscopy. Surg Endosc. 2008;22(4):1042–7.

Part V
Organizations Promoting Safety and Quality

36. Quality and Safety in the American College of Surgeons

David B. Hoyt and Ajit K. Sachdeva

Introduction

The origins of the American College of Surgeons were focused on quality at a time when medicine was united and prosperous and based on a system of autonomy. Control over the environment was essential in early surgery. Our heritage as an organization developed out of the need for education – the Clinical Congress and education model – and subsequently, standards for surgeons. Early programs in the College included defining qualifications for surgeons, initial hospital reviews, and even initial attempts at public reporting [1]. The Committee on Trauma started in 1924 as the Committee on Fractures and the Commission on Cancer started in 1922 as attempts to define standards of care and improve the quality of care and safety of care for surgical patients. Ultimately, these early programs led to the establishment of The Joint Commission, which became an independent organization in 1951. Interest in quality and safety has remained the focus of the American College of Surgeons over the last 50 years and characterizes the development of many newer programs.

New Forces in Medicine Today

Two major forces have shaped our responsibility professionally in the last 30–40 years. The first is the ongoing attempt to control escalating costs, which most recently have affected the national deficit and continues to be of profound economic concern. Effectiveness research has suggested that controlling costs can be done through systematic evidence-based, best practice models and implementation of protocols. Reduction of complications will also affect cost [2].

D.S. Tichansky, J. Morton, and D.B. Jones (eds.), *The SAGES Manual of Quality, Outcomes and Patient Safety*, DOI 10.1007/978-1-4419-7901-8_36, © Springer Science+Business Media, LLC 2012

The second major trend in medicine has been a result of the Institute of Medicine's *To Err is Human* study in 1999 [3] and the subsequent report, *Crossing the Quality Chasm* [4]. This report calls into focus opportunities for quality improvement across medicine and puts quality care in the forefront of the public's eye.

As a result of these two forces (economic and quality movement), many thoughtful analyses of ways to redefine our health care system have occurred. This has been accompanied by a number of quality organizations and quality measurement techniques, which have begun to define the way we will measure quality in the future. This movement has been somewhat overwhelming for organized medicine, but under the recently passed health care legislation, the implementation of quality and the connection of this to cost-effective care will be paramount.

The New Legislation

The Accountable Care Act puts forth as a national priority several new trends which will focus on the experience of care, the health of populations, and reducing per capita cost, the so-called triple aim [5]. A national health care quality strategy will be defined in 2011. This will be based on the four cornerstones of value-driven heath care as articulated in particular by Michael Porter's book, *Re-defining Health Care* [6]. These principles include measuring and publishing quality reports, measuring and publishing price, and creating positive incentives to accomplish these goals.

The Surgeons of the Future

The surgeon of the future is going to be involved in leading a safe, high-performance team, which increasingly integrates surgical and nonsurgical skills. Surgeons will be parts of systems of care and will have their practice based on evidence and outcomes data. Accountability will include public reporting. Similarly, continuous professional development and continuing education will be linked to specific practice and maintenance of certification will be linked to practice and demonstrated new skill acquisition.

The American College of Surgeons' models for disease management in trauma and cancer have existed for over 85 years. The defining thread of our organization is the definition of professionalism. Whereas in the past professionalism defined assertion, authority and control, in the future we will be best defined by collaboration, evidence, measurement, and accountability.

A Learning Health Care System

A recent concept articulated by the Institute of Medicine defines effective quality improvement in the context of a "learning health care system." The American College of Surgeons has promoted a learning health care system for surgery from its start and today has brought these elements together in a model of quality and safety [7].

The model begins with the definition of high quality surgical care standards set through consensus and best evidence collaborating with programs like SAGES defining specific guidelines. The second step in the process is to have outcome measurement systems to evaluate performance against these standards. Databases like NSQIP have created the infrastructure by which quality improvement can occur. There is now important data to suggest that the implementation of a measurement system in a hospital reduces complications, reduces mortality, and improves quality of care overall [2]. In addition, the cost reduction associated with complications is significant and has been estimated to be as high as 25 billion dollars annually if implemented across all of American surgery.

When you measure quality using appropriate risk adjustment and collect data using established methodology, you know how you are doing, you are directly improving care and outcomes and you are contributing to setting the next set of standards and benchmarks. Payers and regulators (both public and private) are carefully evaluating the American College of Surgeons' databases as a way to consider payment in the future.

When standards are developed and measurement is accomplished, the opportunity for verification of these standards and quality improvement efforts is made possible. It has become the basis of verification programs in cancer, trauma, geriatric surgery, breast disease, etc. The process of preparing for verification of a program both improves care in the institution and, at the same time, assures the public that what the program says it is doing, it is in fact doing.

Public Reporting

The ultimate goal of current health care trends will be some form of public reporting. The American College of Surgeons will remain very involved in trying to balance public reporting that satisfies the public's need, while at the same time, does not inhibit the vital importance of quality improvement efforts at the local hospital level.

The elements of learning health care systems are the essential parts of the American College of Surgeons' quality programs. These are probably the most important commitments we can make in the areas of quality and safety on behalf of our patients. To that end, the most recent focus of the American College of Surgeons is our new byline, *Inspiring Quality: Higher Standards, Better Outcomes.*

Quality and Education

Just as setting standards for quality are essential to optimal patient care at the institutional level, educational standards to improve provider skills are essential. Recommendations from prestigious national bodies emphasizing the need to improve quality of patient care have clearly articulated the importance of education and training [3, 4, 8, 9]. As a consequence of these reports, as well as advances in the sciences of continuous professional development (CPD) and surgical education and training, major national efforts are underway to link quality improvement initiatives with innovative education and training interventions. Collection and analyses of outcomes data from registries are only the first step in this process. This helps to identify gaps in patient care as part of the comprehensive needs assessment that is necessary to perform prior to designing specific education and training interventions. These interventions should address the needs of individuals and members of teams, and should be completed with requisite changes in systems and entrenched cultures to achieve the desired outcomes.

Practice-Based Learning

Education and training to improve quality of care should follow the cycle of practice-based learning and improvement, which includes the following four steps: Identifying areas for improvement; engaging in effective education and training; applying the new knowledge and skills to practice; and checking for improvement [10]. Each of these steps is critical and requires involvement of individuals with expertise in surgical education and training. Such efforts should address all six core competencies as defined by the American Board of Medical Specialties and the Accreditation Council for Graduate Medical Education [11, 12]. In view of the special nature of surgical practice, the core competencies need to be addressed in an integrated fashion to facilitate learning and support transfer of new knowledge and skills to real settings. The acquisition of skills and new procedures or technologies presents unique challenges that should be addressed through education and training programs that are based on the following principles.

A comprehensive, disease-based approach should be used rather than a technology-driven approach; participation in a longitudinal educational experience is critical because isolated interventions are not effective; preceptoring should follow participation in experiential courses to ensure safe transfer of skills; and the entire surgical team needs to be trained and credentialed [13]. Simulation should be incorporated into the education and training programs to address specific tasks, offer opportunities for deliberate practice, and support sharing of feedback in controlled settings, without exposing patients to risk. A variety of simulations, including cognitive case simulations, standardized patients, task trainers, simulators, virtual reality, and immersive environments should be used as appropriate to achieve specific learning objectives. Many surgical skills can be effectively addressed through the use of low fidelity and relatively inexpensive simulators [14, 15]. This can facilitate broad implementation of simulation-based surgical education and training in the current environment of health care in which resources are finite.

Verification of knowledge and skills is essential to ensure that learners have achieved pre-established standards. Such verification must involve valid and reliable assessment tools and involve trained surgeon evaluators. Verification and validation of knowledge and skills can permit award of specific certificates of achievement that may be used in processes of credentialing, privileging, and Maintenance of Certification. Efforts to offer competency-based education and training with validation of knowledge and skills should be attractive to captive insurance companies because of the importance of these efforts on reducing the risk of liability.

American College of Surgeons' Programs

The American College of Surgeons (ACS) Division of Education has designed a broad spectrum of innovative surgical education and training programs to improve the quality of surgical care. Comprehensive gap analyses have been used to define the needs of individuals and various groups of learners. These programs are founded on principles of CPD and surgical skill development, and focus on the needs of practicing surgeons, surgery residents, and members of surgical teams. Highlights of several of these programs are provided in the following paragraphs.

The Annual ACS Clinical Congress provides a broad range of educational sessions that include didactic and skills-oriented courses. The *Surgical Education and Self-Assessment Program (SESAP)* remains the premier self-assessment and cognitive skills education program for practicing surgeons. Significant transformational changes have been made in the most recent edition of *SESAP* to ensure robust self-assessments and guided cognitive skills education. The *Selected Readings in General Surgery (SRGS)* is a pre-eminent, evidence-based educational program in surgery and *SRGS* is now available in a variety of formats to enhance its educational impact and improve access. The ACS Comprehensive General Surgery Review Course covers the broad content of general surgery through contemporary educational approaches that include a case-based format and online pre- and post-tests. A spectrum of e-learning resources is available to address various topics and increase access to cutting-edge educational programs of the division. The *ACS Fundamentals of Surgery Curriculum* is a simulation-based interactive online program that focuses on cognitive skills and is primarily directed at surgery residents in the early years of training. The case simulations include a variety of special features that increase the program's fidelity and effectiveness.

The need to address surgical skills of trainees through structured simulation-based education and training has been widely recognized at the national level. The ACS has taken a lead in this regard and is collaborating with a number of national organizations to develop and launch national curricula to address the needs of surgery residents and medical students. The *ACS/APDS Surgical Skills Curriculum* addresses the need to develop and verify the surgical skills of residents in general surgery across all 5 years of training. Also, the needs of residents from across the surgical specialties in the early years of training can be addressed through this curriculum. The curriculum includes 20 modules that address basic surgical skills and tasks, 15 modules that address advanced procedures, and 10 modules that address team-based skills. The first version of this *ACS/APDS Surgical Skills Curriculum* was released 2 years ago. The curriculum is currently being revised and new modules will be added. Also, additional tools for verification of proficiency will be designed and included. The *ACS/APDS/ASE Entering Surgery Resident Prep Curriculum* is being designed to appropriately prepare 4th-year medical students to transition into surgery residency training. This curriculum should provide a solid foundation on which further education and training in residency programs may be built. The *ACS/ASE Medical Student Simulation-based Surgical Skills Curriculum* is being developed for all medical students in years 1–3. The curriculum will address basic areas of cognitive, clinical, and technical skills relative to surgery that medical students should acquire regardless of the intended specialty. Thus, these three national curricula will address the entire continuum of surgical skills education for medical students and surgery residents, and will be linked.

The *Fundamentals of Laparoscopic Surgery* (*FLS*) Program was initially developed by the Society of American Gastrointestinal and Endoscopic Surgeons (SAGES) and ACS subsequently partnered with SAGES to jointly manage, enhance, and disseminate this national curriculum. This has been a very exciting and productive collaboration. *FLS* includes validated assessment tools to ensure achievement of predetermined standards and is now required by the American Board of Surgery for certification.

ACS programs that address the other core competencies include cutting-edge courses on communication skills and a program that focuses specifically on communicating with patients and their families about surgical errors and adverse outcomes. A definitive program on professionalism was designed to address the critical topics in professionalism as they relate to surgical practice. This multimedia program includes interactive case simulations, with critiques of various options selected by the learners. Systems-based practice is being addressed through the *Surgeons as Leaders* Course. An online program to remodel the Morbidity and Mortality Conference is specifically designed to address practice-based learning and improvement and systems-based practice. The strategies articulated in this program should enhance the educational and quality improvement value of these important conferences. Also, an e-learning program on multi-disciplinary approaches to preventing errors and near misses in surgery will be launched soon. In addition, the ACS, in collaboration with the Accreditation Council for Graduate Medical Education, has created a blueprint of a Patient Safety Curriculum for

Surgical Residency Programs based on the results of a national consensus conference [16].

The ACS Division of Education has launched a five-level Program for Verification of Surgical Knowledge and Skills. Level I involves verification of attendance; Level II, verification of satisfactory completion of course objectives; Level III, verification of knowledge and skills; Level IV, verification of preceptorial experience; and Level V, demonstration of satisfactory patient outcomes [14]. All Postgraduate Courses offered at the Clinical Congress are designed based on these levels of verification using pre-established standards. Different certificates are awarded to course participants based on achievement of specific levels of verification.

The ACS Division of Education has been heavily engaged in advancing simulation-based surgical education and training and has provided national and international leadership in this field. The division has developed and launched innovative educational programs and products based on the use of simulation and is pursuing scholarly work to advance this field. In 2005, the ACS Program for Accreditation of Education Institutes (Simulation Centers) was launched following a multi-step process that included thorough gap analyses, followed by development, benchmarking, and pilot testing of the accreditation model. The program continues to grow and currently there are 61 Accredited Education Institutes, including accredited institutes in the USA, Canada, UK, Sweden, Greece, Israel, France, and China. A Consortium of the ACS-accredited Education Institutes has been created to fully realize the potential of this powerful network of simulation centers. A number of Standing Committees have been appointed to pursue lofty goals that are beyond the capabilities of individual accredited institutes.

In summary, the focus on quality must include innovative surgical education and training if the goal of improving quality is to be realized. The science underlying quality initiatives must be coupled with the scientific basis of contemporary education and training in surgery to achieve the best results. Innovative education and training programs must be founded on scientific principles of contemporary surgical education and continuous professional development, skill acquisition and maintenance, human factors, and systems change. Simulations and emerging technologies are central to efforts aimed at offering cutting-edge education and training and improving access to innovative programs. Objective assessment and verification of knowledge and skills through use of valid and reliable assessment tools should be an integral part of proficiency-based education and training. Collaboration across national organizations and professional societies is essential to addressing the many challenges and opportunities to improve the quality of surgical care through state-of-the-art education and training programs that will result in enduring impact.

Selected Readings

1. Codman EA. A study in hospital efficiency as demonstrated by the case report of the first five years of a private hospital. Oakbrook Terrace, IL: The Joint Commission on Accreditation of Healthcare Organizations; 1996.

2. Hall BL et al. Does surgical quality improve in the American College of Surgeons National Surgical Quality Improvement Program. Ann Surg. 2009;250:363–76.

3. Kohn LT, Corrigan JM, Donaldson MS, editors. To err is human: building a safer health system. Washington, DC: National Academy Press; 2000.

4. Committee on Quality of Health Care in America, Institute of Medicine. Crossing the Quality Chasm: A New Health System for the 21st Century. Washington, DC: National Academy Press; 2001.

5. Berwick DM, Nolan TW, Whittington J. The triple aim: care, health, and cost. Health Affairs. 2008;27(3):759–69.

6. Porter ME, Olmsted Teisberg E. Redefining health care creating value-based competition on results. Boston, MA: Harvard Business School Press; 2006.

7. Olsen LA, Aisner D, McGinnis JM. The learning healthcare system workshop summary. Roundtable on evidence-based medicine. Institute of Medicine of the National Academies. Washington, DC: National Academic Press; 2007.

8. Greiner AC, Knebel E, editors. Health professions education: a bridge to quality. Washington, DC: The National Academies Press; 2003.

9. Hager M, Russell S, Fletcher SW, editors. Continuing education in the health professions: improving healthcare through lifelong learning. New York: Josiah Macy, Jr. Foundation; 2008.

10. Sachdeva AK, Blair PG. Educating surgery residents in patient safety. Surg Clin N Am. 2004;84(6):1669–98.

11. ABMS Maintenance of Certification (MOC). http://www.abms.org/Maintenance_of_Certification/ABMS_MOC.aspx. Accessed 1/17/11. American Board of Medical Specialties, Chicago (IL); 2006.

12. ACGME Outcome Project. General competencies. http://www.acgme.org/outcome/comp/compFull.asp. Accessed 1/17/11. Accreditation Council for Graduate Medical Education, Chicago (IL); 2001.

13. Sachdeva AK. The new paradigm of continuing education in surgery. Arch Surg. 2005;140(3):264–9.

14. Sachdeva AK. Acquiring skills in new procedures and technology: the challenge and the opportunity. Arch Surg. 2005;140(4):387–9.

15. Grober ED, Hamstra SJ, Wanzel KR, Reznick RK, Matsumoto ED, Sidhu RS, et al. The educational impact of bench model fidelity on the acquisition of technical skill: the use of clinically relevant outcome measures. Ann Surg. 2004;240(2):374–81.

16. Sachdeva AK, Philibert I, Leach DC, Blair PG, Stewart LK, Rubinfeld IS, et al. Patient safety curriculum for surgical residency programs: results of a national consensus conference. Surgery. 2007;141(4):427–41.

37. The Institute of Medicine: Crossing the Quality Chasm

Kevin Tymitz and Anne Lidor

In an era of medical consumerism such as we are now in, the health care environment in the USA has understandably come under intense scrutiny. Many of the changes we have seen in the US health care delivery system over the past few decades have their origin in the introduction of managed care in the late 1980s. This system promised to increase the quality of health care in the USA while at the same time holding down cost. However, studies have shown that only 54% of adult consumers are receiving adequate and appropriate care [1]. Meanwhile, many deficiencies have been recognized in the US health care system which pose serious threats to the health of the American public. Many of these deficiencies are directly traceable to the lack of widespread implementation of the principles of evidence-based medicine. For instance, it has been estimated that nearly 10,000 deaths from pneumonia could be prevented annually by appropriate vaccination among elderly patients [2]. It is apparent that there is a huge gap between the care patients should receive and the care that they actually do receive.

Driven by the assertiveness of the consumers, a new set of challenges has been presented. This includes the traditional roles of physicians and health care provider organizations in establishing quality standards and in determining quality improvement priorities.

In response to the demand for better quality of health care, a report entitled "President's Advisory Commission on Consumer Protection and Quality in the Health Care Industry" was released in 1998. The commission was created by President Clinton to "advise the President on changes occurring in the health care system and recommend such measures as may be necessary to promote and assure health care quality and value, and protect consumers and workers in the health care system." Members of the commission included representatives of consumers, institutional health care providers, health care professionals, other health care workers, health care insurers, health care purchasers, state and local

D.S. Tichansky, J. Morton, and D.B. Jones (eds.), *The SAGES Manual of Quality, Outcomes and Patient Safety*, DOI 10.1007/978-1-4419-7901-8_37, © Springer Science+Business Media, LLC 2012

government representatives, and experts in health care quality, financing, and administration. The president had asked the commission to develop a "Consumer Bill of Rights" in health care and provide him with recommendations to enforce those rights at the federal, state, and local level.

The Commission developed a consensus on specific aims for improving the quality of health care in the USA. The initial set of aims that was presented included:

- Reducing the underlying causes of illness, injury, and disability
- Expanding research on new treatments and evidence on effectiveness
- Assuring the appropriate use of health care services
- Reducing health care errors
- Addressing oversupply and undersupply of health care resources
- Increasing patient participation in their care

The commission's purpose was to produce high quality effective care with better health outcomes, greater patient functionality, improved patient safety, and a system with easy access for all people [3]. Around the same time, the Institute of Medicine (IOM) had also been convening on topics related to health care quality. The IOM has been instrumental in providing guidance for identifying the contributors to the quality issues within the health care system.

The IOM is an independent, nonprofit organization that works outside of government to provide unbiased and authoritative advice to decision makers and the public. It was established in 1970 and is the health arm of the National Academy of Sciences. The aim of the IOM is to help those in government and the private sector make informed health decisions by providing evidence upon which they can rely. Many of the studies undertaken by the IOM begin as mandates from Congress while others are requested by federal agencies and independent organizations. The IOM forms consensus meetings of experts and also convenes a series of forums, roundtables, standing committees, and other activities to provide unbiased and authoritative advice to decision makers and the public.

Recognizing the urgent need to improve health care quality, the IOM held a series of roundtable discussions which met six times between February 1996 and January 1998 [4]. These discussions led to several conclusions about the quality of health care in the USA:

1. *The quality of health care can be precisely defined.* According to the IOM, quality of care can be defined as "the degree to which health services for individuals and populations increase

the likelihood of desired health outcomes and are consistent with current professional knowledge." There are many implications which accompany this definition. For instance, it emphasizes that health care professionals must stay up-to-date with the vast and dynamic knowledge base in their profession and use that knowledge appropriately. The phrase *desired health care outcomes* pertains to the outcomes that patients desire and also emphasizes that patients and families must be well-informed of their expected outcomes as well as alternative interventions that may be available.

Creating reliable and valid measures to assess the quality of health care may seem like a daunting challenge, however, a number of specific examples of different types of quality measures and their uses were discussed at the September 1996 IOM conference entitled "Measuring the Quality of Health Care: State of the Art." The conclusion formulated at this meeting was that the quality of care for a large variety of specific clinical conditions as well as procedures can be measured with sufficient precision in order to allow judgments to be made and actions taken to bring about improvement.

2.   *Quality problems are serious and extensive.* Health care problems can be divided into three categories: underuse, overuse, and misuse. Underuse is defined as failure to provide a service to a patient that would have produced a favorable outcome. Examples include failure to administer a childhood immunization such as polio or measles, or failure to use effective treatment such as aspirin for acute myocardial infarction. This has been a serious problem with the health care system. The problem is compounded when patients lack health insurance. One study found that patients who lacked insurance had a 25% greater chance of dying within 12 years when controlled for age, race, education, income, and co-morbidity [5].

Overuse is defined as providing a health care service where the potential for harm outweighs the potential for benefit. For example, prescribing antibiotics for a common viral illness such as the common cold. The excessive use of antibiotics in the ambulatory setting has contributed to the emergence of antibiotic-resistant bacteria in our communities. It has been estimated that in 1998, nearly 76 million office visits were for colds, upper respiratory tract infections, and bronchitis. This resulted in 41 million antibiotic prescriptions. When comparing bacterial prevalence estimates to prescribing rates, it was estimated that nearly 55% of the prescriptions were unlikely to be treating actual bacterial infections. This resulted in an estimated total excess cost of $726 million dollars [6].

In an effort to publicize the overuse of antibiotics, several organizations, such as the Centers for Disease Control and Prevention (CDC) and the IOM, have worked diligently to improve antibiotic selection and appropriate use. A report issued by the IOM in 1998 entitled "Antimicrobial Resistance: issues and options" commented on a workshop that was held to discuss the issue of antimicrobial overuse and the development of microbial resistance. Through this report, the IOM concluded that greater effort must be placed on expanding research on the outcomes of antibiotic misuse, nonuse, and prudent use in health care facilities and the communities. This will allow individual health care providers to make rational clinical decisions on the prescription of appropriate antibiotics. Since this report, there have been several studies that have followed the guidelines and recommendations of the IOM. One such study did show that there has been a significant decrease in the use of antimicrobial prescribing for upper respiratory infections among adults and children [7].

Misuse occurs when an appropriate service has been selected but a preventable complication occurs and the patient does not receive the full potential benefit of the service. Misuse is not the same as error: not all errors result in adverse events. Avoidable complications of surgery or medication use are two of the most common areas of misuse in the USA. It is estimated that over 1900 adverse drug events occur per year in each large teaching hospital with around 28% being preventable [8].

3. *Current approaches to quality improvement are inadequate.* It is recognized that this is not a problem at the individual level. In fact, the individuals who represent a vast array of disciplines are among the most highly trained, technically gifted, and best motivated of professionals. It is rather a problem at the systems level. The answers are not simple and involve shortcomings in the complex systems in which health care is delivered.

4. *There is an urgent need for rapid change.* Everyone should be concerned about the issues of quality of health care. The roundtable believes that the lead role should be taken by all health care providers. We must all play an active role in order to assure that patients receive quality care and also have the opportunity and the information they need to participate in their

own care and also to take responsibility for their own health. Meeting this challenge will require radical thinking on how to deliver the best health care and how to assess and improve its quality and safety.

Two landmark reports by the IOM have been instrumental in identifying the type(s) of safety and quality issues that we as a society must recognize and address. "To Err Is Human: Building a Safer Health System" was the first report to be published. This report on patient safety is part of a larger study examining the quality of health care in America. This report publicized the nature of medical errors that, if discussed at all, were only discussed behind closed doors. The committee had focused its attention on medical errors for several reasons including the fact that errors are responsible for an immense burden of patient injury, suffering and death. Errors are readily understandable to the American public and are events that everyone agrees just should not happen.

The report proposes a comprehensive approach for reducing medical errors and improving patient safety. One of the report's main conclusions is that the majority of errors do not occur as the result of the reckless actions of a single individual. More commonly, errors occur due to systems failure. Viewed in this light, it is clear that mistakes can best be prevented by designing a health system with safeguards at all levels of the system. In other words, make it harder for people to do something wrong and make it easier for them to do something right. With this in mind, when an error does occur, it does little good to blame individuals, as this will do very little to make the system safer and prevent someone else from making the same mistake.

The report recommends four ways to approach health care safety and reduce medical errors by "redesigning the system":

1. *Establishing a national focus to create leadership, research, tools, and protocols to enhance the knowledge base about safety.* Recognizing that health care is a decade or more behind many other high-risk industries in its attention to ensuring basic safety, a single government agency needs to be established devoted to improving and monitoring safety of the entire health care system.

2. *Identifying and learning from errors by developing a nationwide public mandatory reporting system and by encouraging health care organizations and practitioners to develop and participate in voluntary reporting systems.* Such systems would hold health care organizations and providers accountable for maintaining

safety, provide incentives to organizations to implement internal safety systems that reduce the likelihood of errors occurring, and respond to the public's right to know about patient safety.

3. *Raising performance standards and expectations for improvements in safety through the actions of oversight organizations, professional groups, and group purchasers of health care.* Performance standards can be regulated through mechanisms such as licensing, certification, and accreditation which are used to define minimum performance levels for health professionals. Professional societies can also be utilized to ensure safety by encouraging and demanding performance standards, communication with members about safety, incorporating patient safety into their training programs and collaborating across disciplines.

4. *Implementing safety systems in health care organizations to ensure safe practices at the delivery level.* Systems must be implemented that incorporate a variety of well-understood safety principles. This may require standardizing and simplifying equipment, supplies, and processes. Systems must also be in place for continuous monitoring of safety.

The second report entitled "Crossing the Quality Chasm: A new health system for the twenty-first century" is the final report on the Quality of Health Care in America by the IOM published in March 2001. With the knowledge that there exists a huge gap or chasm between the health care that we have and the potential health care that we could have, this report focuses more broadly on how the health care delivery system can be designed to innovate and improve care.

Multiple factors have contributed to this chasm that plagues the current health system. Medical science and technology have grown exponentially in the past half-century. So too has the complexity of health care and the amount of knowledge and people involved. Unfortunately, the health care delivery system has fallen short in its ability to translate this knowledge and technology into safe and efficient medical care. The health care needs of patients are also changing. As the population ages, the incidence of chronic illness such as heart disease and diabetes is rising. However, much of today's health system remains devoted to the treatment of acute, episodic care needs.

The health care delivery system is poorly adapted to delivering such care. Care is often overly complex and uncoordinated. Patient "handoffs" only contribute to the lack of quality care as information gets missed, leading to huge voids in coverage. Additionally, health care organizations, hospitals, and physician groups often work separately without much cooperation or communication. This also leads to huge voids in information on the patient's condition, medical history, and medications provided by other clinicians.

Crossing the Quality Chasm focuses on changing the structure and processes of the environment in which health professionals and organizations function. Many of these areas have already seen a great deal of change in the past several years. For instance, the use of information technology has played a large part in helping to transform the health care delivery system. The automation of patient-specific clinical information has made it more organized and easier to manage various illnesses, especially chronic conditions that require frequent monitoring and support. In addition, the use of automated systems for ordering medications can reduce errors in prescribing and dosing drugs.

The report also raises the topic of aligning payment policies with quality improvement. The development of pay-for-performance incentives falls in this category. Glickman et al. compared quality improvement in the management of acute MI between 54 hospitals in a Centers for Medicare and Medicaid Services (CMS) pay-for-performance pilot project and 446 control hospitals without pay-for-performance incentives. They found that the pay-for-performance hospitals achieved a statistically significantly greater degree of improvement compared with control hospitals on two of six process-of care measures (use of aspirin at discharge and smoking cessation counseling), but there was no significant difference between groups in improvements in in-hospital mortality [9]. One can argue that the use of outcome measures in surgery are even more complicated and controversial as case mix adjustments must be made. This will avoid punishing hospitals and surgeons who take on tougher case loads and more complex patients. Case mix adjustments cannot be standardized and there are multiple methods for making these adjustments that have the potential for providing differing results [10].

The response to the IOM reports on improving health care quality has, for the most part, been very positive. Through the efforts of the IOM, health care professionals, organizations, policy makers, and patients are becoming more familiar with the shortcomings of the nation's current system and the importance of finding new and better approaches to meeting the health care needs of all Americans. Although not providing simple solutions to very complex issues, at least a common vision and goal can be established.

Selected Readings

1. McGlynn EA et al. The quality of health care delivered to adults in the united states. N Eng J Med. 2003;348:2635–45.
2. Woolf SH et al. The need for perspective in evidence-based medicine. JAMA. 1999;282:2358–65.
3. Kizer KW et al. Establishing health care performance standards in an era of consumerism. JAMA. 2001;286:1213–17.
4. Chassin MR et al. The urgent need to improve health care quality: institute of medicine national round table on health care quality. JAMA. 1998;280:1000–5.
5. Franks P et al. Health insurance and mortality: evidence from a national cohort. JAMA. 1993;270:737–41.
6. Gonzales R et al. Antibiotic prescribing for adults with colds, upper respiratory tract infections and bronchitis by ambulatory care physicians. JAMA. 1997;278:901–4.
7. Manious AG et al. Trends in antimicrobial prescribing for bronchitis and upper respiratory infections among adults and children. Am J Public Health. 2003;93:1910–4.
8. Bates DW et al. Incidence of adverse drug events and potential adverse drug events: implications for prevention. JAMA. 1997;277:307–11.
9. Glickman SW et al. Pay for performance, quality of care, and outcomes in acute myocardial infarction. JAMA. 2007;297:2373–80.
10. Glance LG et al. Impact of changing the statistical methodology on hospital and surgeon ranking: the case of the New York state cardiac surgery report card. Med Care. 2006;44:311–9.

38. Using Patient Safety Indicators as Benchmarks

Tina Hernandez-Boussard, Kathryn McDonald, and John Morton

Ever since the Institute of Medicine's report *To Err is Human,* patient safety has taken the forefront of quality healthcare delivery. One measure of patient safety is the rate of in-hospital preventable adverse events (PAE), or preventable injuries caused by medical care. PAEs have been linked to higher mortality rates and increased lengths of stay. Adverse events have been associated with most surgical procedures, and range from 2% incidence to almost 20% incidence by surgical procedure. Furthermore, it has been determined that over half of surgical adverse events are preventable.

The Agency for Healthcare Research and Quality (AHRQ) has developed set of quality indicators to measure PAE during hospitalization, known as the patient safety indicators (PSIs). PSIs may be applied to administrative or billing databases. These indicators identify populations at risk for an event based on ICD-9 codes, DRG codes, and type of hospital admission. Each PSI has specific inclusion and exclusion criteria for both the population at risk for the event. Data generated from these quality indicators can help evaluate both hospital performance and patient safety improvement efforts.

In addition to the definitions of the 18 PSIs, AHRQ has also created a software package that enables users to easily apply their capture algorithms to administrative databases. This software is updated on a regular basis and is available for various software programs. Data generated from the AHRQ software include individual patient data flagged with an event, summary statistics on the number of each event within the population, and lastly risk-adjusted rates for each event. The risk-adjusted rates incorporate patient age, gender, payor, and different comorbidities.

D.S. Tichansky, J. Morton, and D.B. Jones (eds.), *The SAGES Manual*   387
of Quality, Outcomes and Patient Safety, DOI 10.1007/978-1-4419-7901-8_38,
© Springer Science+Business Media, LLC 2012

PSIs are becoming an international standard and are now seen in hospital dashboards, federal reports, and in international comparisons. These data are being used to identify potential lapses in quality healthcare delivery and for benchmarking different areas of healthcare delivery. Due to the standardization of the definitions, a patient flagged with failure to rescue (PSI#4) in one state uses the same criteria to flag a patient with failure to rescue in another state.

An example of the use of PSIs as benchmarks is in bariatric surgery. In a recent population-based study performed by Morton et al. in Archives of Surgery, researchers used PSIs to evaluate the quality of surgical care of open gastric bypass patients vs. laparoscopic patients. Laparoscopic surgery had superior patient outcomes including mortality, lengths of stay, complications, and PAE. In particular, laparoscopic surgery had significantly fewer risk-adjusted events for the following: failure to rescue, postoperative hemorrhage or hematoma, postoperative respiratory failure, postoperative pulmonary embolism or deep vein thrombosis, and accidental puncture or laceration.

Discussion

PSI can provide a first-pass examination of hospital-based outcomes. The clear advantages to PSIs are their accessibility, reproducibility, and consistency. By utilizing existing data present in administrative or billing data, AHRQ-provided software allows generation of impactful quality outcomes reporting. Given that the source variables are similar from hospital to hospital, it allows for outcomes that may be benchmarked against other hospitals or population-based benchmarks. The PSIs have been repeatedly validated in numerous settings demonstrating their consistency.

Clearly, there are disadvantages to PSIs. First, PSIs employ data that were collected for purposes other than quality. The data are not clinically derived and may not be as clinically relevant. Previously, present on admission (POA) diagnoses could influence the rate of PSIs. For example, patients may be admitted with a preexisting decubitus ulcer that becomes counted as a PSI. Recent changes in both the designation of POA diagnoses and AHRQ software help account for this implication. In addition, procedure-based coding is considerably more accurate in administrative databases given the incentive for payment for procedures. Diagnoses codes may, as a result, be less often coded which can have direct implications upon comorbidity recognition. Finally, AHRQ PSIs accuracy is directly dependent on the accuracy of the data entered.

In conclusion, AHRQ PSIs present readily available, benchmarked quality outcomes for hospitals. PSIs should be part of any hospital quality dashboard. An important function for PSIs is to help provide a mechanism for prioritization of quality improvement. Hospitals can readily examine their quality performance against population means and determine opportunities for improvement. By finding where gaps in quality performance exist, hospitals can initiate quality improvement. With each initiative, hospitals can track their progress against the same PSI rates. Finally, with each quality improvement initiative, collateral benefit can be entertained when the entire hospital is aware of emphasis and accountability in quality.

Selected Readings

1. Kohn KT, Corrigan JM, Donaldson MS. To Err is Human: building a safer health system. Washington, DC: Institutes of Medicine, National Academy Press; 1999.
2. Zhan C, Miller MR. Excess length of stay, charges, and mortality attributable to medical injuries during hospitalization. JAMA. 2003;290(14):1868–74.
3. Rivard PE, et al. Using patient safety indicators to estimate the impact of potential adverse events on outcomes. Med Care Res Rev. 2008;65(1):67–87.
4. Friedman B, et al. Do patient safety events increase readmissions? Med Care. 2009; 47(5):583–90.
5. Vogel TR et al. Evaluating preventable adverse safety events after elective lower extremity procedures. J Vasc Surg. 2011
6. Kaafarani HM, et al. Validity of selected patient safety indicators: opportunities and concerns. J Am College Surg. 2011;212(6):924–34.
7. Gawande AA, et al. The incidence and nature of surgical adverse events in Colorado and Utah in 1992. Surgery. 1999;126(1):66–75.
8. Kable AK, Gibberd RW, Spigelman AD. Adverse events in surgical patients in Australia. Int J Qual Health Care. 2002;14(4):269–76.
9. Agency for Healthcare Research and Quality. Guide to patient safety indicators. Rockville, MD: Department of Health and Human Services; 2003
10. AHRQ, A.f.H.R.a.Q. AHRQ Quality Indicators Software Download. 2007; Available from: http://www.qualityindicators.ahrq.gov/software.htm
11. NQF, N.Q.F. NQF Endorsed Standards. 2011 [cited 2011 March 11]; Available from: http://www.qualityforum.org/Measures_List.aspx

12. Drosler SE, et al. Application of patient safety indicators internationally: a pilot study among seven countries. Int J Qual Health Care. 2009;21(4):272–8.
13. Agency for Healthcare Research and Quality, A., National Healthcare Disparities Report, U.S.D.o.H.a.H. Services, Editor. Rockville, MD: Agency for Healthcare Research and Quality; 2007
14. Morton JM, et al. Laparoscopic vs open gastric bypass: population-based results in patient safety. Arch Surg. 2011 (in press)

39. Institute for Healthcare Improvement: Best Practices

Atul K. Madan and Julian Omidi

Founded in 1991, the Institute for Healthcare Improvement (IHI) is a nonprofit organization based in Cambridge, Massachusetts with a purpose to help lead the improvement of healthcare throughout the world. The IHI has pioneered and developed many efforts in improving healthcare. Its collaborative approach has allowed simple and proven methods to institute meaningful change. Additionally, its Web site (http://www.ihi.org) gives access to a fund of knowledge in healthcare improvement. While the IHI has developed, refined, and implemented healthcare improvement in numerous ways, herein we sample some of the meaningful and essential program methods of the IHI.

According to IHI's vision and values, their aim is to improve the lives of patients, the heath of communities, and the joy of the healthcare workforce. IHI uses the six improvement aims set forth by the Institute of Medicine: safety, effectiveness, patient-centeredness, timeliness, efficiency, and equity [1]. Additionally, IHI has a "No Needless List" as displayed in Exhibit 39.1. Exhibit 39.2 describes the IHI strategies and values. Inline with their vision, strategies, and values, the IHI has made available 21 white papers online (http://www.ihi.org/IHI/Results/WhitePapers/) representing innovative work in healthcare improvement.

Initially, the IHI helped identify and spread of best practices for healthcare institutions. The goal of best practices is to reduce defects and errors in microsystems. Then, the IHI focused on innovation, R&D, and new solutions on a broader scale working to reinvent multidimensional systems of care. Eventually, this work was utilized to transform entire systems of care.

The IHI has developed and published a collaborative model for healthcare improvement [2]. This model requires the team to answer three questions: (1) What are we trying to accomplish? (Aim) (2) How will we know that a change is an improvement? (Measures) (3) What changes can we make that will result in improvement? (Changes).

D.S. Tichansky, J. Morton, and D.B. Jones (eds.), *The SAGES Manual of Quality, Outcomes and Patient Safety*, DOI 10.1007/978-1-4419-7901-8_39, © Springer Science+Business Media, LLC 2012

Exhibit 39.1. No needless list.

No needless deaths
No needless pain or suffering
No helplessness in those served or serving
No unwanted waiting
No waste
No one left out

Exhibit 39.2. IHI strategies and values.

IHI strategies
Motivate: Build will and optimism for change
Get Results: Drive broad scale adoption of sound changes
Innovate: Invent new solutions
Raise joy in work: Help build the future healthcare workforce
Stay vital for the long haul: Achieve excellence in loyalty, financial stability,
  and worklife for IHI
IHI values
Without boundaries
Speed agility
Focus on subject matter
Valuing volunteers
Customer focus
Honesty
Transparency
Orderliness
Celebration and thankfulness

Changes are implemented with "Plan-Do-Study-Act" (PDSA) cycles of learning [3]. Eventually theories, ideas, and hunches are evolved, with multiple PDSA cycles, into proven clinical pathways.

Best practices alone are often hard and intimidating to implement for an individual or institution. Thus, the concept of "bundles" has been developed by IHI. A bundle is defined as a structured way of improving the process of care and patient outcomes. Usually three to five evidence-based practices, which have been proven to improve patient outcome, are considered a bundle. These practices are meant to be scientifically robust that when performed together create improved outcome. Each practice is considered a change. Each change is necessary and based on Level 1 evidence. Additionally, each change is considered an all-or-nothing measurement so there is no question about what the change is or if there is partial implementation of the change. Each change occurs in the same time and space continuum (at a specific time and in a specific place).

To help determine appropriate healthcare improvements, the IHI employs a 90-day R&D process to help initiate and support innovation efforts. The 90-day R&D Project is based on Proctor and Gamble's method of innovation [4]. IHI has an R&D team that initiates a minimum of five new projects every 90 days. Each project has a specific question, a charter which states a problem, network of innovators to find answers to the problem, a specific time frame for the investigation, and a decision at the end of 90 days. The decision can include recommendations to begin a new program, include content to an existing program, halt any additional development, or perform another R&D Project if needed. Each 90-day R&D Project can be divided in three 30-day phases:

Phase I (Scan): The first phase involves scanning literature and discussing key interviews with appropriate individuals to understand the problem or issue from all directions. At the end of the first phase, the charter is produced. The aim, description of current landscape, methods to potentially solve problems, specification for an effective solution, and bibliography are included in the charter.

Phase II (Focus): The second phase involves testing the theories and developing what works. This involves teaming with the appropriate healthcare organization to test and refine ideas. This phase involves transitioning from a descriptive theory to a normative theory. Basically, developing an early theory to a tested theory is the goal of this phase. A driver diagram helps visual and conceptualize a specific and determine which specific system components are needed to create a pathway to a set-specific goal [5].

Phase III (Summarize and disseminate): The third phase involves finishing tests, summarizing conclusions, creating a final report, and determining the best method to disseminate the information in the appropriate venues such as IHI programs and publications. During this phase, the information learned is given to the appropriate individuals to develop new programs, incorporate into current programs, or conduct future R&D Projects.

Additionally, the IHI launched a nationwide initiative known as the *100,000 Lives Campaign* to significantly decrease morbidity and mortality in healthcare for the USA. The goal was to reduce harm and deaths with six changes as listed in Exhibit 39.3. The success was enumerated by the involvement of 3,100 hospitals and an estimated 122,000 lives in 18 months. This impressive campaign was seceded by another more lofty (and successful) 2-year campaign known as *5 Million Lives Campaign*. Six new interventions (Exhibit 39.4) were added to the six initial interventions from the *100,000 Lives Campaign*.

Exhibit 39.3. 100,000 Lives Campaign.

1. Deploy rapid response teams
2. Deliver reliable, evidence-based care for acute myocardial infarction
3. Prevent adverse drug events
4. Prevent central line infections
5. Prevent surgical site infections
6. Prevent ventilator-associated pneumonia

Exhibit 39.4. 5 Million Lives Campaign.

1. Prevent harm from high-alert medications
2. Reduce surgical complications
3. Prevent pressure ulcers
4. Reduce methicillin-resistant *Staphylococcus aureus* (MRSA) infection
5. Deliver reliable, evidence-based care for congestive heart failure
6. Get boards on board

To help institution and individuals interested in healthcare improvement, the IHI has published an online tool (http://www.ihi.org/imap/tool/) known as the IHI Improvement Map. The IHI Improvement Map allows access to the key process improvements that will lead to exceptional patient care. Over 70 processes are currently accessible online. Exhibit 39.5 gives the elements of two sample processes: central line bundle and pre-operative patient assessment.

The IHI President and CEO summarized another newer IHI agenda as the Triple Aim [7]: better care, better health, at lower cost. Better care was described as safe, effective, patient-centered, timely, efficient, equitable care, which is common to many organizations involved in healthcare improvement. Better health encompasses much more than healthcare; for example, more global issues including but not limited to substance abuse, violence in society, environmental hazards, workplace hazards, etc. The last aim is per capita cost of care. Balancing health, healthcare, and per capita cost is this other agenda.

To help disseminate the knowledge of healthcare improvement, the IHI has an IHI Open School for Health Professions available online at http://ihi.org/IHI/Programs/IHIOpenSchool/. This "school" allows access to an interprofessional educational community. The aim is to help give students the skills to become change agents in healthcare improvement. The focus is patient safety, teamwork, leadership, and patient-centered care. Individuals are able to complete online courses and earn a certificate of completion.

Exhibit 39.5. Sample elements of two processes in the IHI Improvement Map

---

Central line bundle [6]
- Hand hygiene
- Maximal barrier precautions upon insertion
- Chlorhexidine skin antisepsis
- Optimal catheter site selection, with avoidance of using the femoral vein for central venous access in adult patients
- Daily review of line necessity, with prompt removal of unnecessary lines

Pre-operative patient assessment [6]
- Obtain complete medical history, including questions about risk factors
- Establish process for evaluation of history, including criteria and action steps when further assessment is necessary
- Verify critical allergy information, including medications and latex
- Verify all medications, including over-the-counter medications, and ensure process to inform patients about medications that should be taken the morning of surgery
- Define criteria and actions for patients whose ongoing medical conditions are not stable when presenting for surgery
- Ensure that medical history, diagnostic test results, and any other pre-op assessment information are available for anesthesiologist and surgical team to review in advance of surgery

---

The IHI has a remarkable record of instituting change and disseminating knowledge to improve healthcare. Its collaborative approach has helped set best practices for various healthcare providers and institutions. Individuals and institutions interested in patient safety and healthcare improvement should be familiar with the IHI efforts as well as the resources that the IHI has made available.

Selected Readings

1. Institute of Medicine. Crossing the quality chasm: a new health system for the twenty-first century. Washington: National Academy Press; 2001.
2. The Breakthrough Series: IHI's Collaborative Model for Achieving Breakthrough Improvement. IHI Innovation Series white paper. Boston: Institute for Healthcare Improvement; 2003. (Available on http://www.IHI.org).
3. Speroff T, O'Connor GT. Study designs for PDSA quality improvement research. Qual Manag Health Care. 2004;13(1):17–32.

4. Huston L, Sakkab N. Connect and develop. Harvard Business Rev. March 2006:58–66.
5. http://www.ihi.org/NR/rdonlyres/A161C1EC-5C2A-45FA-BD10-B7D1CACC4880/0/
   IHI90DayResearchandDevelopmentProcessAug10.pdf. Accessed September 1, 2010.
6. http://www.ihi.org/imap/tool/. Accessed September 1, 2010.
7. http://www.ihi.org/IHI/About/EvolutionIHIWorkStrategy.htm. Accessed September 1,
   2010.

40. SAGES History and Commitment to Education and Safety

Steven D. Schwaitzberg

Thirty years ago, a small group of visionary surgeons banded together to focus on the idea that flexible endoscopy was important to the practice of gastrointestinal surgeons. They came together at a time when it was unclear whether or not surgeons would continue to do flexible endoscopy or whether these procedures would completely fall in the realm of the gastroenterologists. Under the leadership of Jerry Marks, Ken Forde, George Berci and others, a group committed to preserving the controversial topic of the surgical practice of endoscopy was organized. They crafted a strategy and founded an organization named The Society of American Gastrointestinal Endoscopic Surgeons – SAGES. The founders' meeting was held in Atlanta in 1981. In addition to the struggle for endoscopic privileges, the clarity of SAGES' commitment to education and training has its roots in the early years of the organization. As early as 1982, the fledgling organization formed a resident education committee. This committee still exists today and manages one of the cornerstone activities of the society.

Additional early SAGES accomplishments include:

1982: The organization issued a preliminary statement on instrument cleaning. Began work on the first two major documents to be issued by SAGES.
Guidelines on Resident Training in Endoscopy.
Surgical Privileges for Endoscopy.
1983: SAGES holds its First Scientific Session.
1984: A colonoscopy model is developed, making it easier to teach colonoscopy. A Surgical Residency Guideline for Endoscopy is issued.
1986: SAGES affiliates with its first official journal, the *American Surgeon* (SAGES began it affiliation with Springer-Verlag as the publisher of *Surgical Endoscopy* in 1991).

D.S. Tichansky, J. Morton, and D.B. Jones (eds.), *The SAGES Manual* of Quality, Outcomes and Patient Safety, DOI 10.1007/978-1-4419-7901-8_40, © Springer Science+Business Media, LLC 2012

1987: SAGES issues Guidelines for Granting of Privileges for Surgeons in Flexible Endoscopy.

1988: First World Congress of Endoscopic Surgery takes place in Berlin in June, 1988. SAGES first Postgraduate Course (laser surgery) was presented in 1988 at the San Antonio Meeting. A Video Library was established with the help of CineMed.

In 1989, Lee Smith served as SAGES president (then a society of about 1,000 members) during the first year of the laparoscopic revolution which in some sense began for SAGES at the meeting where Jacques Perissat showed his video on laparoscopic cholecystectomy for the first time in the USA. Out of the necessity that few surgeons were knowledgeable in these techniques, the old precepts of one-on-one teaching from master to student quickly fell by the wayside. To help fill this void, SAGES undertook a "Training-the-Trainers" series of courses in 1990 to teach laparoscopy and laparoscopic cholecystectomy. Furthermore, the SAGES Standards and Practice Committee issued: The role of laparoscopic cholecystectomy (L.C.) Guidelines for clinical application later published in Surgical Endoscopy in 1993 [1].

".... It is the opinion of the Society of American Gastrointestinal Endoscopic Surgeons (SAGES) that for optimal quality patient care this procedure must be performed only by surgeons who are qualified to perform open cholecystectomy. Only such surgeons possess the skill to perform biliary tract surgical procedures; only such surgeons are able to determine the best method of cholecystectomy and only such surgeons can treat complications consequent to Laparoscopic Cholecystectomy...." In many ways this was a seminal event for a young society. At that time it was unclear whether or not endoscopy into the abdomen to treat gastrointestinal disease would be performed solely by surgeons or whether or not this would be an extension of endoscopy to be performed by gastroenterologists as well.

Thus the role of SAGES grew from a small group of committed surgical endoscopists, mavericks in their own right, to the leading organization in the emerging field of minimally invasive surgery. SAGES presidents such as Jeff Ponsky guided SAGES through the hazardous course of creating new guidelines and training criteria for an emerging cluster of procedures, rapidly changing techniques and exploding technology.

Building on a foundation of innovation, successful educational training programs, scientific sessions and a respected peer-reviewed journal, SAGES has evolved to encompass preeminence in surgical education and patient safety as well as leadership in clinical gastrointestinal surgery and endoscopy. One of the critical turning points was the inception of the *Fundamentals of Laparoscopic Surgery* (FLS). This was first suggested by then SAGES Vice President Jonathan Sackier who noted the persistent high degree of variability in laparoscopic training in the USA and around the world. In the summer of 1997, a working group was formed to develop this concept further. This group was comprised of many of the then and current leaders of the society who developed a set of principles: (1) recognized standard "ATLS-like," (2) Cognitive and psychomotor skills, (3) Measurable & validated, (4) High stakes exam, and (5) Surgeon-only exam. This was later refined by the FLS Taskforce and was articulated in 2004 by Jeff Peters [2]. The overall goal of the FLS program was to "teach a standard set of cognitive and psychomotor skills to practitioners of laparoscopic surgery" in the belief that knowledge and application of these fundamentals would help "ensure a minimal standard of care for all patients undergoing laparoscopic surgery." In order to develop the psychmotor component of FLS, the taskforce engaged team and the work published in 1998 by Gerry Fried and a group at McGill University [3]. They developed a set of training tasks for a laparoscopic simulator (then named MISTELS – McGill Inanimate System for Training and Evaluation of Laparoscopic Skills) and demonstrated Content, Construct, Criterion, and Face validity for the FLS program as it related to the performance of laparoscopic skills [2, 4–6]. This commitment to validated training with high stakes examination has become a hallmark of the "Fundamentals" training programs that SAGES has developed. Today, FLS has become the de facto gold standard for validated surgical education and training. In 2009, the American Board of Surgery began to require residents training in general surgery to complete FLS as a requirement for the privilege of sitting for their qualifying board examinations. In development are two more "Fundamentals" programs and version 2.0 of the FLS program: *The Fundamentals of Endoscopic Surgery* (FES) and *The Fundamental Use of Safe Energy* (FUSE). SAGES' commitment to patient safety through *validated* education will continue to evolve as the goal of educating surgeons to perform specific procedures with highest level cognitive and technical expertise, will likely lead to the development of further programs using this paradigm.

Now a society of more than 6,000 surgeons (SAGES) has developed a wide menu of educational programs designed to improve cognitive/technical skills as well as patient safety. The committee structure of the society reflects this dedication (http://www.sages.org/leadership/committees/). More than half of the SAGES committees, working groups, and taskforces are charged with tasks that relate to patient safety, education, or quality. The Program, Continuing Education, and Educational Resource committees develop educational/scientific programs in strict accordance with ACCME guidelines. This allows SAGES the privilege to grant CME directly to program participants. This reflects the highest standards of bias-free education based on needs assessment and follow-up for program impact. To assist with these tasks, the Conflict of Interest Taskforce (CITF) and Ethics committees monitor program development. These groups have produced the annual scientific sessions/postgraduate courses which are attended yearly by more than 2000 surgeons from around the world, and acclaimed educational products such as the SAGES Top 21 video series, SAGES Grand Rounds, and SAGES Pearls. The resident education committee, which has existed since the founding of the society, organizes and manages a series of didactic and hands on courses which are attended by surgical residents from around the USA. These courses allow for an opportunity for trainees to meet, learn from, exchange ideas and receive hands-on training from experts from around the country in MIS and endoscopic procedures often filling in local training gaps. Members of the Guidelines Committee create, update and revise a series of guidelines in the field of MIS, gastrointestinal, and endoscopic surgery. These guidelines are evidence-based and are used by hospitals, payers, clinicians from around the world. More than 32 Guidelines/Statements/Outlines for Continuing Education are currently available (http://www.sages.org/publications/). Clinically oriented committees such as the Bariatrics Liaison Group, Flexible Endoscopy, and Pediatric committees oversee special educational, training, and safety issues related to these procedures. The Bariatrics Liaison group organized an appropriateness conference for bariatric surgical procedures which was the model for further regional/national work such as the Betsy Lehman Center Guidelines for Bariatric Surgery. The Publications committee manages (along the European Association of Endoscopic Surgery) the editorial process of *Surgical Endoscopy* (Springer-Verlag), a highly ranked surgical journal with wide readership. The journal developed and introduced the concept of "the video is the manuscript" and video supplementary material to text manuscripts allowing surgeons for the first time to not only read about procedures but also to watch them in the context of peer-reviewed surgical literature searchable through PubMed [7]. This committee also oversees the SAGES manuals (Springer-Verlag) *The SAGES Manual of Strategic Decision Making: Case Studies in Minimal Access Surgery, The SAGES Manual of Perioperative Care in Minimally Invasive Surgery, The SAGES Manual: Fundamentals of Laparoscopy, Thoracoscopy and GI*

Endoscopy 2/e, and *The SAGES Manual of Bariatric Surgery* which presents a practical "how to" approach to minimally invasive bariatric surgery. The Research and Career Development Committee receives, reviews, and scores grant requests in the field of MIS and awards between 5 and 10 grant awards each aimed at improving the clinical outcome and fostering research in this field. The "Fundamentals" groups as noted above are charged with the task of developing and administering validated surgical training. Greater than 95% of graduating surgical residents complete FLS by the end of their training. Other specialties such as gynecology and urology have shown interest in the FLS program as well. Payers and even malpractice carriers have demonstrated a willingness to direct attending surgeons to the FLS program [8]. The Outcomes, Quality and Safety Committee (QOS) evolved from a committee originally named the Outcomes Committee which was the brainchild of Bill Traverso in the mid-1990s. He recognized the need and the value of surgeons logging their own cases into a secure database in order to evaluate their own outcomes as the basis for improved care [9]. This effort antedated and perhaps was the forerunner of terrific programs such as Surgical Care Improvement Project (SCIP), Self-assessment in surgical Maintenance of Certification (MOC), or Practice-Based Learning introduced by the American College of Surgeons (ACS). In 2007, the Outcomes committee merged its database assets into the ACS case log system which is now the largest surgeon-entered surgical database in existence. Today the QOS committee has expanded its charge by developing patient safety programs in MIS, bariatrics, and was instrumental in developing the FUSE program. SAGES was an early signatory to the World Health Organization Safe Surgery Saves Lives Checklist Project. The most recent work is a collaboration with the Association of Operating Room Nurses (AORN) resulting in the development of a safety checklist of MIS procedures.

Despites its name, SAGES is an international organization. The Global affair committee is charged with creating and managing international outreach programs. Some of them are organized in conjunction with the program committee in the form of symposia conducted with local MIS societies. The SAGES Go Global team has provided on-site hands-on training in MIS and endoscopy in rural locations where equipment and training have traditionally been sparse. The ultimate goals of these programs are to foster self-sufficiency and safe surgery in MIS. Overall SAGES global activities have taken place in Europe, Asia, Central America, the Caribbean, and South America. Some of these activities have been augmented with Internet-based communication technologies such as Skype in order to extend the effectiveness of the outreach [10]. It is not unexpected that a surgical society with deep roots in cutting edge technology to use those skills in education. The Technology Committee developed a series of program entitled *Surgeon in the Digital Age* educating surgeons to use the new array of tools available to enhance their practice, develop educational materials, and troubleshoot in the operating room. In addition this group led the society, thus surgical societies in general, in the conversion from analogue-based educational materials (video tape, paper syllabus, audience response, slide projection) to digitally based cutting edge (IPod, Web-based, smart phone compatible) education materials that are environmentally friendly a more economical method of enduring material creation and a more efficient distribution platform. This group spawned the Web task force. This group led by Dan Herron, Jason Levine, and Ed Rosado has speared headed SAGES' second digital revolution and is converting the society to do its work through a social network framework. SAGES extensive collection of surgical video was placed on the Internet, free of charge on SAGES TV (http://www.sages.org/video/index.php). While anybody can view these videos, SAGES members can upload their own contributions to the site, rate other video and submit reviews. iMAGES at SAGES (http://www.sages.org/image_library/index.php) is the search/ratable/reviewable image repository. Designed as an educational resource, SAGES members can freely upload and download these images for any educational activity within the terms of the use agreement. The SAGES Wikipedia may represent the ultimate evolution of the SAGES manuals. It is a commonly held belief that textbooks are at least in part, out-of-date by the time they arrive on the shelf or e-book reader. The SAGES Surgical Wiki project (www.sageswiki.org) will allow real-time update of the conventional surgical wisdom by SAGES members shortening the time that new information is publically available. Finally, the SAGES Board of Governors and Executive Committee have sustained the educational mission of the society through continuous reinvestment of the society's resources for new and proven beneficial education and safety program throughout its 30-year history.

The diffusion of novel technologies and techniques in the surgical milieu represents unique challenges in education and patient safety. In 2005, the prospect of translumenal endoscopic surgery captured the imagination of surgeons and endoscopists around the world. The techniques were either experimental or theoretical at that point and questions such as "how would this be developed" or "how would this be introduced safely to patients" were raised. To answer these challenges,

SAGES and The American Society of Gastrointestinal Endoscopy (ASGE) under the leader of David Rattner and Rob Hawes organized a joint committee to evaluate this problem. These two societies formed the Natural Orifice Surgery Consortium for Assessment and Research (NOSCAR). The consortium organized international meetings, sought funding, distributed research grants, and developed a human registry to track the adoption of Natural Orifice translumenal Endoscopic Surgery (NOTES) [11]. Of critical consequence was the fact that the NOSCAR working group felt that NOTES was experimental, only to be performed under Institutional Review Board (IRB) protocol. The working group will develop the guidelines for training and credentialing surgeons and endoscopists as these procedures are introduced. This thoughtful, deliberate, and evidence-based approach to the introduction of new procedures will hopefully serve as the model for the safe introduction of surgical innovation.

Summary

SAGES 30+ year history is a story of surgical leadership in innovation, education, and a commitment to patient safety. The next decades will further emphasize that the most secure approach to improving patient safety will be through validated training and evidence-based practice improvement.

Selected Readings

1. The role of laparoscopic cholecystectomy (L.C.). Guidelines for clinical application. Society of American Gastrointestinal Endoscopic Surgeons (SAGES). Surg Endosc. 1993;7:369.
2. Peters JH, Fried GM, Swanstrom LL, et al. Development and validation of a comprehensive program of education and assessment of the basic fundamentals of laparoscopic surgery. Surgery. 2004;135:21.
3. Derossis AM, Fried GM, Abrahamowicz M, et al. Development of a model for training and evaluation of laparoscopic skills. Am J Surg. 1998;175:482.
4. Derossis AM, Bothwell J, Sigman HH, et al. The effect of practice on performance in a laparoscopic simulator. Surg Endosc. 1998;12:1117.
5. Fried GM. FLS assessment of competency using simulated laparoscopic tasks. J Gastrointest Surg. 2008;12:210.

6. Fried GM, Feldman LS, Vassiliou MC, et al. Proving the value of simulation in laparoscopic surgery. Ann Surg. 2004;240:518.

7. Schwaitzberg SD. The future is now Surgical Endoscopy announces the electronic publication of multimedia articles and dynamic manuscripts. Surg Endosc. 2003;17:1173.

8. Derevianko AY, Schwaitzberg SD, Tsuda S, et al. Malpractice carrier underwrites Fundamentals of Laparoscopic Surgery training and testing: a benchmark for patient safety. Surg Endosc. 2010;24:616.

9. Archer SB, Sims MM, Giklich R, et al. Outcomes assessment and minimally invasive surgery: historical perspective and future directions. Surg Endosc. 2000;14:883.

10. Okrainec A, Henao O, Azzie G. Telesimulation: an effective method for teaching the fundamentals of laparoscopic surgery in resource-restricted countries. Surg Endosc. 2010;24:417.

11. Rattner DW, Hawes R. What is NOSCAR? Surg Endosc. 2007;21:1045.

Part VI
Professional Education

41. Standardizing Surgical Education: Implications for Quality of Care

Jo Buyske

Surgical education in the USA has evolved slowly over the last 200 years. Now, in the early part of the twenty-first century, we are in a period of self-examination and change. Standardization has become an important goal: standardization of training; measurable and universal standards of achievement; ongoing measures aimed at preserving a baseline of knowledge; and lifelong learning in a field in which the knowledge base changes seemingly hourly.

In the nineteenth century, both medical education and surgical training in the USA were essentially unregulated. Many medical schools were private, for-profit enterprises with no universal standards. Many surgical "training programs" were simple preceptorships in which the trainee worked for a surgeon for some period of time and was then declared independent, again without any universal standards. Change toward more standardization and accountability occurred at the turn of the last century in both medical and post-graduate training. We are now in another period of change aimed at increasing standardization and, through standardization, increased ability to measure and improve outcomes. Several surgical groups are involved in identifying and documenting these standards: the regulatory bodies of the American Board of Surgery (ABS), the Residency Review Committee in Surgery of the Accreditation Council for Graduate Medical Education (ACGME RRC-S); and the education-focused surgical societies, including the American Surgical Association (ASA), the American College of Surgeons (ACS), the Association of Program Directors in Surgery (APDS), the Association of Surgical Educators (ASE), and the Society of American Gastrointestinal and Endoscopic Surgeons(SAGES).

D.S. Tichansky, J. Morton, and D.B. Jones (eds.), *The SAGES Manual of Quality, Outcomes and Patient Safety*, DOI 10.1007/978-1-4419-7901-8_41, © Springer Science+Business Media, LLC 2012

Standardization of Medical Education

In 1908, the Council on Medical Education (created by the AMA) worked with the Carnegie Foundation for the Advancement of teaching to survey all 155 existing North American Medical schools. The work was carried out by Abraham Flexner, and the result was the now famous Flexner report. Flexner took two full years to do his work, and visited every medical school in the nation. His resulting report was quite harsh, condemning many of the common practices. He did identify some model schools, including Harvard, John Hopkins, and Wake Forest. He made several strong recommendations in the interests of improving and standardizing medical education, and they can be summarized as follows:

- Admission to a medical school should have a minimum requirement of a high school diploma and 2 years of college, preferably devoted to basic science.
- Medical school should last for 4 years, and should have a defined curriculum.
- Medical schools should be part of a university, and not stand alone institutions.

Less known is Flexner's recommendation that medical schools appoint full-time clinical professors. Holders of these appointments would become "true university teachers, barred from all but charity practice, in the interest of teaching." Flexner pursued this objective for years, but was not able to win adoption of this part of his recommendations.

It is useful to note, as we struggle with effecting change in this century, that it took 10 years for Flexner's recommendations to be fully implemented, and the last one never was. Sometimes one needs to compromise in order to get things done!

Standardization of Surgical Training

Flexner's report led to improved and more standardized medical education. Surgical training was also in need of improvement and standardization. Through the 1800s, surgical training was essentially a question of private preceptorships. A potential surgeon apprenticed with a practicing surgeon, did what was asked of him, and after an indeterminant period of time was declared ready for practice, and allowed to work independently. There were no case requirements, time requirements, or tests of skill or knowledge.

Dr. William Halsted, then chief of the department of surgery at Johns Hopkins Hospital, conceived of a new plan for surgical training. Halsted's surgical residency program consisted of an internship, residency, and housemanship. The duration of the internship was left undefined, and individuals advanced once Halsted believed they were ready for the next level of training (this is an early example of competency-based advancement). Internship was followed by 6 years as an assistant resident and then 2 years as house surgeon. In 1889, Halsted took on his first surgical resident.

Halsted's program of mentored graduated responsibility persisted as the model for surgical training for the next 100 years. Thus, by the early part of the twentieth century both medical education and surgical training were on a continuum of a new standard of consistency.

The Board Movement: Standards for the Practicing Surgeon by Way of Certification

The American Board of Surgery was formed in 1937, out of a committee created by the ASA with representatives from other societies. The Flexner report had exposed the discrepancies in medical education; there followed a growing realization in the surgical community that just as there were good and bad medical schools, even with the new Halstedian residencies there were surgeons who were well trained and surgeons who were not. There were essentially no objective standards or hurdles to declaring oneself a fully trained, independently operating surgeon. The charge toward evaluation and certification was lead by Derrick Vail, an opthalmologist, who, in a 1908 speech to the American Academy of Opthalmology and Otolaryngology stated:

I hope to see the time when ophthalmology will be taught in this country as it should be taught. That day will come when we demand…that a certain amount of preliminary education and training be enforced before a man may be licensed to practice ophthalmology. After a sufficiently long term of service in an ophthalmic institution …he should be permitted to appear before a proper examining board for examination…and if he is found competent let him then be permitted and licensed to practice ophthalmology.

That speech inspired the formation of the American Board of Opthalmology in 1917, and in 1937 surgery followed suit. The American Board of Surgery, when formed, committed itself to establish a comprehensive, standardized certification process, which included periodic assessment of individual hospitals as appropriate places of training, the requirement of 5 years of training beyond internship, and the development of an examination process. Those processes endure to this day, in the form of the residency review committee of surgery, surgical residency programs, and the qualifying and certifying examinations of the American Board of Surgery. It is worth noting that the original mission statement of the American Board of Surgery states that it is formed to "protect the public and improve the specialty" and that the path to that goal was the institution of standards of education and knowledge.

Standardizing Training Programs

Directly related to the board movement was the development of residency review committees, or the RRC. The originators of the American Board of Surgery recognized that a separate body was needed to set standards and assess programs, and that the quality of a training program could not be separated from the quality of the trainee. Thus the RRC was developed in parallel to the board process, and programs were assessed by an independent group to ensure that they could provide the training environment needed to train a young surgeon into a surgeon capable of becoming board certified and practicing independently. Simply put, the RRC accredits programs, and the ABS certifies individuals.

The Development of New Standards in this Century

The Six Competencies

In 1999 the ACGME, in concert with the American Board of Medical Specialties (ABMS), endorsed the concept of the Six Competencies as a way of improving quality and increasing standardization across all medical specialties. Each specialty area was responsible for identifying which tools would be used to fulfill training and assessment in each of the six competencies. The Six Competencies are as follows:

- Patient Care and Procedural Skills: Provide care that is compassionate, appropriate and effective treatment for health problems and to promote health.
- Medical Knowledge: Demonstrate knowledge about established and evolving biomedical, clinical and cognate sciences and their application in patient care.
- Interpersonal and Communication Skills: Demonstrate skills that result in effective information exchange and teaming with patients, their families and professional associates (e.g., fostering a therapeutic relationship that is ethically sound, uses effective listening skills with nonverbal and verbal communication; working as both a team member and at times as a leader).
- Professionalism: Demonstrate a commitment to carrying out professional responsibilities, adherence to ethical principles and sensitivity to diverse patient populations.
- Systems-based Practice: Demonstrate awareness of and responsibility to larger context and systems of healthcare. Be able to call on system resources to provide optimal care (e.g., coordinating care across sites or serving as the primary case manager when care involves multiple specialties, professions or sites).
- Practice-based Learning and Improvement: Able to investigate and evaluate their patient care practices, appraise and assimilate scientific evidence and improve their practice of medicine.

Effective implementation and use of the Six Competencies has proved challenging. They have been used as a framework for evaluation in both surgical training and in Maintenance of Certification (MOC), and yet objective measures and effective teaching tools in several of the arenas remain to be developed. The American Board of Surgery In-training Examination fulfills the assessment for Medical Knowledge, the second competency. SCORE (see below) addresses the competency of Patient Care, and may be used to address other competencies as well. MOC collapses the competencies into four, but still addresses each one. To date the greatest value of the Six Competencies has been to force thinking of medical competencies as standard and universal to all physicians, expressed differently in each specialty but still sharing a common responsibility. Curriculum development and assessment in each arena is an ongoing endeavor.

The Blue Ribbon Committee

The Blue Ribbon Committee of the American Surgical Association was formed in 2002. Composed of representatives from the ASA, the ACS, the ABS, and the ACGME RRC-S, the Blue Ribbon Committee was charged with assessing the current state of surgery and surgical education in the USA, and with making recommendations for change. After meeting over 2 years, the Blue Ribbon Committee developed recommendations regarding improving or developing standards as follows:

In the domain of medical student education: that students develop technical proficiency in clinical skills laboratories before encountering patients.

In the domain of residency education in surgery: that the basic topics that all surgical residents should master be defined, and a modular, fundamentals of surgery curriculum be developed.

In the domain of the structure of surgical training: that new teaching technologies and verification of competence at each training milepost should be instituted as these tools are developed and validated.

Surgical Council on Resident Education

At least one charge of the Blue Ribbon Committee was heard and addressed. In 2006 the ABS and five other surgical organizations formed SCORE, the Surgical Council on Resident Education. SCORE's mission is to improve the education of general surgery residents (trainees) through the development of a standard national curriculum for general surgery residency training. SCORE draws upon the Six Competencies to provide a structure, and currently addresses primarily the first competency, Patient Care and Procedural Skills. The Association of Program Directors in Surgery worked closely with the General Surgery Residency Committee of the American Board of Surgery and, using an iterative process, identified the essential cases and diseases that surgical residents should be able to manage to varying degrees. This accomplishment, that of defining the curriculum for surgical training, is a long missing key toward standardization of surgical training. A curriculum is the keystone for ensuing assessment.

Board Certification

The requirements for board certification have so far been few: 5 years of training in an ACGME-accredited training program; a case log documenting 500 cases; and the signature of a program director attesting to satisfactory completion of training were the tickets to taking the qualifying (written) and, if successful, the certifying (oral) examinations. The ABS did not intersect with any individual until the end of residency.

In 2010, for the first time the ABS instituted measurable requirements to be completed during residency in order to be eligible for the qualifying examination. These included successful completion of Advanced Trauma Life Support (ATLS), Advanced Cardiovascular Life Support (ACLS), and FLS (Fundamentals of Laparoscopic Surgery). The case log requirements were expanded and more detail was added, especially in the arena of surgical critical care. It is likely that this is only the first step in instituting standardized requirements and milestones in residency.

Milestones would be in the form of additional requirements in residency. They could be "go/no go" points, meaning that failure to achieve a milestone means nonprogression in residency, or they could be a series of formative assessments used for feedback. The ACGME and the ABS, both jointly and independently, are considering a variety of milestones, which could include things as diverse as objective assessment of technical and operative skills, assessment of patient interactions using standardized tools, passing scores on examinations at various levels of training, case minimums by year, courses and examinations in professionalism and ethics, and participation in institutional review or quality programs. Institution of milestones opens the door to several desirable outcomes: one, it would be possible to move to competency-based advancement in residency training as opposed to the current time-based advancement, and two, residents who were struggling could be more objectively identified earlier in their training, and either remediated or allowed to move into a different career path. As noted by the Blue Ribbon Committee, tools for these measures should be implemented as they are developed and validated.

Maintenance of Certification

Originally, once certified, a surgeon was certified forever. He or she simply walked out of the oral exams, got a letter from the ABS saying they had passed, and that was it for the rest of his or her career unless they got arrested for felony. The directors of the ABS and leadership in surgery were not satisfied with this standard. Starting in 1976, all certificates were time limited. Once every 10 years the diplomats submitted their license and credentials, a case log, recommendation forms, and if these were satisfactory, took a general multiple choice examination. Interestingly, the results of those examinations, called the recertification exams, confirmed that the knowledge base of a surgeon 20 or 30 years out of training was not the same as the knowledge base of surgeons within 10 years of their training; the former group failed the exam in high numbers.

Over time even recertification was deemed inadequate for ongoing certification. In 2000, the 24-member boards of the ABMS voted to adopt MOC across all specialties. MOC changes the timeline for surgeons maintaining certification from once every 10 years to ongoing. MOC requirements fall in four categories, and are based on the ACGME/ABMS Six Competencies. The areas of MOC are as follows:

- Part 1: Professional standing through maintenance of an unrestricted medical license, hospital privileges, and satisfactory references.
- Part 2: Lifelong learning and self-assessment through continuing education and periodic self-assessment.
- Part 3: Cognitive expertise based on performance on a secure examination.
- Part 4: Evaluation of performance in practice through tools such as outcome measures and quality improvement programs, and the evaluation of behaviors such as communication and professionalism.

The ABS MOC requirements are evolving. Parts 1 and 3 are straightforward, and involve documentation of credentials and participating in the recertification examination, as before. Parts 2 and 4 are where lie the challenge and the opportunity. Part 2 is currently fulfilled by a variety of CME activities, including some which require taking a short multiple choice exam to ensure understanding of the material. A goal for Part 2 self-assessment would be to link the self-assessment to practice, such that the self-assessment tools are used in an area that matches the diplomats practice pattern as identified through their case logs. Better still would be an application of self-assessment that actually involves assessing a given surgeon's processes and practice. The ABS has challenged the professional surgical societies to come up with these tools, so that each surgeon has the opportunity to use measures and self-assessment pertinent to his or her practice.

Part 4 is also a challenge and an opportunity. In surgery it seems clear that this measure must be about outcomes, and comparing one's own outcome to a national standard. Although there are excellent outcomes databases available, each suffers from short comings related to either expense, self-reporting, lack of audit, or large time commitments. To date there is not a universally applicable, accessible, affordable, and pertinent database that surgeons can use to compare their own outcomes to others. The ABS, the ABMS, and the ACS are working aggressively to correct this deficiency so that a usable database is available to all surgeons to inform their practice. In the meantime superb databases are available for specific situations: the Society of Thoracic Surgeons database is widely subscribed and highly reliable, as is the National Surgical Quality Improvement Program. Both of these programs are expensive, and demand institutional support, and yet they serve as a model for what can be done. Meanwhile, participation in any of a variety of databases fulfills Part 4, on the theory that the practice of measuring anything is a valuable exercise.

MOC, when mature, will provide both a vehicle and a requirement for surgeons to structure their learning and measure their practices and outcomes.

Summary and Conclusion

It has been a long journey since Flexner and Halsted set about trying to put some structure on medical student and surgical training. We have gone from a wild west of no common standards to an era where medical school curriculum and surgical training curricula are explicitly defined. We are immediately engaged in defining milestones across the six competencies that will help define if and when residents meet their training goals. MOC brings with it the opportunity to use a standard tool to assess outcomes, as well as adding rigor and structure to continuing medical education and professional development. It is our hope and expectation that residents will use SCORE and Milestones as part of a lifelong portfolio, acquainting them with the process of continuous documentation of professional competency and learning. To document in an organized manner is to allow study. Now that education is being brought into a standardized form, and practice is quickly following, the door will be open to studying best practices and outcomes in ways that have not previously been available.

Selected Readings

1. Griffen, W. The American Board of Surgery in the 20th Century-Then and Now. Copyright Ward O. Griffen, 2004.
2. Debas HT, Bass BL, Brennan MF, Flynn TC, Folse JR, Freischlag JA, et al. American Surgical Association Blue Ribbon Committee Report on Surgical Education: 2004. Ann Surg. 2005;241(1):1–8. doi:10.1097/01.sla.0000150066.83563.52.
3. Sachdeva AK, Bell Jr RH, Britt LD, Tarpley JL, Blair PG, Tarpley MJ. National efforts to reform residency education in surgery. Acad Med. 2007;82(12):1200–10.
4. Bell RH. Surgical council on resident education: a new organization devoted to graduate surgical education. J Am Coll Surg. 2007;204(3):341–6.
5. The ABS Booklet of Information. http://home.absurgery.org/xfer/BookletofInfo-Surgery.pdf. Accessed January 28, 2011.
6. SCORE. http://www.surgicalcore.org/about.html. Accessed January 28, 2011.

42. Training Standards/Fellowship Council

Adrian Park and Erica Sutton

Evolution of Quality Standards in Postgraduate Surgical Training

Minimally invasive surgery (MIS) techniques define the most recent era of innovation and discovery in a field known to change slowly and with reservation. Laparoscopic cholecystectomy (LC), first introduced by Dr. Philippe Mouret in 1987 [1], offered a significantly less invasive approach to a commonly performed abdominal procedure, creating widespread public demand that, in turn, necessitated widespread and rapid training of surgeons of all levels [2]. This broad need for training resulted in a new model of surgical education – namely partnerships between industry and stakeholder surgical societies who collaborated to offer short, intensive courses in LC [2]. Academic centers were initially reticent to champion laparoscopic techniques to the youngest of trainees – residents – viewing MIS procedures as unproved and marginal [2]. With the inhomogeneous introduction of LC, however, came a reexamination of the need for quality training in laparoscopic techniques. This need was essentially unmet in the early 1990s in surgical residency programs.

As the limitations, even failings, of the "weekend courses" were recognized, often in the form of suboptimal patient outcomes [3, 4], demand for apprenticeships or "mini-fellowships" with the (relatively) few MIS experts steadily increased, soon evolving into 1- or 2-year fellowships. One of the first postgraduate fellowships in MIS was instituted at the University of Maryland in 1990. In 1997, there were nine such fellowships. That number increased to 80 – nearly ninefold – by 2004 [2]. These fellowships varied in duration, focus, content, and end product. During this period of unprecedented growth, directors of the fellowship programs recognized the need to establish quality, standards, and consistency in the postgraduate training of surgeons. There was also

D.S. Tichansky, J. Morton, and D.B. Jones (eds.), *The SAGES Manual of Quality, Outcomes and Patient Safety*, DOI 10.1007/978-1-4419-7901-8_42, © Springer Science+Business Media, LLC 2012

a growing consensus around the need to bring order to the rather chaotic process by which fellowship program directors and applicants selected one another. Abuses on both sides abounded in these early years of MIS fellowship training. It was unfortunately often a case of "buyer and seller" "beware"! Thus it was that in 2003, the Minimally Invasive Surgery Fellowship Council (MISFC) was founded as a nonprofit organization, governed by an executive committee of fellowship directors along with 40 founding fellowship programs [2]. It was seen, among other things, as a forum for leaders in postgraduate surgical education to discuss issues related to the developing of fellowship training curricula, program administration and funding, and establishing a mechanism (match) for the selection of fellows.

The MISFC conducted its first match process in December 2003 for fellowships beginning in July 2004. Within a year or so, the MISFC joined with representatives of the Society for Surgery of the Alimentary Tract (SSAT), the Society of American Gastrointestinal and Endoscopic Surgeons (SAGES), the American Hepato-Pancreatico-Biliary Association (AHPBA), and in 2005 with the American Society for Metabolic and Bariatric Surgery (ASMBS) to form the organization known, more inclusively, as the Fellowship Council (FC) [5]. The FC now oversees 113 member fellowships, recruits applicants annually, establishes fellowship training standards, and engages an independent accreditation process for postgraduate training programs in minimally invasive, gastrointestinal (GI), bariatric, hepatobiliary, and colorectal surgery.

The guidelines for accreditation established by the FC represent a consensus among sponsoring organizations and relevant thought leaders as to the key components of a high quality fellowship and describe/ illustrate quality standards in postgraduate surgical training within these disciplines. Specific direction is provided by the guidelines as to the necessary qualifications of fellowship directors and teaching staff, the range of academic activity in which fellows are expected to engage, the minimum competencies fellows are expected to demonstrate, and the educational resources that ought to exist for the successful achievement of these educational objectives [6]. Importantly, the guidelines contain a clear imperative to preserve the quality of surgical residency training in programs where both residents and fellows exist. In fact one of the fundamental tenets upon which such fellowships are evaluated is that residency training experience and case load not be compromised in the least by the coexisting MIS fellowship.

Outcomes Related to Training Standards

What is the measurable impact – both for surgeon and patient – of a surgical fellowship? Recent data suggest that the mere intention to participate in a laparoscopic fellowship is associated with having performed higher volumes of laparoscopic cases during the residency training period [5]. A 2009 survey indicated that 19% of minimally invasive fellows had decided to pursue fellowship training in order to gain increased laparoscopic experience [7]. This decision on the part of trainees suggests that residency was not expected to provide adequate exposure to advanced laparoscopy by the end of chief year. Another importance of this finding is the belief on the part of trainees that volume matters. Such a belief is supported in the literature by observational studies relating center volume and patient outcomes after pancreaticoduodenectomy [8, 9]. Of equal importance, Park et al. found that the combination of general surgery residency and MIS fellowship produced case volumes more reflective of competence than residency alone [5]. Thus, when case volume is examined as a surgeon-specific outcome, fellowship training has a favorable impact.

The relationship between fellowship experience and patient outcomes has, importantly, been systematically investigated. Direct supervision by experienced faculty has been noted as a positive contributor to the fellowship experience. Indeed, in a study that demonstrated that laparoscopic gastric bypass (LGB) morbidity or mortality was unchanged by MIS fellowship, Clements et al. attributed having an experienced attending on hand from beginning to end of all cases as a crucial factor permitting fellows to safely concentrate on and accomplish such operations [10]. Both preventative and corrective measures were available as a result of the attending's knowledge and technical facility. The attending was also credited with promoting adherence in regard to proven, step-by-step procedural methods and with able assistance, both understanding and anticipatory.

Seeking to determine whether an advanced MIS fellowship program could be safely established for training, Kothari et al. compared pre- and post-fellowship outcomes in an academic community hospital [11]. The result was a characterization of positive outcomes regarding the impact of fellowship experience on institutional bariatric surgical outcomes: no increase in length of stay or in rates of major [anastomotic leak, deep venous thrombosis/pulmonary embolism (DVT/PE), transfusion, intestinal obstruction, mortality] or minor complications (stomal stenosis, marginal ulcer, wound infection, incisional hernia) as well as comparable percentages of excess weight loss. The only significant difference reported was a 31-min increase in operative time (substantially higher than the 5-min increase described by Clements et al. [10]), which was accounted for by variety of instructional methodology, procedural technique, and fellow skill level.

Ali and associates [12] sought to measure the complication-related outcomes of five fellowship-trained bariatric surgeons for the initial 100 cases performed by each immediately after fellowship completion. The collected data were then compared with the 611 cases that during their fellowships had collectively been performed by all five under the mentorship of experienced bariatric surgeons. The two groups of patients under comparison did not differ statistically with respect to BMI, gender distribution, conversion to open gastric bypass, rates of marginal ulceration, gastrojejunal leak, gastrogastric fistulization, jejunojejunal leak, jejunojejunal obstruction, internal hernia formation, pulmonary embolism, or mortality. Fellowship graduates (FGs) had slightly older patients, more wound infections, and a higher rate of GI hemorrhage. FGs also had fewer gastrojejunal strictures, nongastrojejunal leaks, bowel obstructions, and incisional hernias. The findings of Ali and colleagues [12] support the observations of Oliak, Owens and Schmidt [13] who reported improved perioperative outcomes over the first 75 laparoscopic gastric bypasses performed by a fellowship-trained surgeon when compared with a surgeon who had not completed a fellowship. These studies validate the concept that advanced postresidency training can help surgeons overcome the learning curve for advanced minimally invasive procedures and achieve quality outcomes equal to reported benchmarks.

Training Methods that Promote Patient Safety

As the public demand increases for minimal access techniques and their resultant benefits, including less perceptible scars and quicker recovery, it stands to reason that surgeons want to meet that demand. Identification of which training methods are associated with the safe adoption and implementation of new surgical techniques is increasingly scrutinized [14]. Early experiences with the introduction of LC have demonstrated that the setting in which a surgeon learns a new procedure influences safety. A 2001 survey of 1,661 surgeons conducted by Archer and colleagues [15] demonstrated that those trained to perform LC as part of surgical residency had fewer bile duct injuries in the early performance of the procedure than those who learned to perform LC after residency training. Furthermore, surgeons in the latter group were 39% more likely to report one bile duct injury and 58% more likely to report two or more bile duct injuries than surgeons trained to perform LC during residency. This led the authors to conclude that residency training led to improvements in the safety of LC. As surgical technique and instrumentation continue to evolve and new technologies are introduced, practicing surgeons continue to be faced with the challenges of acquiring new surgical skills and implementing them safely into practice.

Zerey et al. [16] describe two common methods – mini-fellowships and preceptorships – by which the surgeon in practice might acquire MIS skills. Mini-fellowships allow a group of surgeons to attend a short course commonly taught by subject matter experts and consisting of a didactic component followed by a hands-on experience, usually practiced using an inanimate model, in a relevant surgical technique. The preceptorship, in contrast, allows a novice surgeon to be mentored or precepted though a procedure by a more experienced surgeon in the live patient setting. Both methods present challenges and limitations with respect to time away from one's practice and credentialing issues. Yet in studies performed by Heniford and colleagues [17] comparing these two instructional methods, surgeons who participated in a preceptorship were more likely to later perform the procedure taught and were less likely to use an open approach. The authors suggested that in order to safely achieve the goal of acquiring and transferring new skills to an established surgical practice, training would ideally involve a structured preceptorship.

Preceptorships represent a high-fidelity model of surgical education in that they provide the intense expert supervision well matched to the highly skilled and developed learner, specifically the surgeon in practice looking for additional training. In the case of less experienced learners, simulation-based medical education (SBME) appropriately moves training out of the operational environment in favor of increased patient safety. SBME now has many forms, ranging from mechanical models, box trainers, Web-based simulators, and cognitive skill trainers to remotely controlled mannequins capable of replicating human physiology and virtual reality (VR). SBME has improved patient safety among its central objectives – its efficacy in this role is well established. The benefits to patient safety are of dual consequence immediate in that novices are not learning new skills on patients and eventual in terms of resultant skill acquisition that is improved and transferable to the operating room.

A validated example of simulation-based training is the Web-based education module – Fundamentals of Laparoscopic Surgery (FLS) education module – developed by SAGES that includes a cognitive assessment tool as well as a hands-on skills training component and assessment tool. The module presents the basics of laparoscopic surgery – technical as well as cognitive, surgical decision-making skills – in a format that is consistent and scientifically accepted and that facilitates practice and assessment with its concluding purpose being improved quality in relation to patient care. Germane to this chapter is the use of FLS certification as a validated training tool to measure competency in the basic tenets of laparoscopic surgery. In a move signifying the module's importance as a training standard indicative of basic competence and safety in laparoscopy, the American Board of Surgery (ABS) has endorsed FLS. Additionally, FLS certification is now an eligibility requirement for board certification. Certainly, the fact that a central objective of FLS is to provide a validated educational tool measuring both skills and knowledge that are primary to laparoscopic surgical performance speaks to a potential future role for it both in the credentialing process and in application for hospital privileges.

Conclusions

The evolution of quality standards in postresidency training is due in large part to the creation and influence of the Fellowship Council. The benefits of fellowship training have been quantified in bariatric surgery, where surgeon- and patient-centered outcomes appear favorable for fellowship-trained surgeons. Training methods that promote patient safety have begun to rely increasingly on simulation, though they continue to incorporate learner supervision such as that which is part of residency training and proctorships in the operational environment. The use of validated assessment tools as a measure of competence and safety in surgery is increasing.

Selected Readings

1. Mouret P. How I developed laparoscopic cholecystectomy. Ann Acad Med Singapore. 1996;25(5):744–7.
2. Swanstrom LL, Park A, Arregui M, Franklin M, Smith CD, Blaney C. Bringing order to the chaos: developing a matching process for minimally invasive and gastrointestinal postgraduate fellowships. Ann Surg. 2006;243(4):431–5.

3. Zucker KA. Training issues [editorial]. Surg Laparosc Endos. 1992;2:187.

4. Reznick R. Let's not forget that CME has an "E.". Foc Surg Ed. 1999;17:1–2.

5. Park A, Kavic SM, Lee TH, Heniford BT. Minimally invasive surgery: the evolution of fellowship. Surgery. 2007;142(4):505–11. discussion 511–13.

6. The Fellowship Council. Guidelines for Fellowship Council Accredited Fellowships in Surgery. http://www.fellowshipcouncil.org/finalguidelines.php. Accessed April 19, 2010.

7. Grover BT, Kothari SN, Kallies KJ, Mathiason MA. Benefits of laparoscopic fellowship training: a survey of former fellows. Surg Innov. 2009;16(4):283–8.

8. Gordon TA, Bowman HM, Tielsch JM, Bass EB, Burleyson GP, Cameron JL. Statewide regionalization of pancreaticoduodenectomy and its effect on inhospital mortality. Ann Surg. 1998;228:71–8.

9. Birkmeyer JD, Warshaw AL, Finlayson SR, Grove MR, Tosteson AN. Relationship between hospital volume and late survival after pancreaticoduodenectomy. Surgery. 1999;126:178–83.

10. Clements RH, Leeth RR, Vickers SM, Bland KI. Incorporating laparoscopic fellowship does not increase morbidity or mortality in a university-based bariatric practice. J Am Coll Surg. 2007;204:824–8.

11. Kothari SN, Boyd WC, Lambert PJ, Mathiason MA. Can an advanced laparoscopic fellowship program be established without compromising the center's outcomes? Surg Innov. 2008;15(4):317–20.

12. Ali MR, Tichansky DS, Kothari SN, et al. Validation that a 1-year fellowship in minimally invasive and bariatric surgery can eliminate the learning curve for laparoscopic gastric bypass. Surg Endosc. 2010;24(1):138–44.

13. Oliak D, Owens M, Schmidt HJ. Impact of fellowship training on the learning curve for laparoscopic gastric bypass. Obes Surg. 2004;14(2):197–200.

14. Park A, Klein RV, editors. Minimally Invasive Surgery Training: Theories, Methods, Outcomes [e-book]. Washington: Department of Health & Human Services (US), National Institutes of Health, National Library of Medicine; 2010 January. Available from: http://www.mastri.umm.edu/NIH-Book. Accessed August 23, 2010.

15. Archer SB, Brown DW, Smith CD, Branum GD, Hunter JG. Bile duct injury during laparoscopic cholecystectomy: results of a national survey. Ann Surg. 2001;234(4):549–58. discussion 558–9.

16. Zerey M, Harrell AG, Kercher KW, Heniford BT. Minimally Invasive Surgery Training Overview. In: Park A, Klein RV, eds. *Minimally Invasive Surgery Training: Theories, Methods, Outcomes* [e-book]. Washington: Department of Health & Human Services (US), National Institutes of Health, National Library of Medicine; 2010 January. Available from: http://www.mastri.umm.edu/NIH-Book. Accessed April 23, 2010.

17. Heniford BT, Backus CL, Matthews BD, Greene FL, Teel WB, Sing RF. Optimal teaching environment for laparoscopic splenectomy. Am J Surg. 2001;181:226–30.

43. Accreditation Standards: Bariatric Surgery and Beyond

Bruce Schirmer

Introduction

The dictionary defines the word "accreditation" as the process in which certification of competency, authority, or credibility is presented. Authoritative bodies concern themselves with the accreditation of processes or programs. Since the Society of American Gastrointestinal and Endoscopic Surgeons (SAGES) manual is concerned with the areas of patient safety, outcomes, and quality, the focus of this chapter will be to review the relevant history and experience of the accreditation process of surgical programs in this country to date, as a basis for understanding the accreditation process as it currently exists and as it interfaces with patient safety and outcomes. Accreditation in the realm of the broad field of surgery currently occurs for training programs, hospital facilities, and clinical programs as part of large national networks. For clarification, the process of "certification" involves the confirmation of certain characteristics of an organization, object, or person. Professional certification is the confirmation of a level of competency of an individual to perform a task, usually as demonstrated by the passage of an examination. Thus for the purposes of this chapter, certification is the process of confirming individual competency, while accreditation is the process of confirming credibility of programs or facilities. The other process often confused with accreditation and certification is the process of privileging. Privileging in the health care field is the granting of the ability to render health care to patients based on the individual's qualifications. Privileging is a local process, governed by individual hospitals or health care facilities. Privileging often relies on an individual being both certified by a professional certifying body as well as complying with local hospital regulations and meeting quality standards as reviewed by the hospital privileging and credentialing committee. Table 43.1 summarizes the major differences and working definitions and applications between the processes of accreditation, certification, and privileging.

D.S. Tichansky, J. Morton, and D.B. Jones (eds.), *The SAGES Manual of Quality, Outcomes and Patient Safety*, DOI 10.1007/978-1-4419-7901-8_43, © Springer Science+Business Media, LLC 2012

Table 43.1. Accreditation, credentialing, and privileging.

Accreditation	Program	National Corp. Specialty society	Review and inspection
Example	Trauma program	ACS[a]	Inspection, site visit
Credentialing	Individual	Specialty board	Pass examination
Example	Dr. John Smith	ABS[b]	Pass certifying examination
Privileging	Individual	Hospital	Hospital committee review
Example	Dr. John Smith	St. Elsewhere	Passes committee review

[a]American College of Surgeons
[b]American Board of Surgery

Accreditation Processes in Place

Accreditation of Training Programs

In the realm of surgery, there is a well-defined national organization that accredits surgical training programs: the Accreditation Council for Graduate Medical Education (ACGME). The ACGME is the largest and most comprehensive accrediting body of training programs in medicine, dealing with not only surgeons in training but all graduate medical education. Its governing board is composed of representatives from five national associations interested in graduate medical education, and details of the organization of the membership of the ACGME Board are given in Table 43.2.

The ACGME has traditionally been recognized as the authority for regulating graduate medical education in the USA. Recently, however, lay pressure and political pressure have been exerted upon the organization to try to make what the political and public arenas see as improvements in safe practices of medicine. Much of the issue of political pressure has centered about duty work hours for trainees. A report by the Institute of Medicine in 2001 alleging high rates of medically related deaths in US hospitals sparked a public controversy about hospital safety. Some benefit has come from the uproar this report created, including a much more extensive review of inpatient care processes. These would include, in the surgical arena, for example, appropriate antibiotic use, DVT prophylaxis, and preoperative site identification. However, the political influence to limit work hours for trainees initially resulted in the ACGME adopting work hour guidelines across all training programs. The ACGME

Table 43.2. Organization of the board of the Accreditation Council for Graduate Medical Education.

American Board of Medical Specialties:	4 Directors
American Hospital Association:	4 Directors
American Medical Association:	4 Directors
Association of American Medical Colleges:	4 Directors
Council of Medical Specialty Societies:	4 Directors
Residents:	2 Directors
Public:	3 Directors
At-large directors:	1–4

Chair of Council of Review Committees
Federal representative (non-voting)

adopted a set of work hour guidelines in 2003, which have been instituted and enforced by the various review committees of the medical specialty boards. These duty hours were perceived and received with mixed emotions by both trainers and trainees of the various specialties. They have, however, been adopted uniformly and seemed to provide adequate safeguards for residents in training against abuses of overwork and fatigue. Limits were set for hours worked per week, hours worked at any one time, rest periods between work days, number of days on call at night in the hospital, and number of days off per week. Recently, there was further political pressure on the ACGME to further restrict work hours. The ACGME held a very comprehensive review of data and presentations for making any changes in the current rules of work, and recently issued a number of new guidelines for resident work hours, effective July 2011. These new rules further limit the work hours of PGY-1 residents, and provide for increased levels of supervision of residents while in hospital as well as some mild relaxation of strict duty hour times for residents in their last years of residency who are involved in critical patient care functions. The 2003 and 2011 new rules can be found on the ACGME Web site at http://www.acgme.org.

Accreditation of Hospitals

Accreditation of hospitals is currently performed by both state and national organizations. The most of these organizations is the Joint Commission, formerly known as the Joint Commission on Accreditation of Healthcare Organizations (JCAHO). The Joint Commission is a private sector, not-for-profit company that performs accreditation for fees for hospitals and other health care organizations. Hospitals pay such fees because JCAHO accreditation has often been the standard by which state governments recognize licensure and the ability of the hospital to receive federal insurance reimbursement under the Medicare and Medicaid programs. Another national organization which accredits outpatient health care facilities is the Accreditation Association for Ambulatory Healthcare, Inc. (AAAHC). While the process of accrediting hospitals will not be the focus of this chapter, it should be recognized that accredited hospitals and health care organizations are a basis for the appropriate facilities that will help insure quality of surgical programs. The human and physical resources at these hospitals must be of an acceptable standard so as to not compromise the quality of the surgical program that is operating in its realm.

Accreditation of Clinical Programs

Accreditation of clinical programs also has been in place for specific areas in surgery. National surgical societies have taken on the responsibility of accrediting various types of programs in the past. Most medical centers providing trauma care have been reviewed and accredited by the American College of Surgeons (ACS), as have medical centers providing surgical treatment of cancer. The ACS has long been an advocate for the accreditation of surgical care processes. In fact, the original organization of hospital accreditation that has now evolved into the Joint Commission was sponsored in its origin by the ACS.

ACS trauma centers must pass an evaluation that encompasses personnel, process, and facilities. The centers are rated by their capacity to care for the critically injured patient, with level 1 centers offering the most comprehensive and highest level of care. Accreditation for an appropriate level of trauma care becomes essential for a medical center to fit appropriately into a regional network of trauma care. Referrals of injured patients based on severity of injury and center capability is the basic premise of regionalized trauma networks. This allows the optimal care of the patient in a center prepared to treat all the patient's injuries.

Cancer centers also must meet basic criteria for oncologic treatment for patients. Appropriate multidiscipline evaluation, pathologic-based staging tumor registry, and availability of medical, surgical, and radiation therapy are all key elements of the center obtaining accreditation.

Accreditation of Non-ACGME Training Programs

During the last two decades, the number of non-ACGME fellowships in various areas of surgery has dramatically increased. Currently there are fellowships for individuals looking for further and more advanced experience in many areas of surgery, including minimally invasive surgery, bariatric surgery, hepatobiliary surgery, colorectal surgery, flexible endoscopic surgery, advanced GI surgery, oncologic surgery, breast surgery, endocrine surgery, thoracic surgery, and transplant surgery. These various areas of fellowship training are not accredited by the ACGME at present. They are instead offered by individual institutions. The overall monitoring groups for these fellowships, which usually accredit them as well, may be by the various surgical specialty societies which are focused on the various areas. For example, transplantation fellowships are governed by the Transplantation Society, oncology and breast fellowships by the Society for Surgical Oncology, and endocrine fellowships by the Endocrine Society. The rapid rise of fellowships in the late 1990s in the areas of minimally invasive surgery and bariatric surgery led to an association of the program directors involved with such fellowships. This association then joined in a common organization with the representative existing societies interested in the clinical focus of these fellowships, including the SAGES, the Society for Surgery of the Alimentary Tract (SSAT), the American Society for Metabolic and Bariatric Surgery (ASMBS), and the Americas Hepato-Pancreatico-Biliary Associaton (AHPBA). The newly formed organization was called The Fellowship Council, which currently serves as the accrediting society for a large number (over 150 currently) of non-ACGME fellowships. Until recently, these were fellowships focused on advanced GI surgery. However, this past year has seen the addition of other non-ACGME fellowships in colorectal and thoracic surgery. The American Society for Colon and Rectal Surgery joined as a member society of the Fellowship Council in 2010.

The Fellowship Council currently accredits its member fellowships, with the program directors of each fellowship being members of the society. Standards for accreditation and the accreditation process for fellowships by the Fellowship Council have been ongoing since 2004. Programs must satisfy criteria of curriculum, case load, clinical experience, scholarship, faculty, and facilities. The curriculum and case load experience are specific for the individual types of fellowships, and fellowships are listed as being of one of these defined categories.

Current categories include minimally invasive, bariatric, HPB, flexible endoscopic, advanced GI, colorectal, and thoracic. Accreditation involves initial application and acceptance by the Membership Committee of the society, followed by a site visit by a surgeon with expertise in the area of the fellowship. The accreditation cycle is for up to 3 years, with renewal being possible by paper review for programs with no substantial changes who have repeatedly met criteria, or repeat site visit for those with major changes since the last accreditation visit.

The Foundation for Surgical Fellowships was founded in 2010 and serves currently as the main organization for funding for surgical fellowships in the areas under the jurisdiction of the Fellowship Council. Prior to 2010, many of the fellowships accredited by the Fellowship Council received direct support from industry partners to the individual institutions and fellowships. However, concerns on the part of industry regarding conflict-of-interest queries that might arise in the near future regarding this process led to the formation of the non-profit Foundation which could serve as an intermediary for determining funding for the various fellowships and the level of funding on an annual basis.

Accreditation criteria for these non-ACGME fellowships have been set by the various societies, and they include requirements in curriculum, clinical experience, case volumes of operative procedures, facilities, faculty, and scholarly activity. Non-compliance with established guidelines may lead to suspension and then loss of accreditation by a fellowship. These societies have served as a regulatory source for a considerable segment of the current fellowship programs in surgery. It should also be noted that the volume of fellowships has dramatically increased during the past two decades, indicating a desire for graduating residents in surgery to seek further specialization before initiating a surgical practice. Providing appropriate guidelines for training, and ensuring an adequate clinical experience during training, is a current valuable role of the Fellowship Council for turning out surgeons with skill and expertise in the various surgical specialties.

Accreditation of ACGME Fellowships

The ACGME boards perform the same important regulation of quality of fellowships which are sponsored by the ACGME. There are multiple boards which serve as the regulatory bodies for the various surgical specialties, including Surgery, Cardiothoracic Surgery, Urology, Neurosurgery, Orthopedic Surgery, Otolaryngology, Pediatric Surgery, and Vascular Surgery. These boards insure standards of quality in training in the various areas of surgery, and almost certainly have done more over the past decades to promote optimal surgical patient care than any other single regulatory group. The standards of testing and renewal of accreditation of the various surgical boards have continued to improve with the passage of time. The ACGME has now demanded more continuing education for practicing physicians, and this has been enforced for recertification by the member boards, including those of the surgical specialties. Surgeons must demonstrate ongoing educational activity, maintenance of practice privileges, self-assessment of knowledge and of their practice, and periodic confirmation of knowledge as documented by written testing for continued recertification. Some boards assess surgeons on a case review basis as well. The boards are therefore responsible for setting standards of initial training of residents, then of fellows, and also of ongoing practitioners.

Bariatric Surgery Accreditation

Background and Factors Causing the Need for Accreditation

Recently, bariatric surgery programs have been accredited by both the American College of Surgeons as well as the Surgical Review Corporation (SRC), the latter being an organization with ties to the American Society of Metabolic and Bariatric Surgery. As the bariatric surgery process is a recent addition to the accreditation process, and is the first focused area of practice in which accreditation of a program was directly linked to individual procedure reimbursement, it shall occupy a significant focus of the chapter. The lessons learned and being learned in the bariatric arena are significantly applicable to future potential accreditation processes for other focused areas of surgical care.

Why was bariatric surgery the first area in which reimbursement was tied to some form of outcomes? The etiology of this was, unfortunately, not initially a result of a conscientious effort to improve patient safety and outcomes, but more an effort to discourage the actual performance of this group of operations by the payers. Prior to 2000, the number of bariatric operations performed in the USA was a predictable 15,000–20,000 annually. Then, with the advent of laparoscopic bariatric surgery, the number of procedures performed increased by almost ten times that

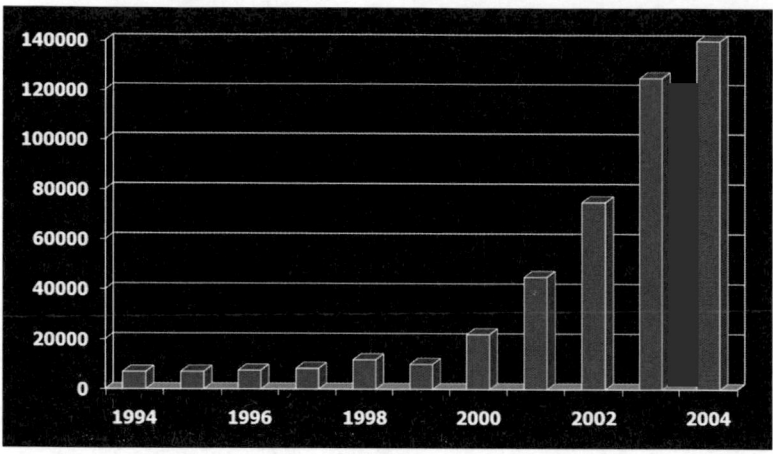

Fig. 43.1. Number of gastric bypass operations performed in the USA by year.

level within 5 years (Fig. 43.1). This sudden surge in the number of procedures put considerable strain on insurance companies, who suddenly faced huge expenses for this category of surgery.

By 2003, most companies suddenly found bariatric surgery to be their single largest expense category for general surgery. Their response at that point was to declare laparoscopic bariatric surgery experimental, despite the fact that there had been numerous articles in the surgical literature documenting its effectiveness and its improvement over traditional open surgery. Such decisions were protested and contested by bariatric surgeons and in particular the ASMBS (then the ASBS), the society representing bariatric surgery. During discussions regarding the decision to limit coverage of bariatric surgery, the insurance companies claimed that there had been an increase in the number of readmissions and complications for bariatric surgery, to an extent that had made them unwilling to continue paying for it. These data were never published. It is certainly possible that, during this time of the start-up of a large number of new bariatric surgical practices in response to patient demand, there were individuals who experienced a higher complication rate for performance of bariatric surgery. This is often the case for any specialty when a surgeon is beginning an experience in a new area. However, the decision to eliminate funding for all bariatric procedures done laparoscopically was a drastic measure unprecedented in the modern era of third party reimbursement for surgical procedures. Such action was probably made less objectionable in the public sector by the still present inherent bias against obesity by the general population, and by the lack of recognition of obesity as a disease.

Lack of recognition by the lay population of obesity as a disease is unfortunately still the norm today in the USA. However, the payer community can no longer adopt such a stance, since CMS (Centers for Medicare and Medicaid Services, the agency which administers the federal funding for these programs) has published their decision to recognize obesity as a disease. CMS has also, with this decision, recommended coverage for medical issues directly stemming from this disease as well as the disease process itself. There is a slow but steady increase in the medical community's awareness of the fact obesity is a disease, but such awareness on the part of the lay public is still lacking. Flagrant abuses against obese individuals still exist. In his last act as governor of Virginia in 2009, Governor Kane balanced the state budget by increasing the waiting period for all state insured employees who desired bariatric surgery from 6 months to 1 year, effectively eliminating that cost item from the budget.

Thus in the setting of such social bias, the actions of the payers against individuals seeking surgical treatment for obesity was not cast in the same negative light as a decision might have been, for example, to stop funding AIDS medications or to stop funding lung resection for lung cancer.

The bariatric surgical community, in 2003, faced the situation of drastic cutbacks in funded procedures for their patients who were deserving of and seeking appropriate surgical treatment for their disease. The response to this situation was on several fronts. First, there was an emphasis by the bariatric surgical community to publish large comprehensive studies demonstrating the success of bariatric surgery, done both laparoscopically as well as using the traditional open approach. Large series in front-line medical journals, meta-analyses, AHRQ funded studies, and population analyses soon were published over the next 2 years. Second, the ASMBS initiated a program of developing centers of excellence, to try and promote optimal performance of bariatric surgery. Such centers were originally designed to be examples of how to achieve optimal outcomes, centers that others could see as an example of best practice and optimal outcome approaches to bariatric surgery. While these centers certainly did achieve that end, the payers quickly adopted a policy that such centers would be the only ones where bariatric procedures would be funded. This led to the necessity of bariatric programs being certified as a center of excellence, a process which continues today.

The approach of the ASMBS to developing centers of excellence was to affiliate with a separate corporation, the SRC, to develop the criteria and methods to determine that a center was indeed a center of excellence. Soon after the establishment of the Surgical Review Organization, the ACS also developed a Bariatric Surgery Center Network, an organization within the ACS for reviewing bariatric centers and including them as centers of excellence. The two competing systems had some intense negotiations during the 2005 era to try and establish a common agency for this process, but a compromise solution was never reached, and the two systems remain intact today.

The two systems of bariatric surgery centers of excellence are most remarkable not for their differences but for their similarities. Both recognize case volume as the initial surrogate for outcomes, with the goal of establishing outcomes criteria once adequate data are accumulated from the member centers. This process is nearing fulfillment for both centers, who now have several years of data accumulated on patient outcomes by their centers. Otherwise, both systems rely on a site visit vetting of the center to become an accredited center. The ACS uses bariatric surgeons as site reviewers while the SRC uses trained nurses. Both systems have minimum requirements for cases performed, as well as types of operations accepted as standard procedures. Facilities, process of evaluating patients, self-assessment of outcomes, support personnel, and ability to report data on all patients are criteria used by both systems to accredit centers. The SRC also accredits individual surgeons while the ACS system limits accreditation to centers. Both systems have developed databases for capturing outcomes data by the centers. Centers must provide personnel time to enter the data for both systems, and the SRC charges a fee for each patient entered as well.

Fortunately, the centers of excellence systems have achieved a remarkable decrease in deaths from bariatric surgery over the past 5 years. When the systems were being established in 2005, a death rate of 1 or even 2%, based on patient population chosen for surgery, was common. Literature reports of such death rates were not surprising. A large review of the patients who had bariatric surgery and were covered by Medicare showed a death rate of 2%, which generated a large amount of negative publicity in the lay press. Now, however, the usual reported rate of deaths for centers applying for new or renewed status as a center is zero. The estimated death rate for bariatric surgery, as evidenced by the data from these systems, is now well below 1% and probably at about 0.3% or lower for gastric bypass and under 0.1% for lap band. No other major abdominal surgery that includes an anastomosis has achieved such a remarkably low mortality rate.

While bariatric surgeons and the centers of excellence concept have achieved, together, an improvement in surgical outcomes, the response from the public and insurers has been not appreciably different in terms of attitude regarding obesity. Most insurance companies, including CMS, require a period of medical dieting before a patient can undergo surgery. This dieting has been shown to not only have no effect, but in some cases have a detrimental effect to only delay appropriate treatment for patients deserving of it. In 2011, most patients contemplating bariatric surgery often have their choice of surgery influenced by their insurance company. For example, in our practice, we do not perform laparoscopic adjustable gastric banding for patients with Medicare because the company that administers Medicare for CMS in Virginia, Trailblazer, will not cover payment for any adjustments to the lap band after it is placed. Thus, while the company can correctly say they cover lap band, the naïve patient is then disappointed to find out that they face paying hundreds of dollars out of pocket for each of many needed band adjustments over the several years following the placement of the band.

Currently bariatric surgery remains the only area of surgery where a surgeon must meet standards of practice encompassed by the centers of excellence system to be reimbursed by third party payers for performing surgery. The unique circumstances associated with the evolution of this situation in bariatric surgery have been explained, and the establishment of the practice probably means that in the future this need for center of excellence status to qualify for reimbursement will continue. Certainly one can make the argument that the centers of excellence systems have improved patient care and outcomes for bariatric surgery. It is feasible that such improvements in the performance of this group of operations would have occurred with the increasing experience of surgeons over the passage of time, but that has not been the case always for other types of surgery where no center of excellence concept exists.

Bariatric Surgery Center Accreditation Criteria

The accreditation standards which arose for the centers of excellence concept are remarkably similar between the two centers' systems. Since the author is very familiar with the ACS system, I shall use the criteria for ACS level 1 center to illustrate these criteria. The ACS system does allow for a two tier approach to centers, with level 1 centers being appropriate for all candidates undergoing bariatric surgery. Level 2 centers are appropriate for lower risk cases, since the volume of cases

Table 43.3. Criteria for eligibility for ACS level 1 center of excellence.

1. Joint Commission-, AOA-, AAHC-, or state-approved hospital
2. Case selection: accepts all cases
3. Facility has performed weight loss operations for more than 1 year
4. Facility performed ≥ 125 weight loss operations in previous 12 months
5. Has a Director of Bariatric Surgery
6. Has a Bariatric Surgery Coordinator
7. Director and active bariatric surgeons are ABS or AOBS certified (if not consider on case by case basis)
8. ≥ 2 surgeons conducted $\geq$ operations over past 24 months
9. Active medical staff in cardiology, intensive care, nephrology, gastroenterology, infectious disease, orthopedics, otolaryngology, psychiatry, pulmonology, and thoracic surgery
10. A full-time board certified anesthesiologist provides coverage for all bariatric cases
11. Full-time Pain service
12. Fully staffed and medically equipped for morbidly obese patients: operating room, recovery room, emergency room, intensive care unit
13. Performs endoscopy procedures for morbidly obese
14. Performs minimally invasive procedures for morbidly obese
15. Radiology equipped to image morbidly obese
16. General accommodations available for morbidly obese
17. Employs practice guidelines and implements clinical pathways
18. Has an established quality improvement program
19. Agrees to report outcomes data
20. Reviews outcomes data as part of the facility review of surgeon's credentialing process
21. Multidiscipline group reviews candidates in the selection process
22. Patient education with printed handouts
23. Extensive explanation of informed consent
24. Surgeons reveal their experience
25. Protocol in place for patient discharge
26. Protocol in place for patient follow-up
27. Protocol for patient counseling regarding rehab, diet, exercise, psychological, and plastic surgery, and long term follow-up

done at such centers is lower by requirement. Requirements for a site to qualify for center of excellence status as a level 1 center are summarized in Table 43.3. Further details as to the specific details of some of these criteria for the ACS system can be found on the ACS Web site at http:// www.facs.org under Bariatric Surgery Centers Network. The criteria for the SRC centers can be found on their Web site at http://www. surgicalreview.org. At the time of writing of this chapter, the SRC site indicates over 400 sites were centers of excellence under their system and the ACS site indicates 134 qualified centers.

Beyond Bariatric Surgery

Payer Issues Impinging on Accreditation

The experience in bariatric surgery should point out several fundamental facts regarding the process of the accreditation process and the practice of surgery. The first is that the individual surgeon may have requirements and demands placed upon him or her by payers at their discretion. The control of such processes is not by the surgeon. In fact, surgeons and other physician health care providers have long ago lost the ability to determine their reimbursement for performing procedures and rendering services, for the most part. Even most private practitioners are subject to the limits, laws, and regulation of third party payers in order to be reimbursed for services. While such limitation on practitioners in the past was usually limited to the amount of reimbursement, the bariatric surgery example shows that it can be altered to represent reimbursement of any type at all.

CMS has recently begun to deny payment to hospitals for avoidable problems felt to represent suboptimal hospital care, such as decubitus ulcers. On the other hand, CMS has also recently issued guidelines for physician compensation for adopting use of the electronic medical record (EMR). Such rewards may not often compensate many practitioners for the expense to convert to the EMR, and potential penalties for not doing so are also likely. It is not a great stretch of the imagination to envision denial of reimbursement to practitioners as well if they fail to meet certain standards, criteria, or other regulations set up by third party payers. Currently the main criteria for assessing physician compliance or competence has been that of practice measures, such as giving antibiotics at the appropriate time before surgery, employing DVT prophylaxis, and so forth. There has been no demand for reporting outcomes, other than for the bariatric surgery community. The expense of performing outcomes reporting for bariatric surgeons had to be borne largely by the surgeons themselves, unless their hospitals were willing to underwrite the cost of this process. In the future, it is not too difficult to imagine that surgeons may be again held responsible for the additional time or expense to meet reporting criteria for a variety of different checklists, outcomes reporting, process evaluations, or other criteria set up by third party payers as a method of attempting to either improve patient care in the best of intentions or to discourage performance of a procedure in the less than best of intentions.

What can be the response of the surgical community to increase accreditation standards looming on the horizon? Certainly those reforms which are likely to improve patient outcomes should be embraced by our profession. The time and expense to meet these criteria, if borne by the surgeon, should also then be compensated to the surgeon as well. No additional compensation would be ethical or indicated, however, and the profession must maintain its high standard of ethics in this realm. Patients still perceive that their surgeon is the person best qualified to determine the number and type of diagnostic tests, therapeutic procedures, and other treatments indicated for surgical disease processes. Payers and third party regulators may and likely will in the future attempt to control the access to such services and procedures. The accreditation process is one form which may be used. Surgeons will then be forced to determine if they wish to undergo future accreditation processes, as have been required of bariatric surgeons, if they wish to continue to practice their specialty.

For the bariatric surgeon community, the additional accreditation processes has not been totally onerous or detrimental to patient care. While increased expense and time of the surgeon have been the negative aspects of the process, there have been positive aspects as well. Centers of excellence have meant improved facilities and resources for patients in many cases. Hospitals which may otherwise have been reluctant to spend money on the resources indicated for optimal care of the morbidly obese patient population have now done so in order to remain competitive in the marketplace for this patient population and for performing bariatric surgery at their institution.

Future accreditation, when it arises, should be viewed with the balanced view of what has happened in bariatric surgery. Patient outcomes have likely improved as a result, and facilities and resources for care of morbidly obese patients have also improved. Surgeons have been burdened with additional expense and time to report outcomes. The latter process may hopefully be made easier as electronic communication systems that are used for the EMR become more capable of interfacing and transfer of data becomes easier. One of the major issues with requirement of outcomes reporting is the accuracy of self-reported data, which is a cheaper and easier process, versus the expense of non-self-reported data. The prime example of the latter type of database system that currently exists is the National Surgical Quality Improvement Program (NSQIP), owned and sponsored by the ACS. This program employs trained nurse reviewers to independently review medical records and determine if a complication did occur, and report it. They also report other data including demographics, preoperative testing data, postoperative testing data, and other outcomes as indicated. A set of preoperative and postoperative variables for all general and vascular surgical procedures has been in place for many years now using the NSQIP.

In the future, the balance of positive aspects of potential improvement in patient care and outcomes will need to be balanced against the potential negative aspects of loss of access to care and loss of reimbursement or compensation for surgeons based on the particular details of any future accreditation system. If the system is set up largely to improve the profits or bottom line of third party payers or the hospital employers of physicians, then the loser will be the surgeons involved. Too great a burden on surgeons could potentially result in such an abandonment of the care of patients needing a particular procedure that there will be a major access problem. The very real possibility exists that such access issues may arise in the near future just on the basis of projected decreased reimbursement for the newly proposed federal insurance option for uninsured individuals. As increased regulation and scrutiny occur of the surgical world, surgeons will hopefully maintain the professional approach that what is best for the patient and insures optimal outcomes and care takes precedent. It is the only area over which surgeons still exert some control. It must be hoped that such an approach will be in turn appreciated and rewarded by the forces that compensate surgeons for their efforts in patient care.

Selected Readings

1. Smith MD, Patterson E, Wahed AS, Belle SH, Bessler M, Courcoulas AP, et al. Relationship between surgical volume and adverse outcomes after RYGB in Longitudinal Assessment of Bariatric Surgery (LABS) study. Surg Obes Rel Dis. 2010;6:118–25.

2. Flum DR, Salem L, Elrod JA, Dellinger EP, Cheadle A, Chan L. Early mortality among Medicare beneficiaries undergoing bariatric surgical procedures. JAMA. 2005;294:1903–8.

3. Schirmer B, Jones DB. The American College of Surgeons Bariatric Surgery Center Network: establishing standards. Bull Am College Surg. 2007;92:21–7.

4. Buchwald H, Avidor Y, Braunwald E, Jensen MD, Pories W, Fahrbach K, et al. Bariatric surgery: a systematic review and meta-analysis. JAMA. 2004;292:1724–37.

5. Centers for Medicare and Medicaid Services (CMS), HHS. Medicare and Medicaid programs: electronic health record incentive program. Final rule. Federal Register 2010;75:44313–588.

6. Jha AK, Orav EJ, Epstein AM. The effect of financial incentives on hospitals that serve poor patients. Ann Int Med. 2010;153:299–306.

7. Neuman HB, Michelassi F, Turner JW, Bass BL. Surrrounded by quality metrics: what do surgeons think of ACS-NSQIP? Surgery. 2009;145:27–33.

Part VII
Safer Surgery Through Simulation and Teamwork

44. Team Training

Philip Omotosho and Dana D. Portenier

Introduction

Lessening the rate of medical errors and improving patient safety are critical components of quality improvement. It has been a decade since the Institute of Medicine (IOM) report *To Err is Human: Building a Safer Health System* laid bare the prevalence of preventable medical errors and the heavy price paid with human life and resources [1]. Errors moreover threaten to diminish public trust in the health care system as well as provider satisfaction, with ramifications that are perhaps impossible to overstate. Positive response followed the IOM report, with action by government agencies, such as the Agency for Healthcare Research and Quality (AHRQ), private sector, and professional agencies. Federal funding was appropriated to support research, new technology, projects, and reporting systems, all targeted at reducing medical errors. Initiatives by professional societies and certification bodies, such as the American College of Surgeons and the American Board of Surgery, include the National Quality Improvement Program (NSQIP) and Maintenance of Certification (MOC), respectively, with goals of measuring and improving the quality of surgical care and engendering continued public trust.

A major recommendation of the IOM report was for a commitment by health care organizations and affiliated professionals to make continued improvement in patient safety a clearly stated goal by establishing patient safety programs with defined executive responsibility. Such stated commitment would include multidisciplinary team training programs that utilize proven methods of team training. Identified high-risk areas where errors often have the gravest consequences include the intensive care unit (ICU), emergency department (ED), and the operating room (OR).

The focal point of surgical care, and consequently surgical training, has long been the technical skill and knowledge of the individual surgeon.

D.S. Tichansky, J. Morton, and D.B. Jones (eds.), *The SAGES Manual*   443
of Quality, Outcomes and Patient Safety, DOI 10.1007/978-1-4419-7901-8_44,
© Springer Science+Business Media, LLC 2012

While these remain key to successful patient outcomes, recent data suggest only weak links between improving a surgeon's technical skills and a diminution in surgical error [2]. More readily associated with error are failure of nontechnical skills, such as communication, decision-making, leadership, and teamwork. Attention to nontechnical skills and teamwork is a relatively new concept, one traditionally not integrated into the training of physicians and other health professionals that compose surgical clinical teams. The complexities of the current health care system have necessitated a paradigm shift evidenced by a new focus on cooperative clinical teams rather than individual expertise. It follows, therefore, that measures taken to diminish error and improve outcome embrace an in-depth evaluation and refinement of clinical team dynamics.

Teamwork

A team may be defined as a group of individuals working toward a common goal. Such is the atmosphere in which surgical care is delivered, where professionals including fully trained physicians, physicians-in-training, nurses, physician assistants, technicians, and other key personnel with varying skills must effectively interact to ensure successful patient outcomes. Yet individually competent professionals constantly work in these clinical teams without previous training in teamwork concepts.

Attitudes toward teamwork appear to vary by discipline. A survey administered to team training participants at eight US academic medical centers revealed that while second-year postgraduate (PGY 2) medical residents agreed that an interdisciplinary team approach is beneficial to patients, they consistently rated their agreement lower than nurse practitioner and masters-level social work students [3]. This suggests preresidency leanings toward individual excellence coupled with a sense of its preeminence over teamwork, and additionally, lack of emphasis on the value of collaboration. The investigators in this study reasonably suggest the integration of team concepts and team training in medical school, as others have argued [4].

Perceptions of collaboration also vary. For example, Makary et al. found physicians rating the teamwork of others as good while nurses perceived teamwork to be mediocre [5]. In this study, OR personnel in 60 hospitals were surveyed using the Safety Attitudes Questionnaire, a tool modified from the Flight Management Attitudes Questionnaire – reliable surveys where elicited attitudes are known to correlate with performance. In addition to perceiving teamwork in the OR to be good overall, surgeons rated teamwork amongst themselves "high" or "very high" 85.2% of the time, while nurses rated collaboration with surgeons "high" or "very high" only 48% of the time. These disparities shed light on an unfamiliarity with team concepts, where collaboration, a defining element and basic metric of effective team functioning, is understood in apparently different terms by individuals composing a clinical team. Professional culture divergence is one possible explanation for this phenomenon. Physicians and nurses are trained to communicate and approach their duties differently. As a result of training, surgeons are apt to give orders and communicate succinct, problem-focused pieces of information to other team members, and are therefore likely to judge a team effectively by the extent to which these ends are satisfied. Nurses tend toward a more holistic approach to information disclosure and service, where a significant component of effective teamwork is reflected in a sense of valued contribution.

The need for effective teamwork is axiomatic, given that most surgical patient care occurs in the context of interdisciplinary teams. Nonetheless, very strong arguments have been made [1, 7, 11]. Surgical care must reflect high-reliability performance, a concept linked with safety [6], as errors in surgery harbor potential for catastrophe. High-reliability organizations are complex institutions (e.g., aviation/aeronautics, nuclear power plants) in which a high penalty is paid for error, but where errors actually occur at an extremely low rate. Effective teamwork is considered an integral component of these organizations [7]. As a starting point, team roles must be clearly defined and agreed upon. Leach et al. define the twofold role of the surgeon in securing a patient's successful surgical outcome [6]. As the agent approached by the patient to procure the resolution of a chief complaint, the surgeon is responsible for applying sound clinical knowledge and technical skill to the attainment of this goal. Second, but no less important, is the surgeon's role in coordinating the efforts of other trained professionals with clearly defined roles within a clinical team. Far from being a theoretical construct, this is an expectation that is implicit in the physician–patient relationship, though it is sometimes explicitly communicated. Strong leadership and communication skills are paramount in fulfilling this obligation. Surgical tradition treasures hierarchy and respect, but this does not preclude effective teamwork. Neither are the surgeon's aforementioned roles diminished by a dedication to teamwork. For example, predetermined role assignments that enable another team member with defined expertise, such as a circulating nurse, to step up and oversee the resolution of an unexpected OR crisis does not constitute a relinquishment of the surgeon's overall leadership. Rather it is affirmed in such a situation, in that it reveals foresight and good communication that makes possible a shift in leadership to the person best equipped to address a crisis, particularly when the surgeon's present task hinders direct involvement. These ideas are embodied in two factors thought to broadly influence successful surgical outcomes: *shared mental models* and *OR environment* [6]. Shared mental models is the notion sometimes referred to as being on the "same page," or in other words, team members possessing a common understanding of the case at hand, including its major steps and points at which challenges are most likely to be encountered. OR environment is simply the nurturing and preservation of a collegial, respectful, and supportive work atmosphere in the OR, where individual contribution is counted on and valued. These factors provide a framework for understanding team dynamics and measuring collaboration.

Team Training

The National Aeronautics and Space Administration (NASA) in the late 1970s made the once astounding discovery that fatal flight crashes more commonly reflected a failure of nontechnical skills, such as communication, which led to ineffective teamwork, rather than technical incompetence or mechanical failure [8]. This led to a concerted effort with the Federal Aviation Authority (FAA) and industry, which revolutionized commercial aviation. Pilot training preceding this focused on the mastery of technical aspects of flight, not unlike most physician training at the present time. The team training program now known as crew resource management (CRM) was developed to address system failures as well as human factors that hinder effective collaboration in a multiperson team that parallels the multidisciplinary clinical teams through which health care is delivered today. Even though there is currently only some evidence of the clinical effectiveness of CRM [9], it is being increasingly embraced by health care delivery establishments. This is largely due to the now recognized association between communication breakdown and medical error leading to patient injury, as well as the long-standing acceptance of CRM by other high-reliability organizations [10, 11]. Additionally, observed improvements in patient outcome may not be easily attributable to CRM, as it is difficult to evaluate in isolation from other programs and changes an organization might institute to improve outcome.

The clinical staff at many hospitals and ORs is required to undergo some form of team training, but what does this entail? Often this is accomplished by a daylong seminar in which a series of lectures and group activities extol the virtues of teamwork. Staffs are then checked off as having completed required training, and the status quo is resumed. Two elements of effective team training have been suggested: a well-defined, *task analysis-oriented curriculum* and *interdisciplinary simulations* [8].

With the discovery that human factors (i.e., unique physical, cognitive, or social properties of individuals which influence their environmental interactions and functionality within systems) played a significant role in aviation errors, the industry in the 1980s created an Advanced Qualification Program (AQP), which incorporated team training with the technical training of pilots [8]. Specific safety-enhancing team training topics were recognized and established within the AQP curriculum. Trainee awareness of the prevalence of system and human error increased, as did the team skills needed to mitigate their effects. A direct parallel can here be drawn to surgical training. While certain team topics clearly apply, such as "communication" (subtopics include briefings and conflict resolution) and "team building and maintenance" (subtopics here include leadership and workload management) [8], there remains a need to study surgical teams and identify exactly how they apply. Topics unique to surgical teams also need to be explored and incorporated into medical student and resident training curricula. Since fully trained surgeons, anesthesiologists, nurses, and technicians usually have not undergone training in specific teams skills, a sustained, well-designed curriculum must be the goal here as well, rather than the more common 1- or 2-day seminar.

The most effective currently available means to achieve these goals is interdisciplinary simulation. Indeed, this constitutes another recommendation of the IOM for combating medical errors. The efficacy of simulation in training and improving individual technical skill is well established [12]. Evidence is now emerging that simulation improves team performance [13]. Simulation has already assumed a critical role in graduate medical education for a variety reasons, including a decreased error tolerance, work-hour restrictions, and OR operating costs. These factors make the OR not an ideal place for initial skill acquisition, although this has been the traditional approach. Moreover, due to logistical and staffing issues, most OR teams form ad hoc for the procedure at hand, and it is commonplace to have a team consisting of different members for different procedures throughout an operative day. Nontechnical skills, such as communication, are therefore learned and put to the test during real-time surgery. This is generally tolerated for routine cases, but can be quite problematic in a crisis situation.

Simulated training modules within a well-designed curriculum provide a solution to this problem. Simulation allows trainees to acquire technical skills in the context of supervised multidisciplinary team operations, while fully trained professionals acquire team skills as well as new technical skills all in an environment in which patient safety is not jeopardized. Focusing on the collaborative necessity that attends even the most straightforward laparoscopic case, Powers et al. recently developed and validated a simulation-based team training tool for minimally invasive surgery [9]. This study utilized a virtual or "mock" endosuite in which a crisis scenario (unexpected hemorrhage) is generated during a simulated elective laparoscopic case. The investigators used the simulated experience to merge instruction in safe practices in laparoscopic surgery with acquisition of OR multidisciplinary team skills in a crisis. Both technical and nontechnical skills of expert and novice surgeons were compared to examine and confirm construct validity. Another recently developed tool is the Legacy Inanimate System for Endoscopic Team Training (LISETT), which evaluates individual technical skills and team skills displayed in the execution of defined laparoscopic tasks in a box trainer [2]. This is reflected in an overall "LISETT score" derived from averaged normalized scores assigned based on the accuracy and speed with which a defined task is completed. These initiatives represent not only a means to accomplish needed training in team skills, but also a reliable means for measuring progress and giving immediate feedback.

Conclusion

In the past decade much deserved attention has been directed toward reducing medical errors with the goal of improving the quality of care and patient outcome. Emphasis on building and maintaining high-reliability clinical teams is key to ensuring the success of these endeavors, particularly in the OR and other high-risk areas within the health care system. Resources of health care organizations, professional societies, government agencies, and the private sector are needed. Lastly, success will also depend partly on efforts by professional schools (medical, nursing, and technical) to embrace curriculum changes that establish foundational training in team skills. Graduating professionals then enter into a career-long perfection of these skills utilizing a simulation-based task analysis-oriented curriculum. Excellent tools for achieving these goals have now begun to emerge.

Selected Readings

1. Kohn LT, Corrigan JM, Donaldson M. To Err is human: building a safer health system. Washington, DC: Institute of Medicine; 1999.

2. Zheng B, Denk PM, Martinec DV, Gatta P, Whiteford MH, Swanström LL. Building an efficient surgical team using a bench model simulation: construct validity of the Legacy Inanimate System for Endoscopic Team Training (LISETT). Surg Endosc. 2008;22:930–7.

3. Leipzig RM, Hyer K, Ek K, et al. Attitudes toward working on interdisciplinary healthcare teams: a comparison by discipline. J Am Geriatr Soc. 2002;50:1141–8.

4. Lerner S, Magrane D, Friedman E. Teaching teamwork in medical education. Mt Sinai J Med. 2009;76:318–29.

5. Makary MA, Sexton JB, Freischlag JA, et al. Operating room teamwork among physicians and nurses: teamwork in the eye of the beholder. J Am Coll Surg. 2006;202:746–52.

6. Leach LS, Myrtle RC, Weaver FA, Dasu S. Assessing the performance of surgical teams. Health Care Manage Rev. 2009;34:29–41.

7. Baker DP, Day R, Salas E. Teamwork as an essential component of high-reliability organizations. Health Serv Res. 2006;41:1576–98.

8. Hamman WR. The complexity of team training: what we have learned from aviation and its applications to medicine. Qual Saf Health Care. 2004;13 Suppl 1:i72–9.

9. Powers KA, Rehrig ST, Irias N, et al. Simulated laparoscopic operating room crisis: An approach to enhance the surgical team performance. Surg Endosc. 2008;22:885–900.

10. Grogan EL, Stiles RA, France DJ, et al. The impact of aviation-based teamwork training on the attitudes of health-care professionals. J Am Coll Surg. 2004;199:843–8.

11. Anderson M, Leflore J. Playing it safe: simulated team training in the OR. AORN J. 2008;87:772–9.

12. Seymour NE, Gallagher AG, Roman SA, et al. Virtual reality training improves operating room performance: results of a randomized, double-blinded study. Ann Surg. 2002;236:458–63.

13. Falcone Jr RA, Daugherty M, Schweer L, Patterson M, Brown RL, Garcia VF. Multidisciplinary pediatric trauma team training using high-fidelity trauma simulation. J Pediatr Surg. 2008;43:1065–71.

45. Training to Proficiency

Daniel J. Scott and Michael J. Lee

Introduction

"See one, do one, teach one," the paradigm ingrained in surgical minds for the past century since the days of Halsted, has helped to mature generations of well-trained surgeons. Many contemporary issues such as advances in technology, restrictions in training work hours, expensive operating room costs, safety, and ethical concerns challenge this ideology. Today, there are significant concerns that question the efficacy of the traditional paradigm particularly in the realm of technical skills acquisition. Newfound interest in simulation now cultivates progression of novel training equipment and training methods for the modern era.

Background

Cadaver and animal models have long been used to teach surgical skill; while cadaver tissue may be noncompliant and animate anatomy may differ from humans, these models have proven useful for both open and laparoscopic operations. The advantages are obvious. The simulated environment creates a consequence-free setting in which the learner may try different techniques with tactile feedback from biological tissue. However, the immense cost and resource consumption are major drawbacks in the widespread use of these models as cost-effective simulators. Initial bench top inanimate models have been limited in complexity compared to biological tissue to simulate entire operations. Due to the limitations of the early simulators, the operating room remained the major training ground where surgeons in training learned and practiced their skill.

In comparison to its use in aviation and military, simulation development in surgery lacked much momentum. The advent of laparoscopy and demand

D.S. Tichansky, J. Morton, and D.B. Jones (eds.), *The SAGES Manual
of Quality, Outcomes and Patient Safety*, DOI 10.1007/978-1-4419-7901-8_45,
© Springer Science+Business Media, LLC 2012

for minimal access surgery in the 1990s, however, revolutionized surgical practice [1, 2]. Laparoscopic operations for cholecystectomies, bariatrics, and antireflux procedures soon became commonplace. The subsequent increase in early complications for laparoscopic cholecystectomies questioned safety and training quality in surgical trainees and surprisingly surgeons in practice. Quality and safety measures soon became practical concerns and challenged physicians to re-examine the fundamental way we learn and perform.

The Theory and Practice of Expert Performance

Many of the lessons regarding skill acquisition and optimal performance as studied in psychology are applicable to medicine. Ericsson's theories and experiments on expertise have had wide application in sports, medicine, and related domains [3]. He challenged traditional thought that achievement in a given domain is limited by innate factors. He devised a method by which expertise is rather obtained through specific training and experiential learning.

By arbitrary default, educational protocols have often been based on training duration or number of repetitions [1–3]. Simple activities generally take less than 50 h to reach an acceptable standard of performance and a subsequent performance plateau [3]. In contrast, expert level skill often requires 10 years of practice [3]. Currently, the ACGME requires completion of 750 major cases and 85 endoscopies approximating 5 years for general surgery residents. In Ericsson's argument, experts seem to acquire extensive experience; however, extensive experience does not always create experts. He cites examples of computer programmers, wine discriminators, stockbrokers, and clinical psychologists who are able to outperform their counterparts with much greater experience. He deduced that experience is not always related to efficiency and success.

By examining learning and skill acquisition in expert performers, he realized that there existed a pattern that cultivated expert performance. A training regimen that provides coaching for improvement, detailed immediate feedback, and opportunities to improve produced expert performance, a process which he defined as deliberate practice [3].

Expanding on the principles of deliberate practice, Moulton et al. studied the effects of massed (1 day) compared to distributed (weekly) interval practice and its application to an animal-based model; 38 junior surgical residents were randomized and subsequently tested in their microvascular anastomotic skill in a live anesthetized rat [4]. The distributed practice group outperformed the massed practice group in most outcome measures including time, motion economy, and expert global ratings, and convincingly outperformed the massed group in all expert-based measures on the live rat model [4].

Although deliberate and distributed practice have long been used in other performance fields, its direct use in medicine has developed more slowly [3, 4]. The demanding cognitive component adds much to the complexity of efficient training [3, 4]. The practitioner must have extensive background knowledge in addition to the skill set to perform manual tasks; decision-making skills are also needed to ensure development of sound judgment. In procedure-related specialties, deliberate and distributed practice play an important role in maximizing efficiency while minimizing risk [3, 4]. What constitutes the most efficient and effective standard training method, however, is still evolving.

Simulation as a Training Tool

With advancement in technology, simulation evolved into a powerful training tool in the acquisition of both cognitive and psychomotor skill. Simulator training has already had extensive utility in training personnel working in high-risk environments. Laparoscopic simulator training has flourished since the MIS revolution, and its model is applicable to other fields of procedure-based medicine. Laparoscopic skill is especially difficult to acquire because of the diminished tactile feedback, the fulcrum effect, limits in range of motion, and loss of depth perception [1, 2]. Training in a controlled environment allows the learner to practice and obtain fundamental skill without distraction. Ultimately, the learner should become proficient in skill so that the performance is automatic and more attentional resources can instead be used for planning and problem solving in the real environment [1, 2]. In addition to skill and scenario training, the simulator may also provide assessment. Virtual reality simulators may provide immediate and detailed feedback whereas proctors may be used in other environments. Although there are wide varieties, simulator systems share commonalities in achieving goals related to the principles of construct validity and skills transferability, as described later [1, 2]. The power of simulation in achieving both of these goals has led the American College of Surgeons (ACS) and the Society of American Gastrointestinal and Endoscopic Surgeons (SAGES) to incorporate simulation-based training into the Fundamentals of Laparoscopic Surgery (FLS) program and endorsement by the Residency Review Committee in Surgery (RRC-S), the American Board of Surgery (ABS), and the Association of Program Directors in Surgery (APDS).

Construct Validity

Construct validity in the context of simulation refers to the ability to distinguish levels of performance by individuals with differing levels of experience [1, 2]. For example, an experienced laparoscopic surgeon should perform better than a novice at a given task in a significantly quantifiable manner. Many studies have demonstrated such differences, confirming construct validity [5–7, 9–12]. Numerous laparoscopic simulators exist from video training modules with basic object manipulation to complex computer-generated virtual reality simulators. Various simulators such as the MIST VR, LapSim, Southwestern Videotrainer, and MISTELS range in economy and technological complexity [1]. Each has advantages and disadvantages that vary in cost, tactile feedback, assessment ability, need for human supervision, and consumption of resources. Regardless of the mode, the effectiveness of the simulator as a training tool in part stems from its construct validity, which is an indicator that the metrics employed are measuring what they purport to measure, i.e., surgical skill in a given domain area [1, 2]. This is a critical aspect if expert performance goals are to be used for training purposes, or if simulators are intended for assessment purposes.

Skill Transferability

Skill transfer refers to acquiring skill in one situation that effectively allows a trainee to apply it to another situation. Initial studies that evaluated newly created simulators essentially proved that simulator practice directly improved simulator performance. Early data from Scott, Grantcharov, and Seymour confirmed evidence that skills obtained through simulator practice could also transfer to better operative performance and fewer intraoperative errors [6, 7, 9].

In a randomized blinded prospective trial, Scott et al. examined a laparoscopic bench model using the Southwestern Videotrainer Stations to determine if skills obtained would translate into improved operative performance [6]. Twenty-two junior surgery residents were randomized to either a training or a control group and supervised by a blinded faculty surgeon during an elective laparoscopic cholecystectomy. Additional blinded observing faculty surgeons performed global assessments. The trained group practiced 30 min a day for 10 days on the five box-trainer tasks. The trained group not only improved in time reduction in all simulator task compared to controls, but they also improved in operative performance criteria and subjective self-scoring and overall confidence.

In a study using the MIST VR system, Grantcharov et al. randomized 16 surgical residents to a training group who received MIST VR training or to a control group who received no VR training [7]. Both groups performed a baseline laparoscopic cholecystectomy in which the test subjects were evaluated once clips were placed at both cystic artery and duct with a blinded supervising faculty surgeon and were then randomized. The experimental group completed 10 repetitions of 6 tasks of the MIST VR which included manipulating objects in a computer-generated virtual space on a two-dimensional display monitor. Posttesting revealed that the trained group performed laparoscopic cholecystectomy significantly faster than the control group and with greater improvement and economy. These findings were consistent with the works of Seymour who previously published results with improved performance after training on the MIST VR to a proficiency measure of performance [9].

In contrast to previous studies, Ahlberg's investigation did not show skills transfer after MIST VR training [8]. Similar to the previous study designs, 29 medical students were randomized into a MIST VR trained versus a control without VR training. The students then performed a simulated appendectomy on a porcine model after 3 h of supervised MIST VR training. In contrast to other studies, MIST VR training did not improve surgical performance [8]. The authors questioned whether the length of training or high complexity of the required task may have factored in the difference of outcome and perhaps the novices did not have enough time to reach a performance plateau.

Differences in study results suggest that there is no singular measure that will ultimately predict performance. Learners vary in innate ability and motivation. Training methods should be individualized to the trainee and specific performance goals. Construct validity and skill transfer are important principles of effective simulator systems. The best way to use simulators to ultimately improve patient care remains under investigation. Endpoints other than duration or repetition may be necessary to maximize efficient learning.

Establishing Proficiency

Early studies used time, error, and repetition as training endpoints. Although convenient, these metrics were unfortunately arbitrary endpoints and did not sufficiently account for individual differences with respect to skill acquisition [1, 2]. Because individuals differ with a given set of innate skills and experience, as well as speed of skill acquisition, subjecting all participants to a uniform training program denies efficient training [1, 2]. Many variables determine whether it may take an individual 30 min or another individual 30 attempts to perform a task proficiently. Thus, the question still remains how someone should optimally train on a simulator.

Seymour et al. examined virtual reality skill transferability to the OR in a prospective, randomized, blinded study with a standard training group of PGY 1–4 surgical residents vs. a group additionally trained in VR [9]. In contrast, these investigators chose proficiency in each task as an endpoint for training. To establish the proficiency performance criterion level, four laparoscopic surgeons within a single institution completed 10 trials on MIST VR on the difficult setting. The training goal consisted of three to eight training sessions for an hour until each individual completed two consecutive repetitions at or beyond the expert-derived proficiency level for the manipulate/diathermy task. Once the proficiency criterion for training was met, blinded attendings observed dissections of the gallbladder from the liver after division of cystic duct and artery in elective laparoscopic cholecystectomies. The results were remarkable. Gallbladder injury/nonintended burn were five times more likely in standard group. Lack of progress was nine times more likely and overall errors were six times more likely compared to VR group.

Korndorffer et al. also observed similar results elaborating on Seymour's method. To obtain proficiency criterion level, four expert surgeons with more than 250 basic and 50 advanced laparoscopic cases performed 11 consecutive reps on each of the 5 Southwestern Station tasks [10]. Outlier scores deviating from two standard deviations from the mean were removed and the trimmed mean was then defined as the proficiency level. Using this proficiency criterion, only 6% of trainees (medical students, PGY 1–5 residents) could achieve this performance level during the course of three baseline repetitions. In addition, 73% of individuals who reached the proficiency level at baseline were PGY5 residents, supporting the influence of experience on performance. In this study, two pilot novice-level (medical students) subjects were able to reach proficiency for all five tasks in a mean time of 163 min and 90 repetitions, which supported the feasibility of the training protocol.

Applying this model to the validated FLS program, Scott et al. established expert-derived proficiency levels for the five MISTELS tasks [11]. Twenty-one novices (medical students) at two institutions underwent proficiency-based training which required a mean time of 9.7 h and 119 repetitions. Although baseline testing revealed that no one was proficient, all participants acquired sufficient skill to surpass the minimum threshold score required to pass the certification exam criteria for the manual skills portion of the FLS program.

Training to proficiency has proven to be an effective method of acquiring skill and also for maintaining skills. In a 2-year follow-up of 33 surgical residents who successfully completed the proficiency-based FLS curriculum, retention tests were completed at regular intervals [12]. Retention testing at 6 months revealed that half of the trainees did not achieve the proficiency standards and required retraining. After a 2-year program of structured ongoing proficiency training founded in deliberate and distributed practice, retention tests demonstrated over 91–100% retention of complex laparoscopic suturing tasks and 92% for all five tasks. Importantly, 22 PGY4-5 residents who took the certification examination passed the manual skills portion with a wide comfort margin. These data indicate that clinical training alone may be insufficient to maintain some technical skills and that ongoing proficiency training may be necessary.

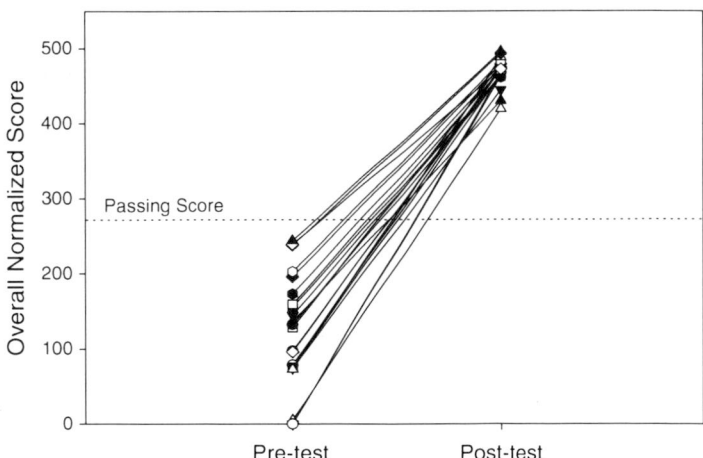

Fig. 45.1. The overall normalized score showed significant improvement (468 ± 24 vs. 126 ± 75; $p < 0.001$) after training, with all participants exceeding the score (270) required to pass the Fundamental Laparoscopic Surgery (FLS) certification examination.

Thus, work to date supports proficiency-based training as an important tool. This training practice utilizes many of the best methods identified by psychomotor learning investigations. Importantly, these practices tailor the educational experience to the specific needs of the individual leaner. In doing so, efficiency and efficacy are maximized. Further work is still needed as protocols undergo refinement and change as needed to ensure that maximum learning and skill transfer are achieved. Additionally, protocols which result in direct benefit in terms of patient outcomes, quality, and safety will need to be established and validated.

Conclusion

As proficiency-based training gains more acceptance, the development of national and international benchmarks may create a more accurate representation of the proficient population [1, 2, 11]. It may seem obvious in the sense that one needs to practice to proficiency in order to become proficient. However, the common theme borrowed from other performance fields is that maintaining motivation and systematic overtraining improve outcomes. Perhaps perfect practice does make perfect, but we have yet to determine what exactly constitutes perfect practice. Further investigations in other complex metrics such as team training performance, attentional capacity, automaticity, and motion economy will also elucidate what constitutes optimal training [1, 2]. Although not yet perfected, proficiency-based training using expert-derived performance goals is highly effective and extensively evidence based. In addition to deliberate and distributed practice, we now know that structured training to proficiency efficiently prepares those in training as well as those already in practice to effectively acquire and maintain expertise in technical skills.

Selected Readings

1. Scott DJ. Proficiency-based training for surgical skills. Sem Colon Rectal Surg. 2008;19:72–80.
2. Gallagher AG, Ritter EM, Champion H, et al. Virtual reality simulation for the operating room: proficiency based training as a paradigm shift in surgical skills training. Ann Surg. 2005;241:364–72.

3. Ericsson KA. Deliberate practice and the acquisition and maintenance of expert performance in medicine and related domains. Acad Med. 2004;79:S70–81.

4. Moulton CA, Dubrowski A, Macrae H, Graham B, Grober E, Reznick R. Teaching surgical skills: what kind of practice makes perfect? A randomized controlled trial. Ann Surg. 2006;244:400–9.

5. Fried GM, Feldman LS, Vassiliou MC, et al. Proving the value of simulation in laparoscopic surgery. Ann Surg. 2004;240:518–25.

6. Scott DJ, Bergen PC, Rege RV, Laycock R, Tesfay ST, Valentine RJ, et al. Laparoscopic training on bench models: better and more cost effective than OR experience? J Am Coll Surg. 2000;191:272–83.

7. Grantcharov TP, Kristiansen VB, Bendix J, et al. Randomized clinical trial of virtual reality simulation for laparoscopic skills training. Br J Surg. 2004;91:146–50.

8. Ahlberg G, Heikkinen T, Iselius L, et al. Does training in a virtual reality simulator improve surgical performance? Surg Endosc. 2002;16:126–29.

9. Seymour NE, Gallagher AG, Roman SA, O'Brien MK, Bansal VK, Anderson DK, et al. Virtual reality training improves operating room performance: results of a randomized double-blinded study. Ann Surg. 2002;236:458–64.

10. Korndorffer JK, Scott DJ, Sierra R, et al. Developing and testing competency levels for laparoscopic skills training. Arch Surg. 2005;140:80–4.

11. Scott DJ, Ritter EM, Tesfay ST, Pimentel EA, Nagji A, Fried GM. Certification pass rate of 100% for Fundamentals of Laparoscopic Surgery skills after proficiency-based training. Surg Endosc. 2008;22:1887–93.

12. Mashaud LB, Castellvi AO, Hollett LA, Hogg DC, Tesfay ST, Scott DJ. 2-Year skill retention and certification exam performance following FLS training and proficiency maintenance. Surgery. 2010;148:194–201.

46. Fundamentals of Laparoscopic Surgery-FLS

Ian Choy and Allan Okrainec

Introduction

Ever since Erich Muhe performed the first laparoscopic cholecystectomy (LC) in 1985, training laparoscopic surgery to new and established surgeons has been a major and complex issue. Spurred on by industry, patient demand, physician competition, and hospital administrations, the rapid adoption of laparoscopic surgery preceded many of the studies of its efficacy and safety. However, as reports of increased rates of complications and steeper than expected learning curves started to appear in the literature, the surgical community began to develop a greater awareness of the distinctiveness of the knowledge and skills necessary to safely incorporate laparoscopy into practice.

The Society of American Gastrointestinal and Endoscopic Surgeons (SAGES) was one of the first organizations to address this issue and in 1990 published the first guidelines outlining the basic educational goals required to learn and perform LCs. Shortly thereafter, the National Institutes of Health published a consensus statement supporting these developments stating that while the overall morbidity and mortality rates for LCs was sufficiently small to justify its use for the treatment of symptomatic gallstones, "strict guidelines for training in laparoscopy surgery, determination of competence, and monitoring of quality should be developed and implemented promptly."

Ultimately, however, it was often the responsibility of the individual hospitals to decide whether a surgeon was capable of performing laparoscopic procedures, with training usually consisting of short weekend-long courses. Unfortunately, such training often proved to be inadequate and it became clear that laparoscopic surgery required a new training paradigm to meet its unique knowledge and skills requirements.

D.S. Tichansky, J. Morton, and D.B. Jones (eds.), *The SAGES Manual of Quality, Outcomes and Patient Safety*, DOI 10.1007/978-1-4419-7901-8_46, © Springer Science+Business Media, LLC 2012

Guiding Principles of FLS

In the mid-1990s, SAGES formed a Fundamentals of Laparoscopic Surgery (FLS) committee charged with the development of a training curriculum that would cover the basic skills and knowledge required to perform laparoscopic surgery. This committee was guided by four major principles: (1) the curriculum should provide comprehensive coverage of both the cognitive and psychomotor domains of laparoscopic surgery, (2) the curriculum should only cover material specific to laparoscopy, (3) the curriculum should be generally applicable to all laparoscopic surgery, and not focus on any specific anatomic location or laparoscopic procedure, and (4) the program should contain mechanisms for assessment along with instruction. The ultimate goal of the FLS program, however, was to respond to the contextual problems outlined above by teaching "a standard set of cognitive and psychomotor skills to practitioners of laparoscopic surgery" and to "ensure a minimal standard of care for all patients undergoing laparoscopic surgery."

Cognitive Component

Development

In developing the cognitive component of the FLS curriculum, the FLS committee identified 13 major content categories of laparoscopic surgery:

1. Equipment and tools of laparoscopic surgery
2. Energy sources
3. Patient considerations (patient selection, contraindications, preparation)
4. Anesthesia (types and complications)
5. Patient positioning
6. Establishment and physiology of pneumoperitoneum (gas biologic characteristics, pressure and flow characteristics)
7. Abdominal access and trocar placement (techniques and complications)
8. Tissue handling, exposure, and examination of abdomen and pelvis
9. Biopsy techniques
10. Hemorrhage and hemostasis

11.   Tissue approximation (indications, techniques)
12.   Exiting the abdomen (drains, site closures)
13.   Postoperative care.

Within these major content categories, they then developed 66 subject areas that were defined and submitted as a survey to the participants of the 2001 SAGES annual meeting. The survey asked respondents to rank the importance of each of the subject and content categories. They were also asked to add any content areas or concepts they felt were necessary but were missing from the original set. In total, 117 surveys were evaluated, 28% of which were completed by surgeons whom performed basic and intermediate laparoscopic surgery, while the remaining 72% also performed advanced laparoscopic surgery.

The content of the cognitive curriculum was then revised accordingly and the 13 content categories were then arranged into five modules: (1) preoperative considerations, (2) intraoperative considerations, (3) basic laparoscopic procedures, (4) postoperative care and complications, and (5) manual skills practice instructions. Initially, the course material was distributed on two CD-ROMs, but in 2009 the course was ported over to an online version with its content unchanged.

The assessment component of the cognitive curriculum was designed specifically to test the understanding and application of the didactic material. As such, emphasis was placed on designing questions that would focus on clinical judgment and intraoperative decision-making. To that end, a small group of laparoscopic surgeons from academic, private urban, and rural practices developed two types of questions: 203 single multiple-choice questions and 138 scenario-based multiple-choice question sets. Seven review sessions were held in total during which the laparoscopic surgeons were asked to attempt to answer the question and rate its relevance. Questions were considered appropriate for beta-testing if they were answered correctly by at least 60% of the reviewers, if at least 70% of the reviewers agreed they were highly relevant to laparoscopic surgery, and if at least 70% of the reviewers felt that the question required clinical problem solving skills rather than simple recall of information.

Validation

To validate the assessment component of the FLS cognitive curriculum, the test questions were then divided into two groups of 21 questions each, and field-tested at eight centers in the United States and Canada. Each center randomly selected 10–15 participants ranging in level of training from resident to practicing laparoscopic surgeon. Data from these field tests demonstrated that experienced laparoscopic surgeons performed similarly on each test, with an average score of 81%. Seventy-three percent of the questions from the first test and 77% from the second test were judged as requiring problem solving skills rather than simple recall. And the projected score for a "minimally qualified" laparoscopic surgeon was estimated to be 67 and 68% for the two tests, respectively.

Construct validity for the questions was assessed across several domains. The first assumed that the performance of the participants would correspond to their level of training and so the results of the tests were separated into three groups – junior residents, senior residents, and a combined group of fellows and practicing surgeons – which demonstrated a significant difference in cognitive performance between them.

The second domain that was examined looked more closely at the laparoscopic experience of the participants. Since the purpose of the FLS program was to focus on laparoscopic skills and knowledge exclusively, it was important to distinguish whether the differences in test scores were a result of an increase in general surgery knowledge of the participants, or an increase in specific knowledge of laparoscopic surgery. This was achieved by grouping the test results based on self-reported numbers of various laparoscopic procedures performed. Again, this grouping demonstrated a significant difference in cognitive performance, with a correlation between these two variables of 0.81. Furthermore, when controlled for the amount of laparoscopic experience, the difference in cognitive performance across training levels was no longer statistically significant.

For the third domain, the test scores were then compared with self-ratings of competence. Participants were asked to rate their competence in performing basic and advanced laparoscopic procedures independently, and in performing general laparoscopic technical skills. All three of these were shown to correlate significantly with performance on the cognitive assessment.

Finally, the different components of the cognitive assessment were analyzed against each other. Multiple-choice questions were found to correlate well with the scenario questions although not to such an extent that they overlapped each other.

Psychomotor Component

Development

The other key dimension in laparoscopic surgical training is the manual skills component. Performing laparoscopy requires a different skill set from conventional open surgery due to the unique optics and instrumentation involved. Surgeons must learn how to perform complex technical skills while looking at a monitor instead of the actual tissues they are operating on. Furthermore, their depth perception is limited by the monitor, requiring surgeons to learn other depth cues such as touch and shading. Laparoscopic instruments present another set of unique challenges. The long shape amplifies tremors and limits the length and width of the operating mechanism. Additionally, the placements and fixed position of the trocars limit the instrument's range of motion and create a fulcrum effect, mirroring the surgeon's movement. A number of different techniques and approaches to teaching laparoscopic surgical skills had already been developed by the time the FLS committee began their work, and so for the manual skills component of their curriculum the committee turned to the work of Gerald Fried's team at McGill University.

In 1998, Fried et al. published the first results of their McGill Inanimate System for Training and Evaluation of Laparoscopic Skills (MISTELS) laparoscopic simulator. The simulator itself consisted of a laparoscopic trainer box measuring $40 \times 30 \times 19.5$ cm covered by an opaque membrane. The membrane contained two fixed holes for trocar placement that were placed at convenient working angles on either side of a freestanding zero-degree camera. A light source was installed within the trainer box and the video camera was connected to an external monitor.

The development of the tasks themselves involved a systematic process that began with the identification of skills that were unique to laparoscopic surgery. A panel of five experienced laparoscopic surgeons reviewed a series of video recordings of laparoscopic cholecystectomies, appendectomies, inguinal hernia repairs, and Nissen fundoplications. Based on these videos, they identified a number of skill domains that they felt to be specific and necessary for the training and evaluation of laparoscopic surgery. These included operating with a magnified two-dimensional monocular vision, using long instruments that diminished tactile feedback and amplified tremors, and the need to work through

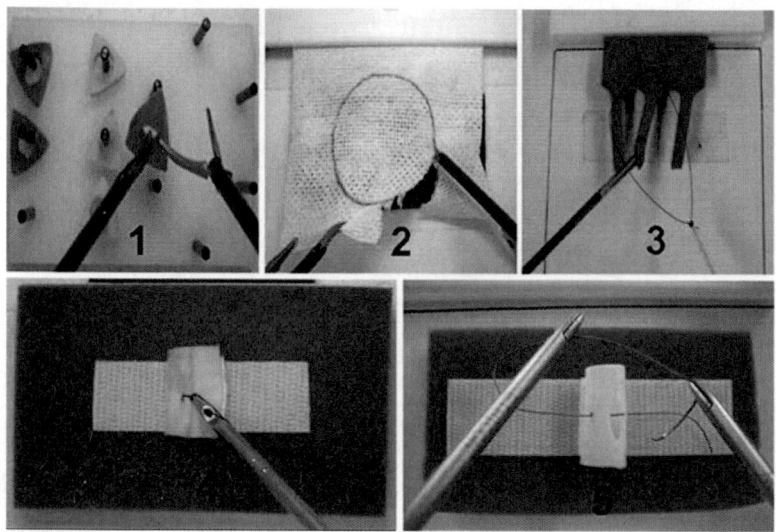

Fig. 46.1. FLS tasks. (1) Peg transfer, (2) Pattern cut, (3) Ligating loop, (4) Extracorporeal knot tying, (5) Intracorporeal knot tying.

trocars with fixed access in the abdominal wall. In addition, skills specific to minimally invasive surgical devices were identified such as using pre-tied looped sutures, clip-appliers, knot-pushers, and staplers for mesh placement.

From these domains, the MISTELS group developed seven tasks along with a brief accompanying video that demonstrated proper performance. These tasks included: (1) peg transfer, (2) pattern cutting, (3) clip application, (4) ligating loop, (5) mesh placement, (6) suturing with extracorporeal knot tying, and (7) suturing with intracorporeal knot tying. However, early analysis of these tasks demonstrated that the clip application and mesh placement models were expensive and did not substantially add to the evaluative ability of the other five tasks, and so they were removed from the curriculum. Scoring for all tasks involves a combination of time and accuracy measures. The original five tasks are described below (Fig. 46.1):

Task 1: Peg Transfer

This task involves the transfer of six rubber triangular rings across a board with 12 pegs fixed into it. The surgeon would begin by picking up the plastic rings with their nondominant hand, transfer them to their dominant hand, and then place them onto a peg on the opposite side of the pegboard. Once completed, the surgeon would then reverse the process, returning the rings to their original positions. This task was designed to exercise depth perception in a two-dimensional environment as well as bimanual coordination.

Task 2: Pattern Cut

In this task, a 4×4 in. gauze with a circular pattern printed on it is suspended within the box trainer. Using a grasper and a pair of laparoscopic scissors, the surgeon is then required to cut out the circle as closely as possible along the line. The purpose of this task is to develop precise cutting skills while using the nondominant hand for countertraction and positioning.

Task 3: Ligating Loop

In this task, the surgeon must place a ligating loop onto a foam appendage and secure it at a premarked position. Once completed, the surgeon then has to cut the free end of the suture with a laparoscopic scissor. The purpose of this task is to mimic similar tasks that involve the ligation of a tubular structure such as a blood vessel, cystic duct, or appendix.

Task 4 and 5: Suturing with Extracorporeal and Intracorporeal Knot Tying

In these two tasks, a curved needle and suture are introduced into the simulator through a trocar, and a stitch is placed through target points marked on either side of a slit penrose drain. The suture is then tied using either an extracorporeal tie with a knot pusher, or an intracorporeal tie.

The scoring metrics for the FLS tasks also underwent extensive study during their development. In order for FLS to be used as a high-stakes assessment tool, a minimum passing score had to be determined. In 2003, Fraser et al. tested 165 individuals on FLS and grouped their results according to their clinical competency in laparoscopic surgery. The noncompetent group was defined as medical students and residents within their first 2 years of training, while the competent group consisted of chief general surgical residents, laparoscopy fellows, and practicing laparoscopic surgeons. The participant's scores were then normalized by dividing each individual's score by the maximum score achieved by a chief resident for that task. A total score was then calculated by summing the scores for each of the five tasks. A frequency distribution was then plotted for these scores, and using a receiver-operator curve from these data, a cutoff passing score of 270 was determined.

Table 46.1. Performance-based proficiency levels.

Task	Task name	Time (s)	Allowable errors	Repetitions
1	Peg transfer	48	No drops outside field of view	2 Consecutive + 10 nonconsecutive
2	Pattern cut	98	All cuts within 2 mm of line	2 Consecutive
3	Ligating loop	53	Up to 1 mm accuracy error allowed. Knot must be secure	2 Consecutive
4	Extracorporeal suture	136	Up to 1 mm accuracy error allowed. Knot must be secure	2 Consecutive
5	Intracorporeal suture	112	Up to 1 mm accuracy error allowed. Knot must be secure	2 Consecutive + 10 nonconsecutive

One criticism of this scoring system, however, has been that the rubric was too complicated for practical use during everyday practice. It was argued that participants required an easier method to measure progression and gauge their competence. As a result, in 2007 Ritter and Scott proposed an alternative proficiency-based training curriculum that avoids cumbersome calculations and requires only that participants time themselves and keep track of their errors (Table 46.1). They noted that should participants achieve these proficiency levels for all five tasks, they would achieve a cumulative FLS score of 454, resulting in a 100% passing rate for the manual skills portion of the FLS.

Validation

Given the high-stakes nature of the FLS program, establishing the reliability and validity of FLS was particularly important. Over the 10 years following the introduction of FLS, numerous studies have been conducted to address these issues.

Analyzing the FLS test results of 10 volunteers including medical students, residents, and attending surgeons, three aspects of reliability were addressed by Vassiliou et al. in 2006: interrater reliability, test–retest reliability, and internal consistency. Intraclass correlation coefficients (ICCs) were used to calculate the interrater and test–retest reliability of FLS, which demonstrated high rates of correlation in both cases 0.988 (95% CI, 0.985–1.00) and 0.892 (95% CI, 0.665–0.968), respectively. To analyze the internal consistency of FLS, Cronbach's alpha was calculated on the means of the scores for the tasks and was found to be 0.86, exceeding the threshold level of 0.8 required for high-stakes evaluations. Furthermore, each task correlated highly with the total score (0.62–0.81), and internal consistency could not be improved with the elimination of any task.

Construct validity, the ability for a test to measure what it is purportedly able to measure, has been evaluated by multiple studies by looking at correlation between training level and FLS score. The most recent of these studies looked at a total of 215 participants from five countries. They were divided into three levels of experience – PGY one half residents, PGY three-fourth residents, and chief residents/fellows/attending surgeons. Analysis of their test scores demonstrated a clear and statistically significant step-wise improvement with increasing level of experience for both the individual task score and the normalized total score.

Given that the psychomotor component of the FLS program was developed at McGill University, and that the majority of the validation studies were conducted at this institution, it was also important to demonstrate that the results were generalizable. To address the external validity of FLS, Fried et al. compared the results from 135 McGill surgeons with 80 surgeons from other institutions. Multiple regression analysis demonstrated that only training level ($p < 0.0001$) and not test site ($p = 0.87$) was an independent predictor of total FLS score.

One of the most important validation measures, however, is concurrent/predictive validity. While FLS may be able to demonstrate good reliability and construct validity for its own tasks, in order for it to be relevant it had to demonstrate that its scores correlated well with intraoperative measures of technical skill in laparoscopy. While a number of preliminary studies were conducted to look at this issue, a direct comparison of FLS psychomotor scores with measures of intraoperative laparoscopic skill would have to wait until Vassiliou et al. developed and validated a separate objective evaluation tool for laparoscopic cholecystectomies called the Global Operative Assessment of Laparoscopic Skills (GOALS). When Fried et al. (2004) compared FLS scores with GOALS scores for 19 surgeons using multiple regression, FLS psychomotor scores and training level were both found to be independent predictors of intraoperative technical skill, with total FLS score correlating highly with GOALS score ($r = 0.81$, $p < 0.001$).

Current Uses of FLS

Since the first FLS participants were tested and certified in 2004, the FLS program has become hugely successful, gaining widespread adoption throughout North America and internationally. Its value, not only as an evaluation tool, but also as an educational program has been clearly demonstrated in a recent study by Sroka et al. in 2010 showing improved laparoscopic performance in the operating room following FLS training. Sixteen surgical residents with no previous FLS training were randomized to either FLS training or control. The FLS group was enrolled in a supervised proficiency-based FLS curriculum developed by Ritter and Scott in 2008, during which time both groups continued their regular residency training. After completion of the FLS curriculum, both groups were evaluated using the GOALS assessment tool during elective laparoscopic cholecystectomies and the FLS group demonstrated a statistically significant improvement in score compared with the control group (6.1 ± 1.9 vs. 1.8 ± 2.2, $p = 0.0005$). In the same year, Rosenthal et al. also demonstrated that an FLS proficiency-based curriculum resulted in a high level of skill retention. Even in the absence of ongoing simulator-based training or clinical experience, 21 novice medical students were able to achieve a high level of performance on the psychomotor component of the FLS up to a year after their training.

As a result of these findings, philanthropic groups such as the Covidien Educational Fund and malpractice insurance companies have provided financial support to surgeons to encourage training with FLS. Furthermore, the educational value of the FLS program has been recognized by a number of licensing bodies. In 2008, the American Board of Surgery (ABS) announced that applicants would be required to obtain FLS certification before taking the ABS examination. And more recently, the Royal Australasian College of Surgeons has also required FLS certification of its surgical residents.

In 2010, Okrainec et al. conducted a review of the FLS program and found that in just 5 years, a total of 2,689 participants took the FLS exam, with a yearly increase in the number of individuals seeking FLS certification. The vast majority of these participants were senior residents or fellows (69%), while attending surgeons made up 19% and junior residents 12%. This study also found that the overall pass rate of these participants was 88%, approaching the target pass rate of 90% established during the initial test-setting process.

The broad appeal and applicability of the FLS program was also highlighted in these results. As mentioned previously, the FLS program was designed specifically to be applicable to all surgeons and procedures requiring laparoscopy. This was highlighted by the fact that 12% of the FLS participants were from surgical specialties other than general surgery. Furthermore, the FLS program had attracted participants from 14 different countries, including an increasing interest from surgeons in the developing world. This trend is likely to continue as MIS equipment becomes increasingly available in these contexts and novel instructional tools such as telesimulation allow for cost-effective remote training.

Conclusion

The FLS program is a training curriculum and evaluation tool that covers the fundamental cognitive and psychomotor components necessary for surgeons to perform laparoscopic surgery. The generalizability of its content and skills exercises has made it broadly applicable to a number of surgical specialties and countries. Furthermore, the FLS program's proven validity and reliability have made it the gold standard for teaching the unique knowledge and fundamental skills required for surgeons to perform laparoscopic surgery.

Selected Readings

1. Peters JH, Fried GM, Swanstrom LL, et al. Development and validation of a comprehensive program of education and assessment of the basic fundamentals of laparoscopic surgery. Surgery. 2004;135(1):21–7.
2. Fried GM, Feldman LS, Vassiliou MC, et al. Proving the value of simulation in laparoscopic surgery. Ann Surg. 2004;240:518–28.
3. Scott DJ, Ritter EM, Tesfay ST, Pimentel EA, Nagji A, Fried GM. Certification pass rate of 100% for fundamentals of laparoscopic surgery skills after proficiency-based training. Surg Endosc. 2008;22(8):1887–93.
4. Sroka G, Feldman LS, Vassiliou MC, Kaneva PA, Fayez R, Fried GM. Fundamentals of Laparoscopic Surgery simulator training to proficiency improves laparoscopic performance in the operating room – a randomized controlled trial. Am J Surg. 2010;199(1):115–20.

47. Fundamentals of Endoscopic Surgery

Brian J. Dunkin

Introduction

It surprises many young surgeons to learn that a number of advances in therapeutic flexible gastrointestinal (GI) endoscopy were first described by surgeons. These include polypectomy, control of hemorrhage, variceal banding, percutaneous endoscopic gastrostomy, and radiofrequency ablation of esophageal mucosa. Despite a history of leadership in the field, many surgeons have not learned or maintained skills in GI endoscopy and this is creating problems in the modern era of surgery.

First, surgeons practicing in rural areas are not being prepared to perform endoscopy in these settings. In a national survey of rural and urban surgeons, Heneghan et al. showed that rural surgeons working in communities of <50,000 population performed an average of 220 endoscopies per year as opposed to 77 by urban surgeons [1]. Despite this, the American Board of Surgery reports that 62% of rural general surgeons sitting for the recertification examination feel more endoscopy training is needed during surgical residency.

Second, the natural progression of minimally invasive surgery is to move toward use of the flexible endoscope. GI bleeding, pancreatic pseudocyst drainage, and establishment of enteral access are just a few examples of procedures that were once a mainstay of general surgery and are now managed almost exclusively with a flexible endoscopic approach. The management of GI leaks and fistulas with stents, radiofrequency ablation of Barrett's esophagus, and intragastric surgery for managing tumors in the stomach are more recent developments which are obviating surgery and on the horizon are endoscopic management options for gastroesophageal reflux disease, obesity, and type II diabetes. The minimally invasive surgeon who does not believe flexible endoscopy will be important in their practice is not paying attention to current trends in the field.

D.S. Tichansky, J. Morton, and D.B. Jones (eds.), *The SAGES Manual*
of Quality, Outcomes and Patient Safety, DOI 10.1007/978-1-4419-7901-8_47,
© Springer Science+Business Media, LLC 2012

Current State of Assessing Endoscopic Competence

A board certified general surgeon just out of residency may have a difficult time gaining privileges to do GI endoscopy in their hospital. This is because the current state of assessing procedural competence relies on case numbers. Most endoscopic units in the USA use case numbers recommended by the American Society of Gastrointestinal Endoscopy (ASGE) whose training guidelines suggest that a trainee needs to perform 130 EGDs and 140 colonoscopies before he or she should even be evaluated for procedural competence [2]. These numbers are based on a published abstract by Cass et al. in which the performance of 135 trainees in 14 different GI fellowships were evaluated demonstrating that it took 130 EGDs and 140 colonoscopies for this group to achieve a 90% success rate in intubating the esophagus and pylorus or the splenic flexure and cecum, respectively [3]. Large, prospective evaluations of the performance of surgical endoscopists, however, do not support such numbers. Reed et al. evaluated 3,525 EGDs performed by surgeons and found no correlation between experience and completion or major complication rates [4]. Surgeons who had performed only 11–49 prior EGDs were able to successfully complete the procedure at the same rate as more experienced endoscopists and required, on average, only 5 more minutes to do so. Wexner et al. prospectively analyzed 13,580 colonoscopies performed by surgeons and found that prior colonoscopic experience and annual volume did have an impact on completion rate and was inversely proportional to the time to completion [5]. However, only 50 prior colonoscopies and 100 annual colonoscopies were necessary to achieve over a 90% rate of completion. Based on Reed's and Wexner's work, the American Board of Surgery requires 35 upper endoscopies and 50 colonoscopies for graduating general surgery residents wishing to take their qualifying examination – a number which may not allow them privileges in their hospital's endoscopy suite.

Why Do We Need the Fundamentals of Endoscopic Surgery Program?

The variability in the literature about the use of procedure numbers as an indicator of competence illustrates the need for a validated assessment tool of knowledge and skill in flexible GI endoscopy. Such a "test" could verify the requisite knowledge and technical skill to do these procedures and establish a baseline by which all endoscopists can be measured. Fundamental of endoscopic surgery (FES) is such an assessment tool.

What Is the Fundamentals of Endoscopic Surgery Program?

FES is a test of knowledge and skills in flexible GI endoscopy developed by the Society of American Gastrointestinal and Endoscopic Surgeons (SAGES). It includes didactic material available in web-based format for review, an online written examination, and a hands-on skills test. The entire examination can be completed in less than 2 h and it serves as a benchmark for demonstrating an understanding of the fundamentals of flexible GI endoscopy and competence in basic endoscopic skills. The minimally qualified candidate who is expected to pass the FES exam is a second- or third-year general surgery resident at the end of their flexible endoscopy rotation or a GI fellow at the end of their first year of training. FES has been developed using rigorous validation methods so that it can serve as a high-stakes examination. Its components and the validation process are described below.

Web-based didactic material. FES provides web-based didactic material to help learners gain the knowledge required to understand the basics of GI endoscopy. This material is written in the form of book chapters and focused on the level of understanding required by the minimally qualified candidate. An outline of the content of the chapters is shown in Table 47.1. The content of this material was derived from interviewing expert surgical endoscopists, colorectal surgeons, and gastroenterologists about the basic knowledge required to perform GI endoscopy. Each chapter was reviewed by these experts for accuracy of content and appropriate scope and then edited by one of two editors assigned to the FES project. SAGES used a web-based learning content and proficiency expert to put the didactic material in an online format with rich illustrations and pictures.

Written examination. SAGES used a testing consultant (Kryterion, Phoenix, AZ, USA) with expertise in creating validated high-stakes exams for the FES written examination. Under Kryterion's guidance, a test definition document was developed defining the scope of the examination and a survey was created to assess the test document content

Table 47.1. FES didactic content (abbreviated).

1. Technology and equipment
   A. Characteristics of endoscopes
   B. Equipment setup
   C. Trouble shooting
   D. Equipment care
2. Patient preparation
   A. Informed consent
   B. Anesthesia risk assessment
   C. Prophylactic antibiotic therapy
   D. Management of anticoagulation
3. Anesthesia/conscious sedation/monitoring/recovery
   A. Monitoring
   B. Conscious sedation
   C. Recovery
   D. Alternative anesthesia
   E. Unsedated endoscopy
4. Upper endoscopy
   A. Indications/contraindications and surveillance/screening
   B. Patient positioning/room setup
   C. Performance of diagnostic EGD
   D. Complications – prevention/recognition/correction
   E. Normal anatomy
   F. Pathology recognition
5. Lower GI endoscopy
   A. Indications/contraindications and surveillance/screening
   B. Patient position/room setup
   C. Performance of diagnostic colonoscopy
   D. Normal anatomy
   E. Pathology recognition
6. ERCP
   A. Indications/contraindications and surveillance/screening
   B. Patient position/room setup
   C. Performance of diagnostic ERCP
   D. Complications – prevention/recognition/correction
   E. Normal anatomy
   F. Pathology recognition
   G. Interventions-tissue sampling, sphincterotomy, stone removal,
       relief of obstruction
7. Endoscopic therapies
   A. Hemostasis – variceal/nonvariceal
   B. Polypectomy
   C. Dilation/stent
   D. Foreign body removal
   E. Enteral access
   F. Combined laparoendoscopic procedures

Table 47.2. Deconstructed task list for performing flexible GI endoscopy.

1. Scope navigation
   A. Tip deflection
   B. Scope traversal
   C. Torque
   D. Use of two-handed technique
2. Loop reduction
3. Retroflexion
4. Traversing a sphincter
5. Management of insufflation
6. Mucosal evaluation
7. Targeting

and weight the content areas according to importance. This survey was distributed to general surgeons, colorectal surgeons, and gastroenterologists to ensure completeness and, based on this definition document and the survey, a comprehensive test objectives outline was created specifying the exact content of the written FES exam and reflecting the weighted importance of each area.

Subsequent to developing the test objectives outline, multiple question-writing sessions were conducted with the oversight of Kryterion to monitor the accuracy and congruency of the questions. It was envisioned that the written exam would contain 75 questions and take 90 min to complete. As a result, at least 225 questions (3×75) were required to ensure there would be two complete exams from which to randomize questions, and an additional 75 questions to fill-in anticipated drop out of poorly performing questions discovered during beta testing. The performance of the written examination was beta-tested at multiple venues such as the SAGES national meeting, the international meeting of the Natural Orifice Surgery Consortium for Assessment and Research (NOSCAR), and the annual meeting of the American College of Surgeons (ACS). It was also taken by physicians from multiple specialties, types of practice, and levels of training. From this beta testing, test question performance was confirmed and a pass/fail rate determined.

Hands-on skills test. The first step in developing the skills test for FES was to ask expert surgical endoscopists to define the skills required to expertly perform flexible endoscopy and create a deconstructed task list of these skills (Table 47.2). This list was used as the basis for designing the FES hands-on examination.

After careful analysis by the FES Task Force, it was decided that a computer-generated (a.k.a. virtual reality or VR) platform would be best

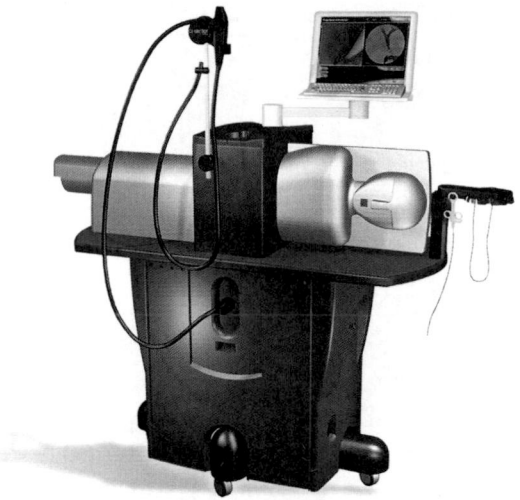

Fig. 47.1. The GI Mentor II.

for the FES skills test. Such a platform has a number of distinct advantages. First, it does not require a testing program to own any flexible endoscopy equipment since it uses a proprietary endoscope. Second, the test can be administered with web-support to standardize administration and eliminate the need for an on-site expert proctor. Third, a VR platform allows for centralized collation of results with secure reporting and easy dissemination of software upgrades. Finally, the manufacturers of the VR GI endoscopy platform voiced a commitment to developing a desktop version that would be significantly less expensive that existing VR training platforms. After a thorough vetting of proposals from multiple vendors, SAGES partnered with Simbionix (Simbionix Ltd., Israel) – manufacturers of the GI Mentor II (Fig. 47.1) – to build and validate the FES hands-on skills test.

The test consists of five separate modules created from the deconstructed task list and is administered on the Simbionix GI Mentor II platform. Because of the cost of this platform, it is envisioned that the test will initially be given at regional testing centers around the world. In time, a desktop testing platform will be developed which could be

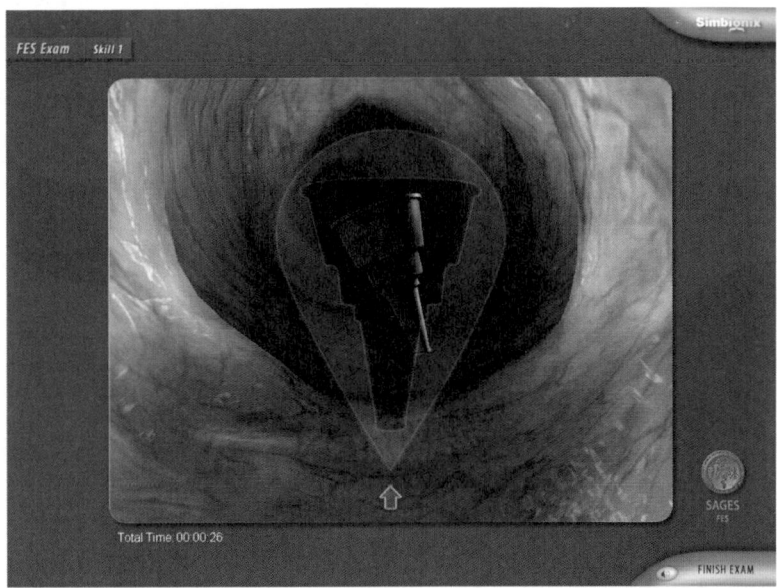

Fig. 47.2. Navigation sample image.

more easily distributed to individual training programs. The five testing modules are: Module 1 – navigation (traversal, tip deflection, and torque). The module requires navigation through a simulated colon by advancing the scope and using torque and tip deflection. It is necessary to use two-handed scope manipulation (one hand on the deflection wheels; the other on the scope shaft) to successfully complete the task. There are multiple floating targets, all pointing at different angles. When the testee reaches a target, the endoscope must be torqued and deflected to line up the "viewfinder" on the screen and the target and make it disappear while avoiding touching the wall (Fig. 47.2).

Module 2 – loop reduction. This module requires reduction of three separate random loops. Each loop differs in anatomic configuration and level of difficulty and if not successfully reduced, there is paradoxical movement of the scope without advancement. All three loops must be reduced to complete the task (Fig. 47.3). Module 3 – upper GI endoscopy with retroflexion, sphincter traversal, and use of insufflation. The simulated environment consists of the sectional anatomy of the upper GI tract including the esophagus, stomach, pylorus, and first portion of the duodenum. The endoscope must be passed into and through the stomach to locate the pylorus which is traversed using a combination of tip control

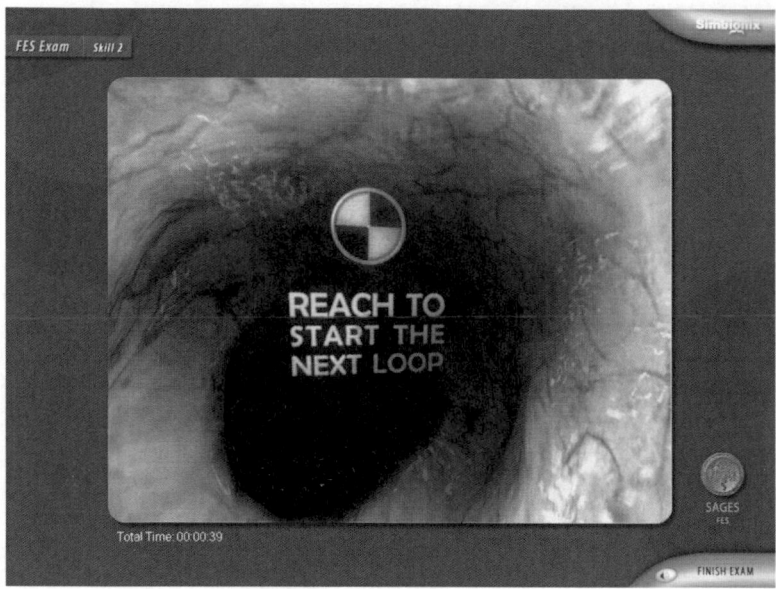

Fig. 47.3. Navigation sample image.

and insufflation. The endoscope is then brought back into the stomach and a combination of insufflation and retroflexion is used to identify targets on the incisura and in the cardia. The task is completed by straightening the endoscope, evacuating insufflation, and pulling back into the esophagus (Fig. 47.4). Module 4 – mucosal evaluation. A thorough evaluation of the colonic mucosa is required to identify multiple targets hidden behind folds (Fig. 47.5). Module 5 – targeting. While advancing the endoscope, the testee must identify a target and deliver a biopsy forceps to its center without colliding with the side walls or touching outside the target area. The position of the targets is randomized. The biopsy tool must be reintroduced into the working channel for each target (Fig. 47.6).

Validation of the metrics used for the hands-on skills test is a cornerstone of the FES project and one that has proved challenging. The tasks and their metrics have undergone a series of iterative changes to improve performance. After each change, the modules were retested at multiple centers in North America to establish construct validity – i.e. verifying that performance on the simulator separates expert endoscopists from beginners. Once construct validity is established, receiver-operator

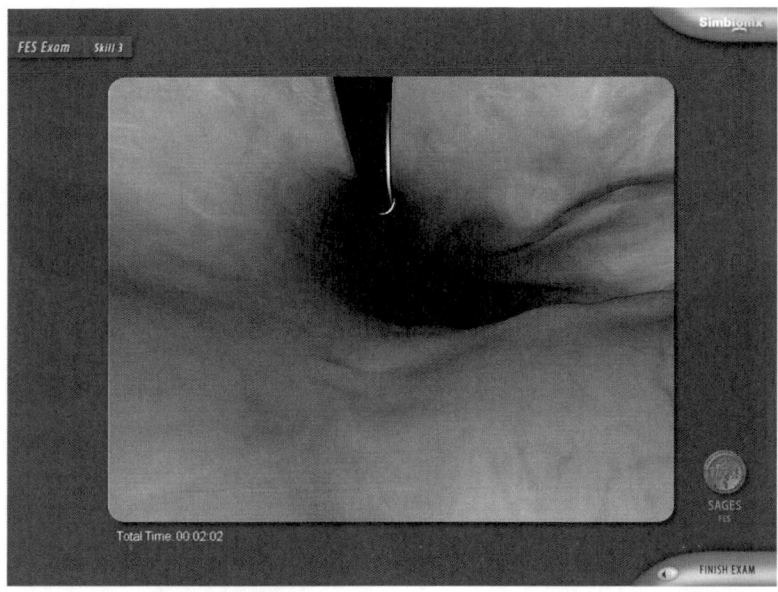

Fig. 47.4. Navigation sample image.

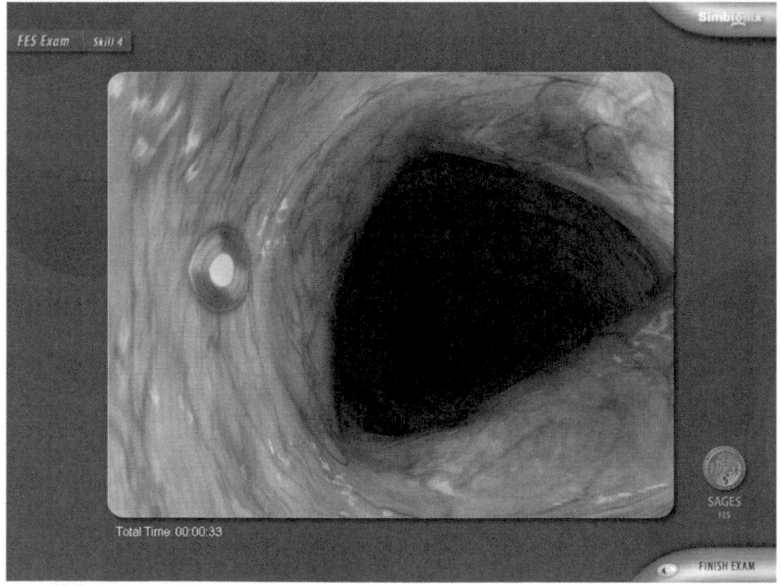

Fig. 47.5. Navigation sample image.

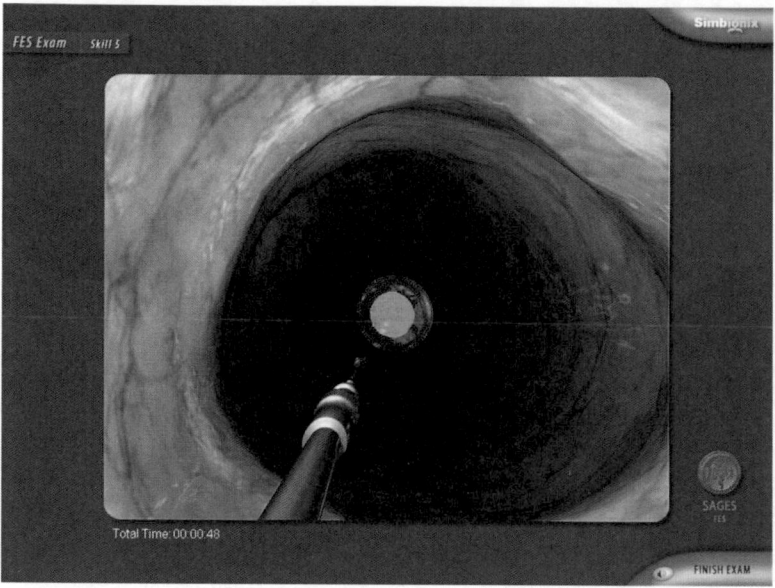

Fig. 47.6. Navigation sample image.

curves plotting the performance of endoscopists with all levels of experience are created to guide choosing the "passing score" for the exam. A score is chosen to maximize the test's ability to separate the minimally qualified candidate from the unqualified candidate. Completion of this validation work is anticipated by the fall of 2011.

The Future of FES

When the validation work for FES is complete, it will be the first high-stakes assessment program of knowledge and skills in flexible GI endoscopy and will serve as a benchmark for both surgeons and gastroenterologists to assure basic competency. It is planned that this assessment tool will become a routine part of surgical endoscopy training and perhaps even adopted by the American Board of Surgery as a necessary certification for taking the qualifying exam. Practice programs for the hands-on component of the FES program will also be developed both on the Simbionix platform and others. Such work has already begun with the development of the Surgical Endoscopy Training Program (STEP) – the SAGES initiative developed in partnership with industry to deliver a flexible endoscopy tower and endoscope to every surgery training program in the country. STEP can serve as a method for gaining hands-on endoscopy experience that could translate into better performance on the FES exam.

It is also anticipated that FES performance will be linked to clinical performance. This is called predictive validity and is the highest form of validation for a simulation platform. Predictive validity means that performance on the simulator will predict real clinical performance. It requires a validated test of clinical performance – something that had never been developed in GI endoscopy until now. In anticipation of this type of validation work for FES, SAGES has developed a clinical assessment tool for GI endoscopy called GAGES (Global Assessment of Gastrointestinal Endoscopic Skills) [6]. This tool allows an experienced endoscopist to watch a physician perform flexible GI endoscopy (either esophagogastroduodenoscopy or colonoscopy), complete the GAGES questionnaire, and report a valid score indicating whether the performance was done at a beginner, intermediate, or expert level. With such a clinical assessment tool, predictive validity for FES testing will be established.

Summary

FES and GAGES are powerful tools for assessing knowledge and skill in flexible GI endoscopy. Using these validated measures, individual practitioners can be assessed more accurately on whether or not they are clinically ready to perform endoscopic procedures making the use of case numbers as a surrogate marker of procedural competence during residency training obsolete.

Selected Readings

1. Heneghan SJ, Bordley J, Dietz PA, et al. Comparison of urban and rural general surgeons: motivations for practice location, practice patterns, and education requirements. J Am Coll Surg. 2005;201:732–6.
2. Sharma VK, Coppola AG, Raufman JP. A Survey of Credentialing Practices of Gastrointestinal Endoscopy Centers in the United States. J Clin Gastro. 2005;39(6): 501–7.

3. Cass OW, Freeman ML, Cohen J, et al. Acquisition of competency in endoscopic skills (ACES) during training: a multicenter study. Gastro Intest Endosc. 1995;41(4):317 (abstract).
4. Reed WP, Kilkenny JW, Dias CE, et al. A prospective analysis of 3525 esophagogastroduodenoscopies performed by surgeons. Surg Endosc. 2004;18:11–21.
5. Wexner SD, Garbus JE, Singh JJ, et al. A prospective analysis of 13,580 colonoscopies. Reevaluation of credentialing guidelines. Surg Endosc. 2001;15:251–61.
6. Vassiliou MC, Kaneva PA, Poulose BK, et al. How should we establish the clinical case numbers required to achieve proficiency in flexible endoscopy? Am J Surg. 2010; 199:121–5.

48. Fundamentals for Use of Safe Energy

Liane S. Feldman, Daniel B. Jones, and Steven D. Schwaitzberg

Heat has been applied to tissue therapeutically for thousands of years to treat symptoms, ablate tumors, and control bleeding. In the 1920s, biophysicist William Bovie and neurosurgeon Harvey Cushing produced a widely adopted electrosurgical generator that could cut and coagulate tissue during surgery. The basic principles underlying Bovie's machine have changed very little since then, and electrosurgery is ubiquitous in operating rooms, endoscopy suites, and clinics around the world. In the last decades, there has been a dramatic rise in the number and complexity of energy devices available, including radio frequency-based systems (e.g., bipolar devices, argon beam, and radiofrequency ablation) and ultrasonic energy systems. These devices often facilitate or even enable complex procedures. It is difficult to imagine modern surgery without energy devices, yet despite their frequent use, they remain poorly understood. The combination of electrical current, heat generation, the wide variety of devices, and the complex environments in which they are used can result in complications. Surgical burns and fires are not rare and remain in the ECRI institute's Top 10 Health Technology Hazards for 2011 (https://www.ecri.org/Forms/Documents/Top_10_Health_Tech_Hazards_2011.pdf. Accessed January 6, 2011). Yet there is no standardized curriculum widely promulgated through surgical training or postgraduate education especially as it applies to emerging devices.

To use energy devices to their fullest potential, prevent complications, and improve the outcomes and safety of surgery, users should understand the principles underlying the function of each device, how it is setup, how it interfaces with other devices, and potential pitfalls. Despite the fact that the majority of surgical procedures in every specialty performed throughout the world involve the use of some device that applies energy to tissue, there is little available information in standard surgical

D.S. Tichansky, J. Morton, and D.B. Jones (eds.), *The SAGES Manual of Quality, Outcomes and Patient Safety*, DOI 10.1007/978-1-4419-7901-8_48, © Springer Science+Business Media, LLC 2012

textbooks. As a result there is a need for a standard curriculum for surgeons and allied health personnel that addresses the physics, safe use, and complications associated with these devices that promotes the best outcomes for patients. This curriculum should include the underlying principles but be flexible in order to maintain relevance in this rapidly changing field.

Fundamentals for the safe use of energy (FUSE) is an educational program/curriculum being developed by the Society of American Gastrointestinal and Endoscopic Surgeons (SAGES) that includes both didactic and hands-on training approaches to the use of energy in interventional procedures. The FUSE program strives to develop both curricula and validated assessments to verify learning. The FUSE program disseminates information in the form of live courses and digital media.

The targeted learners include:

- Surgical residents and fellows enrolled in an accredited program of surgical education.
- Board eligible/certified practicing general surgeons.
- Residents and fellows in an accredited program of gynecology, urology, surgical oncology, colorectal surgery, thoracic surgery, endoscopic surgery, or other programs that incorporate energy devices.
- Board eligible/certified practicing gynecologists, urologists, thoracic surgeons, or other surgeons or physicians that use energy devices for interventions.

FUSE will provide objective evidence to residency program directors, certification and privileging bodies that the trainee or surgeon possesses the basic knowledge and skills fundamental to the use of energy devices for surgical procedures.

The general topics covered by FUSE will include:

(1) Fundamental physics of electrical energy applications.
(2) Safe use of electrical/laser/ultrasonic/plasma and future forms of energy and electrical tools in the OR.
(3) Recognition of faulty equipment and application of correct settings.
(4) Appropriate indications of energy tools and technology in the OR.

FUSE consists of three components:

1. Didactic information.
2. Hands-on stations.
3. An assessment tool to measure knowledge and know-how.

1. The FUSE didactic curriculum
    Fundamentals of Electro-Surgery – Part 1
    Fundamentals of Electro-Surgery – Part 2
    RF-Based Electrosurgical Systems – Monopolar Devices
    RF-Based Electrosurgical Systems – Bipolar Devices
    RF-Based Electrosurgical Systems – Argon Beam and RFA
    RF-Based Electrosurgical Systems – Flexible Devices for Endoscopy
    Ultrasonic Energy Systems – Part 1
    Ultrasonic Energy Systems – Part 2
    Microwave Energy Systems
    Energy Devices in Pediatric Surgery
    Integration of Energy Systems with Other Medical Devices

2. The FUSE Hands-On stations
    Monopolar Devices
    Bipolar Devices
    CUSA/Argon Beam Devices
    Ultrasonic Devices
    Fundamentals and Safety of Electrosurgery
    RFA Devices
    Microwave Devices
    Endoscopic Energy Devices

3. The FUSE Assessment tool
    The assessment tool for FUSE will include a two-part exam to evaluate knowledge and hands-on skills. The testing is proctored and the FUSE certificate will document basic proficiency with the knowledge and specific tools fundamental to the use of energy devices.

After completion of FUSE one should be able to:

*   Describe available energy sources and applications for use in the OR.
*   Understand the physics of energy applications in the OR.
*   Demonstrate correct and safe usage of energy sources in OR.
*   Identify errors of usage, faulty equipment, and malfunction before and during application of energy equipment in the OR.

- Describe potential clinical and operative indications for use of energy sources. Identify correct assembly and testing of energy equipment.

FUSE is an education service, namely, providing on-line and hands-on programs in the field of safe surgical technique. It is designed to communicate and promote best practice for the use of electromechanical, ultrasonic, and microwave energy sources in the OR. Any healthcare professional who has ever picked up an energy device in the OR such as a "Bovie" pencil or ultrasonic dissector will better understand how it works, when to apply it, and what possible hazards and errors in use exist. FUSE establishes a template methodology that allows for the incorporation of new devices into the FUSE program as they emerge in a manner consistent with SAGES white paper on industry relations.

Selected Readings

1. O'Connor JL, Bloom DA. William T Bovie and electrosurgery. Surgery. 1996;119: 390–6.
2. Smith CD, MacFadyen BV. Industry relationships between physicians and professional medical associations: corrupt or essential? Surg Endosc. 2010;24:251–3.
3. Smith TL, Smith JM. Electrosurgery in otolaryngology-head and neck surgery: principles, advances and complications. Laryngoscope. 2001;111:769–80.
4. Ulmer BC. Electrosurgery: history and fundamentals. Perioper Nurs Clin. 2007;2: 89–101.
5. Wu M-P, Ou C-S, Chen S-L, Yen YET, Rowbotham R. Complications and recommended practices for electrosurgery in laparoscopy. Am J Surg. 2000;179:67–73.

49. Simulation and OR Team Performance

John Pawlowski and Daniel B. Jones

Unsafe surgery results from a combination of technical and non-technical errors. These errors, when unrecognized or when combined with latent systemic failures, can lead to significant injury to the patient and even death. The recognition that human error is inevitable in complex tasks has been slow to reach the medical community. In an early paper, Dr. Lucien Leape describes the scope of the problem of medical errors and the difficulty of the culture of medicine in adding to these problems. Twenty percent of all hospitalized patients suffer an iatrogenic illness and 69% of medical errors are preventable. In the Harvard Medical School Institutions, for example, 44% of claims in the perioperative period are for technical reasons (Table 49.1).

The remainder of claims is from nontechnical reasons such as wrong-site surgery, retained objects, abnormal blood loss, and hematoma, which may have had technical components to the error but were all associated with communication breakdowns. In the analysis of these closed claims, the Harvard-affiliated insurance company, CRICO, recognized some common features of these communication gaps: they were verbal; there was status asymmetry; there was ambiguity as to responsibility, and there were multiple handoffs and transfers. To remedy these communication errors, CRICO proposed several solutions: a surgical safety checklist, closed loop communication, and assertiveness in communication (i.e., speaking up). The following chapter will address the use of simulation and OR Team Training as a possible vehicle to train operating room teams, with the final goal being to reduce surgical error and improve the safety of surgical inpatients.

Adverse events occur when errors happen at an inopportune moment. Far more common than adverse events are near misses or slips – those examples of risky behavior that do not result in injury. If one million adverse events occur each year in the USA, it is estimated that the number

D.S. Tichansky, J. Morton, and D.B. Jones (eds.), *The SAGES Manual of Quality, Outcomes and Patient Safety*, DOI 10.1007/978-1-4419-7901-8_49,
© Springer Science+Business Media, LLC 2012

Table 49.1. Perioperative closed claims for CRICO.

Category	Percent
Technical error/injury to adjacent organ	44
Wrong site/level/organ/procedure	21
Retained object	15
Large blood loss	12
Hematoma	8

CRICO Controlled Risk Insurance Company

of near misses would be five million. Therefore, any training of medical personnel should include careful review of performance to identify such risky behavior.

In an observational study of operating room safety, Christian et al. reviewed 63 h of surgery and had over 4,500 observations. They observed a number of critical system failures that had impact on patient safety. All of these critical events involved either communication and information flow or workload and competing tasks. This group recognized at least one close-call during each surgical procedure. All members of the OR team also had periods of decreased activity. A strategy to recognize times of task overload and share the workload were suggested. Thus, multidisciplinary teams that are performing complex tasks can be observed and assessed for specific parameters of patient safety and team performance.

Simulation

The advantage that simulation has over a performance review of actual surgeries is that comparison of time-adverse events can be generated with great frequency and the resultant discussion and intervention can be documented and reviewed in a timely fashion. The scenarios can be constructed from actual events that have occurred, can be taken from closed-claim archives, or can even be constructed to predict future operations. The tasks performed by the operating team can be reasonably realistic. For example, surgeons can incise, sew anastomoses, control bleeding and practice wound closures. Anesthesia personnel can intubate, transfuse, draw laboratory samples, and administer medications. Nurses can assemble and arrange equipment, facilitate communication, and count remaining sponges and needles, for example. The tasks are both familiar and validated. While some "suspension of disbelief" is required, most operating room teams report substantial face validity and can adapt to the simulation environment to perform the operative plan and to participate in their usual role on the team.

The Imperial College in London published their seminal experience with procedures in a simulated operating theater with a standardized OR team in 2005. Their group observed OR crisis and used a checklist and global assessment to record technical skills and communication during femoral arterial hemorrhage. All team members participated in a debriefing session after the scenario and rated the face validity of the simulated environment. Darzi et al. sought a high degree of realism in order to better understand team interactions and performance (Figs. 49.1 and 49.2).

The Carl J. Shapiro Simulation and Skills Center at Beth Israel Deaconess Medical Center expanded this concept and built a mock MIS endosuite for team simulation. Multiple camera mountings, directional microphones record all communication and activity. Models of intraabdominal organs were created that bleed and, behind a one way mirror, staff control simulation, bleeding, vital signs and signal confederates. Powers et al. demonstrated face and construct validity of the mock operating endosuite with laparoscopic crisis scenarios.

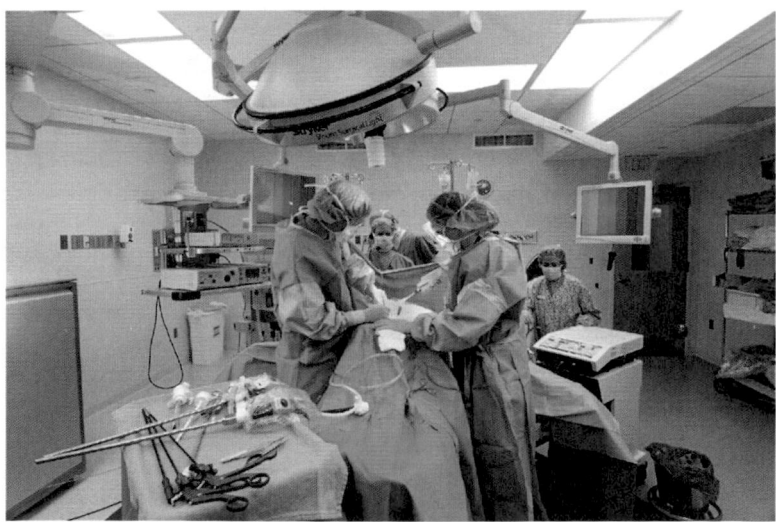

Fig. 49.1. Carl J Shapiro Simulation and Skills Center mock endosuite.

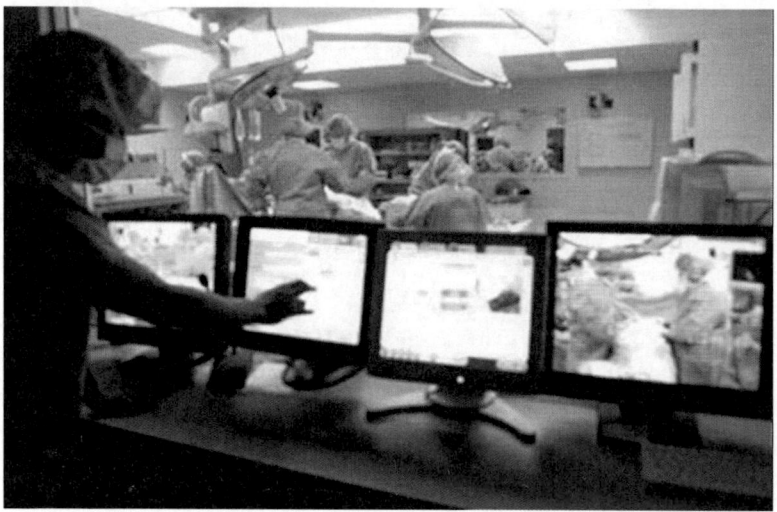

Fig. 49.2. Control room for mock endosuite.

Performances of FLS-certified and non-FLS-certified surgeons were placed in a laparoscopic crisis scenario and recorded the time to diagnose intraoperative bleeding following Veress needle entry, time to inform the operating team for the need to convert to an open procedure, and the actual time to conversion. Technical and nontechnical skills were assessed (Table 49.2). This scenario was recreated at the SAGES 2007 Annual Meeting Learning Center.

The American College of Surgeons recognized the value of simulation with the release of the American College of Surgeons/Association of Program Directors in Surgery National Skills Curriculum (Table 49.3).

Team Training

Team training is an organizational approach that attempts to identify and practice the essential aspects of teamwork and communication in certain endeavors that by their nature show high activity, potential for disaster, or high stress. Therefore, much of the early team training

Table 49.2. Nontechnical skills.

Category	Question
Communication and interaction	Instructions to assistant/scrub nurse; clear and polite Awaits acknowledgment from the assistant/scrub nurse Assistance sought from team members
Vigilance/situation awareness	Monitored patient's parameters throughout procedures Awareness of anesthetist Actively initiates communication with anesthetist during crisis periods
Team skills	Maintains a positive rapport with the whole team Open to opinions from other team members Acknowledges the contribution made by other team members Supportive of other team members
Leadership and management skills	Adherence to best practice during the procedure, e.g., does not permit corner cutting by self or team Time management, e.g., appropriate time allocation without being too slow or rushing team members Resource utilization, i.e., appropriate task-load distribution and delegation of responsibilities Authority/assertiveness
Decision-making crisis	Prompt identification of the problem Informed team members; promptly, clearly, and to all team members Outlines strategy/institutes a plan, i.e., asks scrub nurse for suction, instruments, suture materials Anticipates potential problems and prepares a contingency plan, e.g., asks to order blood, calls for help Option generation; takes the help of the team (seeks team opinion)

efforts have focused on military operations, aviation, and the nuclear power industry. Effective teams adapt a "shared mental model" and work to balance the effort, anticipate problems, seek relevant data, resolve conflicts, and communicate effectively. In addition, such team training can identify stressors such as fatigue, work overload, and crises that can test any team. Most team training performance reviews include a comprehensive debriefing. A full review of this can be found in Chap. 50.

Table 49.3. ACS-APDS simulation modules.

Teamwork in the trauma bay
Postoperative pneumonia (hypoxia, septic shock)
Postoperative hypotension
Laparoscopic crisis
The preoperative briefing
Laparoscopic troubleshooting
Postoperative pulmonary embolus
Postoperative myocardial infarction (cardiogenic shock)
Latex allergy anaphylaxis
Abdominal compartment syndrome (hypotension)
Patient handoff
Retained sponge on postoperative chest radiograph

Medical Disciplines

The use of simulation to teach effective team training has been demonstrated in a number of medical disciplines. All of these disciplines have a high acuity environment and require the use and interpretation of complex and technical monitors and instruments. In a multicenter study involving Emergency Medicine clinicians, for example, high-fidelity simulation was used to construct a team training course that improved clinical performance, increased patient safety, and decreased liability. The Emergency Room Team was asked to care for two patients who presented with significant acuity and hemodynamic instability (anaphylaxis and splenic rupture). The tasks were appropriate and time critical (vital sign assessment, abdominal ultrasound) and the treatments were monitored not only for timeliness and efficiency but also for appropriate safety checks (identification of patient, labeling of tubes, checking blood). In an area of medicine where the cost of teamwork failure is high, such team training was shown to improve outcomes and reduce liability.

Another area of medicine where simulation-based team training has proven to be effective is the discipline of Pediatric Trauma. In one report, an initial simulation exercise showed that the trauma team appropriately completed tasks 65% of the time. These tasks were defined prior to the study as essential and included airway management, management of pelvic fracture, and cervical spine care. A repeat of the team training exercise a year later, however, showed an improvement to 75% of appropriately completed tasks. Thus, the team training exercise using simulation was able to demonstrate an improvement over time of the performances of the pediatric trauma team. The simulations employed were rated as useful and realistic, and consisted of an infant with a head injury, a child with a penetrating wound to the back, and an adolescent with multitrauma that included an unstable pelvic fracture. The tasks were also realistic, such as establish an airway, establish intravenous access and recognize Cushing's signs. In pediatric trauma teams, there are many more team members such as pediatric surgeons, emergency medicine physicians, nurses, paramedics, respiratory therapists and residents, and critical care fellows. Thus, even large medical teams show improvement for simulation-based team training in a longitudinal program.

In a discipline of medicine that is often adjacent to the operating room, the endovascular suite, the use of simulation-based team training has been shown to improve teamwork and communication, clarify roles, and offer examples of conflict resolution. This simulation used trainees to perform procedures that were beyond their abilities and were done without mentoring or supervision. In this case, carotid artery stents were performed by surgical residents and medical students provided technical surgical support. The simulated endovascular suite was able to provide a safe area for trainees to practice and debrief both complex technical skills as well as elements of team training and communication. Learning objectives included both content learning as to the indication and technique of endovascular stent placement as well as concepts of effective team training and crisis management.

Nontechnical Skills

The essential characteristics of exemplary leadership and effective teamwork and communication are described by surgeons as "nontechnical skills." This deflating term includes a number of cognitive and interpersonal skills that are central to team training exercises. The cognitive skills include situational awareness, anticipation, and flexibility. The interpersonal skills focus on planning, advice, and feedback. In each category of skills, there are suggested behavioral markers that indicate both good and poor performance. Unlike many of the validated assessments of technical skills, these cognitive and interpersonal behaviors are not always visually apparent and often require verbal responses. There is always a bias toward the participant who "thinks out loud," even if those thoughts are not always cogent and organized.

Measurement of OR Team Performance

A number of assessment tools have been developed to measure the performance of operating teams in a simulated-OR environment. Most of these tools utilize the taxonomy of crisis management principles and have a graded assessment of each item in the taxonomy. Assessment of leadership, delegation, workload distribution, data collection, avoidance of fixation, utilization of resources, and recognition of limitations are included in most assessment tools. All of these tools suffer from time constraints during the scenario, the clipped phrases during crises, the undeclared thoughts or concerns, and the performance anxieties of being in the spot-lighted, videotaped, artificial environment of a simulation. Often, the most revealing moments come during the debriefing, yet that has only recently been analyzed for content and used in the performance assessment.

One interesting method to provoke the need for effective communication is through the use of "probes." These probes consist of clinical information that is given to one or several members of the operating room team and is usually important information for someone else on the team. For example, an anesthesiologist might hear about a latex allergy, or a nurse might hear about a prior anesthetic reaction. The extent of group sharing was assessed using these probes. This form of provocative probe may be useful in demonstrating the utility of sharing information and might also justify some routine duplication such as site and side and patient identifiers.

In addition to trained rater evaluations of team training performance, there have also been descriptions of self-assessments that use a Likert-type scale rating to evaluate the effectiveness of team training exercises using simulated operating room scenarios. One report cited significant improvements in role clarity, anticipation, cross monitoring, and team cohesion/interaction. Thus, self-assessment tools exist to demonstrate a perceived improvement in the cognition and interpersonal skills required for successful team training.

In order to codify the use of team training throughout the surgical suites at the teaching hospitals at Harvard Medical School, a unique program has been advanced by the insurance company that indemnifies Harvard, the Controlled Risk Insurance Company (CRICO). The CRICO/Harvard Operating Room Team Training with Simulation is an adventurous pilot program. In this program, the CRICO team will identify the major simulation instructors and the surgical education leaders at each of the four major teaching hospitals, identify the nurses and anesthesiologists for the various surgical teams, coordinate the design of ten scenarios using simulation, and organize a systematic evaluation of the pilot program. CRICO has provided funds to secure time for personnel and has promised a discount in the premium charged to surgeons who participate in this simulation-based team training session. Several requirements are included in this CRICO project: a surgical checklist must be designed and implemented in the scenarios and communication skills that practice closed loop (read back) and assertiveness (speaking up) must be included. There are two required scenarios: hemorrhage and cardiac arrest outside the operating room. The course must be 4–6 h in length and must contain no more than 20% didactic sessions, leaving time to focus on hands-on workshops and simulation exercises. During the pilot program, there is a required interim report as well as a final report with the availability of participants for follow up interviews.

This innovative program is, at this time, in the planning and early pilot stage, but promises to be a productive and campus-wide initiative that may lead to other insurance companies becoming involved in similar programs using simulation to help to improve surgical patient safety.

Future Directions

Any new surgical procedures will require an evaluation of techniques along with reevaluation of patient selection and perioperative management. Minimally invasive procedures are being supplanted by robotic procedures, endoscopic procedures, or natural orifice surgeries. Few of these techniques undergo the rigorous scrutiny of a randomized-controlled trial. Instead, surgeons rely on a solid surgical research background and, then, open discussion of the results and professional discussion. The surgical research, however, seldom involves the other members of the operating room team.

One proposed future strategy may be to use simulation to perform team training on new surgical procedures. Not only would surgeons be allowed to practice without potential patient harm, but nurses and anesthesia personnel could also anticipate the requirements for anesthetic management such as muscle paralysis, position pressure ventilation, and also predict possible complications such as airway compromise using esophageal stents, for example. Simulation-based team training could help refine and develop these new procedures and, perhaps, shorten the early portion of the learning curve, or, at least, remove patient harm from that part of the curve.

In conclusion, OR team training using simulation has been shown to improve these skills of teamwork and communication that are so often deficient in episodes of patient injury. The simulated operation room provides a safe environment not only for the patient but also for the practitioner. The surgeon can rehearse necessary technical skills as well as prepare for rare but known complications. The current level of simulation has adequate face validity and provides sufficient challenges to engage the fully trained surgeon. Team training reinforces a set of cognitive and interpersonal skills that are essential to competent crisis management. Surgeons and surgical training programs should embrace the use of high-fidelity simulation to teach OR team training to its trainees and as a periodic refresher course to its graduates.

Selected Readings

1. Anderson M, Leflore J. Playing it safe: simulated team training in the OR. AORN J. 2008;87(4):772–9.
2. Blum RH, Raemer DB, Carroll JS, Dufresne RL, Cooper JB. A method for measuring the effectiveness of simulation-based team training for improving communication skills. Anesth Analg. 2005;100:1375–80.
3. Christian CK, Gustafson ML, Roth EM, Sheridan TB, Gandhi TK, Dwyer KD, et al. A prospective study of patient safety in the operating room. Surgery. 2006;139: 159–73.
4. Cooper JD, Clayman RV, Krummel TM, Schauer PR, Thompson C, Moreno JD. Inside the operating room – balancing the risks and benefits of new surgical procedures: a collection of perspectives and panel discussion. Cleveland Clin J Med. 2008;75(6): S37–54.
5. Falcone RA, Daughterty M, Schweer L, Patterson M, Brown RL, Garcia VF. Multidisciplinary pediatric trauma team training using high-fidelity trauma simulation. J Pediatr Surg. 2008;43:1065–71.
6. Leape LL. Error in medicine. JAMA. 1994;272(23):1851–7.
7. Leape LL. Reporting of adverse events. NEJM. 2002;3(20):1633–8.
8. Moorthy K, Munz Y, Adams S, Pandey V, Darzi A. A human factors analysis of technical and team skills among surgical trainees during procedural simulations in a simulated operating theatre. Ann Surg. 2005;242:631–9.
9. Nestel D, van Herzeele I, Aggarwal R, O'Donoghue K, Choong A, Clough R, et al. Evaluating training for a simulated team in complex whole procedure simulations in the endovascular suite. Med Teach. 2009;31:e18–23.

10. Paige JT, Kozmenko V, Yang T, Gururaja RP, Hilton CW, Cohn Jr I, et al. High-fidelity simulation-based interdisciplinary operating room team training at the point of care. Surgery. 2009;145:138–46.

11. Powers KA, Rehrig ST, Irias N, Albano HA, Feinstein DM, Johansson AC, et al. Simulated laparoscopic operating room crisis: approach to enhance the surgical team performance. Surg Endosc. 2008;22(4):885–900.

12. Powers K, Rehrig S, Schwaitzberg SD, Callery MP, Jones DB. Seasoned surgeons assessed in a laparoscopic crisis. J Gastrointest Surg. 2009;13:994–1003.

13. Small SD, Wuerz RC, Simon R, Shapiro N, Conn A, Setnik G. Demonstration of high-fidelity simulation team training for emergency medicine. Acad Emerg Med. 1999;6(4):312–23.

14. Sundar E, Sundar S, Pawlowski J, Blum R, Feinstein D, Pratt S. Crew resource management and team training. Anesthesiol Clin. 2007;25:283–300.

15. Tsuda S, Scott D, Doyle J, Jones DB. Surgical skills training and simulation. Curr Probl Surg. 2009;46(4):261–372.

16. Tsuda S, Scott DJ, Jones DB, editors. ASE textbook of simulation: technical skills and team training. Woodbury, CT: Cine-Med Inc; 2010.

17. Yule S, Flin R, Paterson-Brown S, Maran N. Non-technical skill for surgeons in the operating room: a review of the literature. Surgery. 2006;139:140–9.

50. Debriefing After Simulation

Neal E. Seymour

Definitions of the term "Debriefing" generally describe a process to elicit information pertaining to an experienced event in order to gain a better understanding of it. This process is further distinguished by the requirement that the information elicited be from the event's participants. Systematic debriefing models have been employed as both therapeutic interventions (e.g., after traumatic events) and as educational tools (e.g., post-mission reviews). In medical education, debriefings have become a critical component of simulation training, particularly training that involves simulated patient care rendered by individuals or health care teams. After implementation of such training, all simulation scenarios ought to be debriefed, focusing on things that went well, things that did not go well, and opportunities for improvement.

In order to appreciate the essential nature of debriefing in this setting, it is helpful to consider it in the context of basic human pedagogical models. Learning in simulation is experiential in the same way it would be for real world experiences. Several taxonomies, most notably Kolb's learning cycle [1], describe cognitive consolidation of recent experiences by a process of reflection (Fig. 50.1) in the timeframe immediately following the experience. This process is a personal one and can involve cognitive and perceptual challenges that might color a participant's reflective account of the experience. Participants new to simulation or to the experience being simulated, who have little or no prior experience with debriefings, may find this especially challenging, and may require significant help and support to initiate the reflective process. The best post-simulation debriefing models call for a skilled debriefer to help compensate for this. This person does not behave as a traditional teacher in post-simulation debriefing. Rather, it is his or her responsibility to serve as (a) a prompter when reflective process stalls or stops, (b) as an objective contributor to help define the record of actual events when it is appropriate to do so, and (c) to guide the process in an ongoing fashion toward achievement of the stated educational goals. Hence, this role is

D.S. Tichansky, J. Morton, and D.B. Jones (eds.), *The SAGES Manual of Quality, Outcomes and Patient Safety*, DOI 10.1007/978-1-4419-7901-8_50, © Springer Science+Business Media, LLC 2012

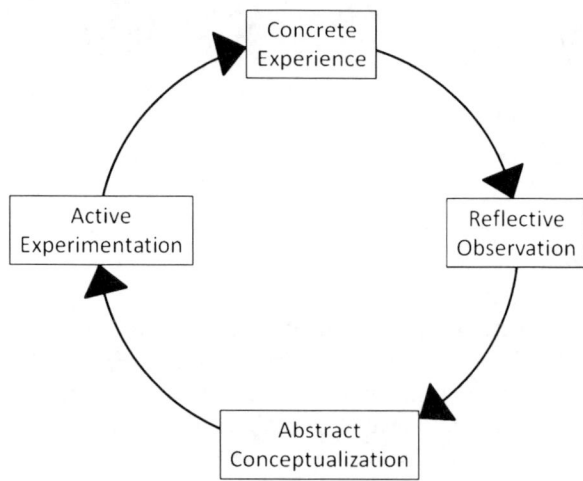

Fig. 50.1. Kolb's learning cycle is one way to view the process of experiential learning such as that might occur in a simulation training environment. The reflection-conceptualization components describe the principle opportunities offered during debriefing. Irrespective of the pedagogical model by which learning might be thought to occur during a session of simulated patient care, the importance of a high-quality debriefing cannot be overemphasized.

Table 50.1. Example facilitator open-ended questions.

How did you feel when you noticed that?
What were your other options at that point?
How did you think things went during…?
What do you think was right/not right about that decision?

more commonly described as "facilitator," given the nature of the responsibilities. There are numerous commentaries on these basic requirements that provide a generally consistent view of the facilitator's role [2–5].

Many standard and situation-specific prompts are available to a facilitator. These often take the form of questions (Table 50.1) that are open-ended and stimulate learner engagement in reflective process. The process should not become facilitator-centric, however, and must remain focused on the participant(s) and development of an understanding of their role in the simulation event in order to be effective. Although the term "structured" is often used to describe high-quality debriefing methods, this does not suggest the need for rigidity in either facilitator prompting or sequencing of questions. One debriefing expert stated that "our belief in the importance of debriefing and in the utility of the structured variety led us to the construction of various debriefing protocols. This approach frequently resulted in undesirable rigidity on the part of the facilitator and unmitigated boredom on the part of the participants" [6]. Structure in the form of general strategies, goal-directed phases, and a systematic plan for assessment [3] are all compatible with effective debriefing.

In the final analysis, debriefing is a tool of fundamental importance to stimulate reflection as an aid to experiential learning. There are several options to ensure learner reflection. Debriefings can take the form of discussion among participants in the course of reviewing the simulation, with the facilitator taking steps to direct discussion only if the process stalls or deviates from an educationally valuable direction. Alternatively, the facilitator can specifically direct individual participants to present aspects of their performance, working toward an understanding of good (or bad) performance. The degree of comfort and prior experience of the learners can be a major determinant of the degree of input made by the facilitator. Ideally, reflection would be spontaneous and complete, and no facilitator would be required. This is rarely the case with student or resident learners in medical simulation, although there are numerous examples of self-debriefing and written debriefing models that do not involve external facilitation. Irrespective of the degree of direction provided, participants are given the opportunity to critically analyze and discuss their actions, decisions, and emotional states.

Rudolph et al. [7] used a phasic description of debriefing in order to better define how it fits into a formative assessment methodology (Table 50.2). Of particular interest is the "analysis" phase, which provides the critical information for assessment by defining the gap between actual and desired performance during the simulation. This performance gap is revealed through facilitated discussion of the simulation, which is also the principle means to ensure a good reflective learning experience. An opportunity to address knowledge gaps with "brief didactics targeted

Table 50.2. Phases of debriefing (Rudolph et al.).

Reactions phase	Learner expresses initial emotional reactions to simulation
Analysis phase	Discussion process directed to close performance gap between actual and desired performance
Summary phase	Distill lessons learned into discrete concepts that can be used in practice

Table 50.3. Pitfalls of debriefing.

Facilitator lecturing
Close-ended questions
Inadequate emotional safety (recriminations, accusations)
Interruptions to find relevant video segments

to immediate learning needs" is also defined. Although it is important not to allow this to pre-empt other debriefing dialog, overall learning objectives ought to accommodate this type of information flow.

Ensuring learner engagement during debriefing is arguably the most difficult challenge facing the facilitator [5]. An actively engaged participant has the best opportunity for a solid learning experience and presumably the best opportunity for retention and transfer of what is learned to clinical care. The common facilitator pitfalls are all detriments to effective learner engagement (Table 50.3). In addition to facilitator "lecturing," ineffective use of audiovisual (A-V) recordings can be problematic. Systems to deliver recorded video represent significant investments for simulation centers, and are now widely available. A-V records of the simulated event may be used as an aid to the debriefing process, provided there are appropriate annotations to guide access to relevant sites in oftentimes lengthy recordings. Excessive time spent scanning videos for segments that are worth reviewing can be a significant distraction and break the flow of the debriefing. If the video is not well annotated, it is probably more effective to use participants recall than to risk losing participant engagement. At present it is not clear that the inclusion or omission of video is a major determinant of the quality of debriefing [8].

Most simulation training events occur in a training lab, a simulation suite, or an actual clinical environment ("in situ" simulation). There is no single successful formula for the site of debriefing and issues of convenience and feasibility often help determine where the debriefing takes place. The site should be quiet, and distraction free, and should accommodate all participants in the simulation session in a way that permits face-to-face discussion. Sometimes access to the simulation environment can be helpful for focused re-enactment, but most debriefings occur outside the simulation suite in a classroom setting with access to audiovisual recordings of the simulation event, which can be referred to as an aid in the reflective process.

Irrespective of the physical site in which debriefings occur, the environment must be the one that ensures emotional safety for the learner [2, 5]. A variety of factors pertinent to the learners, the simulation, and/or the facilitator may potentially compromise this sense of safety, and cause a debriefing situation to become emotionally charged to the detriment of effective education [9]. The learner may be new to clinical care or to the problem being managed and may become defensive, especially if they feel that their performance might be viewed by others as inadequate. The learner's sense of vulnerability may be increased by the impression of having been "deceived" by the manner in which a difficult simulation problem was presented [10]. If other participants are critical or even overbearing, this problem may be accentuated. An unskilled facilitator may provoke the same response by either being excessively critical or expounding their knowledge of good performance at the cost of good learner reflection. The facilitator essentially adjusts the level of supportiveness that a learner encounters in the debriefing environment.

Improving the effectiveness of debriefing may require careful observation of the process by experienced personnel and then a second debriefing for the facilitator. The Center for Medical Simulation developed the Debriefing Assessment for Simulation in Healthcare (DASH©), a tool to assess the effectiveness of debriefing using global ratings applicable to any medical discipline [11]. This is an example of systematic quality improvement in simulation, focusing on development of the educator's skills. Ultimately, experience through repeated trials coupled with feedback from both learners and expert debriefers is the best formula for improvement of debriefing skills. The degree to which debriefing can be made a positive learning experience, can very well be the most important single determinant of the success of a simulation training effort.

Selected Readings

1. Kolb D. Experiential learning: experience as the source of learning and development. Englewood Cliffs, NJ: Prentice-Hall; 1984.
2. Salas E, Klein C, King H, et al. Debriefing medical teams: 12 evidence-based best practices and tips. Jt Comm J Qual Patient Saf. 2008;34:518–27.
3. Lederman LC. Debriefing: toward a systematic assessment of theory and practice. Simul Gaming. 1992;23:145–60.
4. Petranek C. A maturation in experiential learning: principles of simulation and gaming. Simul Gaming. 1994;25:513–22.
5. Fanning RM, Gaba DM. The role of debriefing in simulation-based learning. Simul Healthcare. 2007;2:115–25.

6. Thiagarajan ST. Gameletter. http://www.thiagi.com/pfp/IE4H/august2008.html (2008). Accessed 12 Sept 2010.

7. Rudolph JW, Simon R, Raemer DB, Eppich WJ. Debriefing as formative assessment: closing performance gaps in medical education. Acad Emerg Med. 2008;15:1010–6.

8. Savoldelli GL, Naik NV, Park J, et al. Value of debriefing during simulated crisis management. Anesthesiology. 2006;105:279–85.

9. Savoldelli GL, Naik VN, Hamstra SJ, et al. Barriers to the use of simulation-based education. Can J Anesth. 2005;52:944–50.

10. Stewart L. Ethical issues in postexperimental and postexperiential debriefing. Simul Gaming. 1992;23:196–211.

11. DASH© – Debriefing Assessment for Simulation in Healthcare: The Center for Medical Simulation. http://www.harvardmedsim.org/debriefing-assesment-simulation-healthcare.php. Accessed 10 Nov 2010.

51. Using Simulation for Disclosure of Bad News

Limaris Barrios

Educating the medical community with regard to disclosure of medical errors, unanticipated outcomes, and/or bad news has become a priority for physician educators; and a popular topic over the last decade [1–6]. Unfortunately, physicians and surgeons are not well equipped to deliver this difficult news due to inadequate training. It is not surprising that litigation, humiliation, and stress burden those charged with this responsibility [1, 3–6]. Today, patients, accreditation standards, laws, and hospital policies require explicit and candid communication after such events are recognized [1–3, 6, 7].

Training of physicians in this field has become critical. Seven states have passed laws that mandate notification of patients after an adverse event – Nevada, Florida, New Jersey, Pennsylvania, Vermont, Oregon, and California [1, 8] and the Joint Commission on Accreditation of Healthcare Organizations (JCAHO) and National Quality Forum (NQF) have created standards that require disclosure [1, 7, 9–15]. Similarly, Australia and the United Kingdom have launched pilot programs which promote full disclosure after an adverse event has occurred [3].

Moreover, aggressive disclosure policies developed by health care organizations aim to improve patient satisfaction, decrease litigation costs, and create safe practice protocols [1]. The University of Michigan Health System Program, the Dana Farber Cancer Institute in Massachusetts, and the Johns Hopkins Hospital in Maryland, are among others who have created disclosure policies with positive results thus far [1–3, 5, 9, 10, 12–14, 16]. Since the implementation of these programs, a number of claims and law suits have diminished, and the annual litigation costs were noted to be decreased as well.

Apology immunity laws whereby admission to fault is inadmissible in court have been passed in five States – Nevada, Florida, New Jersey, Pennsylvania, and Vermont; and are under development in four others [1, 4, 5, 13, 14]. Twenty-nine States have enacted laws excluding

D.S. Tichansky, J. Morton, and D.B. Jones (eds.), *The SAGES Manual*
of Quality, Outcomes and Patient Safety, DOI 10.1007/978-1-4419-7901-8_51,
© Springer Science+Business Media, LLC 2012

expressions of sympathy after accidents as proof of liability [14]. More importantly, patients are demanding full disclosure during adverse events. They want to understand how the adverse event occurred, and want to ensure that future events will be prevented [1, 14].

Medical students and resident physicians are also required to prove competency in disclosure of adverse events. The United States Medical Licensing Examination (USMLE), sponsored by the Federation of State Medical Boards (FSMB) and the National Board of Medical Examiners (NBME), includes questions focused on full disclosure and public reporting under the topics of medical ethics, jurisprudence, and physician/patient relationship [17]. Medical students need to pass the USMLE, and therefore correctly answer questions regarding disclosure of adverse events, before qualifying for a medical license to practice in the USA.

The Accreditation Council for Graduate Medical Education (ACGME) has taken similar steps, whereby physician residents need to prove competency in this area before graduating from accredited residency programs in the USA. Unfortunately, many residents do not get an opportunity to lead or even witness such disclosures during their training [1, 17–19]. Most surgeons have learned this difficult task by observing their mentors, and have not had an opportunity to practice and improve this skill before using it in their professional career. This limited training will likely result in poor communication between the surgeon and patient, patient dissatisfaction, and perhaps a greater number of malpractice claims and law suits [19].

Simulation-based training is an integral and essential part of surgical residency training in this era. No one will deny its effectiveness in the acquisition of technical and non-technical skills [20–24]. Different scenarios are recreated to assess and improve communication, team skills, and the ability to react under stress, providing the opportunity to practice and develop a variety of skills in a controlled, risk-free environment [20–24]. The simulated environment is the modern tool whereby learners acquire the skills required for real medical practice, decreasing potential injury to the patient [21, 22]. Simulation-based training has been studied and applied for the training of surgical residents in the disclosure of bad news [1].

One such study was conducted at Beth Israel Deaconess Medical Center in Boston from June of 2007 to March of 2008 [1]. The study aimed to use simulation to evaluate disclosure of bad news among surgical residents who performed a laparoscopic cholecystectomy on a virtual reality simulator in a mock operating room. The surgical residents were randomized into two different scenarios: one in which there was a bile duct injury during the procedure, and the second included incidental findings of metastatic gallbladder cancer. The residents were asked to deliver the bad news to a scripted family member after the procedure. The disclosure encounters were videotaped, and the residents were rated by independent reviewers using a modified SPIKES protocol as an assessment tool [25].

The study found that in general, trainees are ill prepared for conversations that involve disclosure of adverse or unexpected outcomes. Senior residents were more comfortable with disclosure of bad news and obtained better ratings with the modified SPIKES protocol; likely secondary to their increased exposure to these difficult conversations. However, a minority of residents had led or even observed disclosures of iatrogenic injury or incidental operative findings during any portion of their training [1]. This study illustrates how simulation can be applied to the disclosure of bad news, and incorporated into medical school, residency, or physician training. Using a simulation-based module, the learner's responses during difficult conversations can be evaluated, and feedback provided to improve future disclosure encounters.

The American College of Surgeons and the Association of Program Directors in Surgery (ACS/APDS) have recognized the importance of training in disclosure of bad news and have incorporated simulation into a new training module. The surgical skills curriculum for residents (Phase III) developed in the summer of 2008, includes an Apology Module which integrates simulation for the practice and acquisition of skills required in disclosure of bad news [6]. In this module, the surgical resident goes through a scenario where a sponge is inadvertently left in the patient's abdomen during surgery. The resident is asked to disclose the bad news to the patient's husband, who is a confederate (trained actor). The disclosure is videotaped and debriefed, mainly evaluating the quality of the disclosure and the resident's communication skills [6].

To sum up, policies, standards, and laws have been implemented in the USA and abroad which require open disclosure of adverse events and unanticipated outcomes to patients. It is evident that both physicians in training and practice are not prepared or adequately trained for these difficult conversations. Simulation provides the learner with a venue to practice and perfect their skills, including the disclosure of bad news.

Acknowledgments: I thank all the authors of "Framing family conversations after early diagnosis of iatrogenic and incidental findings" published in Surgical Endoscopy April 2009. Their invaluable contributions to the article served as the foundation for this chapter.

Selected Readings

1. Barrios L, Tsuda S, Derevianko A, et al. Framing family conversation after early diagnosis of iatrogenic injury and incidental findings. Surg Endosc. 2009;23:2535–42.
2. Gallagher TH, Levinson W. Disclosing harmful medical errors to patients: a time for professional action. Arch Intern Med. 2005;165(16):1819–24.
3. Gallagher TH, Studdert D, Levinson W. Disclosing harmful medical errors to patients. N Engl J Med. 2007;356(26):2713–9.
4. Kowalczyk L. Doctors say they need protection to apologize. Boston, MA: The Boston Globe; 2007.
5. Lazare A. Apology in medical practice: an emerging clinical skill. JAMA. 2006;296(11):1401–4.
6. ACS/APDS Skills Curriculum for Residents: Phase 3, Module 10-retained sponge on a postop chest X ray. http://elearning.facs.org/course/view.php?id=10&topic=12 (2008). Accessed 29 Jun 2009.
7. Joint Commission Resources. Hospital accreditation standards. Oakbrook Terrace, IL: Joint Commission Resources; 2007.
8. http://www.aon.com/risk_management/default.jsp. Accessed 21 Jan 2008.
9. Kraman SS, Hamm G. Risk management: extreme honesty may be the best policy. Ann Intern Med. 1999;131(12):963–7.
10. Gallagher TH, Waterman AD, Garbutt JM, et al. US and Canadian physicians' attitudes and experiences regarding disclosing errors to patients. Arch Intern Med. 2006;166(15):1605–11.
11. The Leapfrog Group: The National Quality Forum safe practices leap. http://www.leapfroggroup.org/media/file/Leapfrog-National_Quality_Forum_Safe_Practices_Leap.pdf (2007). Accessed 18 Jan 2008.
12. Joint Commission on Accreditation of Healthcare Organizations: Health care at the crossroads: strategies for improving the medical liability system and preventing patient injury. http://www.jointcommission.org/NR/rdonlyres/3F1B626C-CB65-468B-A871-488D1DA66B06/0/medical_liability_exec_summary.pdf (2005). Accessed 18 Jan 2008.
13. Clinton HR, Obama B. Making patient safety the centerpiece of medical liability reform. N Engl J Med. 2006;354(21):2205–8.
14. Wojcieszak D, Banja J, Houk C. The Sorry Works! Coalition: making the case for full disclosure. Jt Comm J Qual Patient Saf. 2006;32(6):344–50.
15. National Quality Forum: National Quality Forum updates endorsement of serious reportable events in healthcare. http://www.qualityforum.org/pdf/news/prSeriousReportableEvents10-15-06.pdf (2006). Accessed 18 Jan 2008.
16. Lamb RM, Studdert DM, Bohmer RM, Berwick DM, Brennan TA. Hospital disclosure practices: results of a national survey. Health Aff (Millwood). 2003;22(2):73–83.
17. United States Medical Licensing Examination: http://www.usmle.org. Accessed 29 Jun 2009.
18. Hutul OA, Carpenter RO, Tarpley JL, Lomis KD. Missed opportunities: a descriptive assessment of teaching and attitudes regarding communication skills in a surgical residency. Curr Surg. 2006;63(6):401–9.

19. Rider EA, Hinrichs MM, Lown BA. A model for communication skills assessment across the undergraduate curriculum. Med Teach. 2006;28(5):e127–34.

20. Chang L, Petros J, Hess DT, Rotondi C, Babineau TJ. Integrating simulation into a surgical residency program: is voluntary participation effective? Surg Endosc. 2007;21(3):418–21.

21. Dunkin B, Adrales GL, Apelgren K, Mellinger JD. Surgical simulation: a current review. Surg Endosc. 2007;21(3):357–66.

22. Park J, MacRae H, Musselman LJ, et al. Randomized controlled trial of virtual reality simulator training: transfer to live patients. Am J Surg. 2007;194(2):205–11.

23. Passman MA, Fleser PS, Dattilo JB, Guzman RJ, Naslund TC. Should simulator-based endovascular training be integrated into general surgery residency programs? Am J Surg. 2007;194(2):212–9.

24. Powers KA, Rehrig ST, Irias N, et al. Simulated laparoscopic operating room crisis: an approach to enhance the surgical team performance. Surg Endosc. 2007;22(4):885–900.

25. Baile WF, Buckman R, Lenzi R, Glober G, Beale EA, Kudelka AP. SPIKES-A six-step protocol for delivering bad news: application to the patient with cancer. Oncologist. 2000;5(4):302–11.

52. Teleproctoring in Surgery

Shawn Tsuda

Introduction

The discussion of teleproctoring in surgery requires defining the taxonomy of various telemedical applications. Telemedicine is the umbrella term describing the use of audio-visual technology, at any distance, to facilitate patient care, administration, or education related to the field of medicine. Many variations or modes of telemedicine have been described, such as telerobotics, telestration, telediagnoses, teleoncology (Table 52.1). However, the most significant modalities describe the most pertinent applications to surgery: teleproctoring, telementoring, and telesurgery [1]. Teleproctoring is the use of audio-visual technology at any distance to offer examinations or certifications between proctors and examinees. Telementoring refers to using the same technology to provide mentoring or teaching, such as an expert laparoscopist taking a less experienced surgeon through a laparoscopic Nissen fundoplication between two different countries. Telesurgery refers to the remote performance of an operation at a distance, usually through robotic technology. Although these terms are often used interchangeably, they deserve distinction. This chapter describes telemedical applications that utilize these and other modalities to improve surgical education, patient safety, and quality.

Challenges of Telemedicine

Integral to the discussion of telemedicine is to describe the need for such technology, and relate them to capability. The need for either telesurgery, teleproctoring, or telementoring leans primarily on the lack of expertise – whether it is expert surgeons, teachers, or examiners – in any given area. Economics and other logistics may dictate that in-person

D.S. Tichansky, J. Morton, and D.B. Jones (eds.), *The SAGES Manual*
of Quality, Outcomes and Patient Safety, DOI 10.1007/978-1-4419-7901-8_52,
© Springer Science+Business Media, LLC 2012

Table 52.1. Described telemedical terms.

Telesurgery	Telemanipulation
Telementoring	Telefollow-up
Teleproctoring	Telepresence
Telerobotics	Telecollaboration
Teleconsultation	Teletriage
Telestration	Teleoncology
Telediagnosis	Telepathology

presence may not be feasible, and therefore wired or wireless technology may be a more cost-effective alternative. A number of demonstration studies have sought to prove that besides adequate technology, the effectiveness of telemedical applications are adequate for patient care, or to perform simulated patient-care related tasks.

For telemedical applications, capability is embedded with the progress of audio-visual, wired, and wireless technology. For the most part, this will be a consistent challenge of telemedicine, as the technology will always approach, but never be equivalent to, the non-teleapplied version of the event. In other words, there may be a need for an expert laparoscopist to proctor a surgeon in a less developed country thousands of miles away, but the limitations of the information technology will always, at least in the foreseeable future, be inferior to some degree than an in-person proctorship. As we will see, however, the exponential progress of information technology makes this gap smaller and smaller. In some cases, it is not necessarily the cost or quality of the technology that is used, but the choice of technology and how it is applied. Luttman, Jones, and Soper were one of the first to show that inexpensive off-the-shelf technology could be used to "teleproctor" laparoscopic operations [2]. In this light, it is foreseeable that the outcome measures may be met to an adequate degree as long as telecommunications are appropriately matched for the activity.

Telemedical Examples in Surgery

The use of video, audio, and digital annotation has been demonstrated over impressive distances including continent to continent, ship to land, and even through an unmanned aerial vehicle to a surgical robot on the ground [3–5]. These are noted primarily for their novelty as impressive feats of both wired and wireless telecommunications technology to allow either telementoring or telesurgery. Cubano et al. in 1999 demonstrated that laparoscopic inguinal hernia repairs could be mentored to land-bound surgeons from the USS Abraham Lincoln. In 2002, Marescaux et al., utilizing robotic technology, performed a laparoscopic cholecystectomy between New York and France, via a high-speed wired connection. They demonstrated a minimal amount of data lag and the operation was performed in 45 min. In 2007, Lum et al. demonstrated the performance of surgical tasks within a training box via an unmanned aerial vehicle through a field deployed surgical robot. All of these examples may not by themselves confer immediate wide-spread applications in medicine, but were impressive feats of how telecommunication technology could be harnessed to perform surgery or simulated surgery, either directly or through mentoring.

Teleproctoring Examinations

In 2008, the Fundamentals of Laparoscopic Surgery (FLS) came to the forefront of surgical technical skills training when it was made a prerequisite for the American Board of Surgery (ABS) Qualifying Examination. With a self-directed didactic digital content followed by a cognitive exam and manual skills exam, FLS has become the most rigorously studied surgical task curriculum. However, directed training, both with didactic lectures and manual skills training, has been shown to confer consistent past rates, as with the 2009 insurance-underwritten course for Harvard teaching staff [6]. In 2010, Okrainec et al. described the gap in laparoscopic skills among surgeons in Botswana, Africa coupled with the high costs of sending experts to the region for in-person mentoring and proctoring [7]. They described using Skype software and off-the-shelf hardware to both mentor and proctor surgeons across continents to train them and perform proctoring of the FLS certification exam. They described this process as telesimulation – and showed that the telesimulation group achieved a pass rate of 100% versus a self-practice group in the same region. This impressive study remains the best example of using cost-effective wireless technology, coupled with a need to provide a practical feat of both telementoring and teleproctoring.

Telemedicine and the Simulation

Okrainec et al. showed that "telesimulation" can have real-world applications for a validated skills training curriculum. The concurrent rise of simulation in surgery with emerging technology such as

Table 52.2. Nomenclature for telementoring.

Term	Definition
Up	Screen up
Down	Screen down
Right	Screen right
Left	Screen left
In	Instrument further into trocar
Out	Instrument further out of trocar
Stop	Freeze

telemedicine may provide a unique and ideal opportunity to refine telesurgery, telementoring, and teleproctoring in the simulation environment [8]. Others have hypothesized that telementoring may be as effective as a local mentor for surgical skills training. Mentoring of medical students performing surgical simulator training exercises between Romania and the United States yielded similar results compared to local on-site mentors in one study [9]. Tsuda et al. showed that telementored laparoscopic cholecystectomies on a virtual reality simulator could improve technique versus non-mentored participants with telestration and voice instruction alone [10]. Key to this example was defining the special challenges of teaching and learning without hands-on interaction or non-verbal human cues. Specific on-screen definitions and voice instruction nomenclature needed to be defined prior to the simulated activity (Table 52.2). Defining and practicing the elements of telementoring may be the key to extending the technology further for real-world applications. This is especially true when ethical issues surrounding adequate supervision in patient care regarding telemedicine applications – particularly in high-stakes fields like surgery – have yet to be addressed.

Conclusion

Telecommunication allows interaction over distances to overcome logistical constraints. In medicine and surgery, high band-width technology has allowed impressive feats of long-distance mentoring, proctoring, consultation, and remote procedures. Feasibility has been shown in controlling robotic arms or providing consultation between continents, between ship and land, and between air and land. However, the exact role of telecommunication in everyday medical practice is unclear. Providing expert consultation where none is available is a clear application of telemedicine. However, as minimally invasive surgical techniques rapidly grow, trainee work hours shorten, and demand for quality patient care heightens, a greater role for telesurgery, teleproctoring, and telementoring will come to the forefront.

Selected Readings

1. Rosser J, Young SM, Klonsky J. Telementoring: an application whose time has come. Surg Endosc. 2007;21(8):1458–63.
2. Luttmann DR, Jones DB, Soper NJ. Teleproctoring laparoscopic operations with off-the-shelf technology. Stud Health Technol Inform. 1996;29:313–8.
3. Marescaux J, Leroy J, Rubino F, Smith M, Vix M, Simone M, et al. Transcontinental robot-assisted remote telesurgery: feasibility and potential applications. Ann Surg. 2001;235:487–92.
4. Cubano M, Poulose BK, Talamini MA, Stewart R, Antosek LE, Lentz R, et al. Long distance telementoring. A novel tool for laparoscopy aboard the USS Abraham Lincoln. Surg Endosc. 1999;13:673–8.
5. Lum MJ, Rosen J, King H, Friedman DC, Donlin G, Sankaranarayanan G, et al. Telesurgery via Unmanned Aerial Vehicle (UAV) with a field deployable surgical robot. Stud Health Technol Inform. 2007;125:313–5.
6. Derevianko A, Schwaitzberg S, Tsuda S, Barrios L, Brooks D, Callery M, et al. Malpractice carrier underwrites fundamentals of laparoscopic surgery training and testing: a benchmark for patient safety. Surg Endosc. 2010;24(3):616–23.
7. Okrainec A, Henao O, Azzie G. Telesimulation: an effective method for teaching the fundamentals of laparoscopic surgery in resource-restricted countries. Surg Endosc. 2010;24(2):417–22.
8. Tsuda S, Scott DJ, Doyle J, Jones DB. Surgical simulation and skills training. Curr Probl General Surg. 2009;46(4):271–370.
9. Panait L, Rafiq A, Tomulescu V, et al. Telementoring versus on-site mentoring in virtual reality-based surgical training. Surg Endosc. 2006;20(1):113–8.
10. Tsuda S, Barrios L, Derevianko A, Irias N, Schneider B, Schwaitzberg S, et al. Does telementoring shorten the pathway to proficiency in the simulation environment? Surg Endosc. 2008;22 Suppl 1:S228.

Part VIII
Medical–Legal Considerations

53. Informed Consent

Timothy A. Plerhoples and James N. Lau

Introduction

Informed consent is a concept that tends to be overlooked by many healthcare practitioners. It often is treated as but a step when it should be viewed as an important preface to the procedure and subsequent relationship with the surgical patient. Currently, patients have "the right to consent to or refuse healthcare *and* that they (must) be provided with all information material to a decision to consent to or to refuse healthcare" [1]. It has reframed the physician–patient relationship in terms acceptable to the individualist values of the USA [1]. Informed consent is a concept that has evolved over the past century, and its interpretation varies from state to state, from locality to locality. However, the basic components remain the same. Informed consent is not just a "legal requirement" but, more importantly, it is an ethical standard that "enhances the surgeon/patient relationship," and may in fact improve a patient's outcome [2]. This chapter describes the historical events that shaped the current iteration of informed consent, the legal issues surrounding it, its most agreed-upon current definition, advice to practitioners wishing to comply with the standard, and finally to discuss future directions.

History

The responsibility for health care decision making has shifted from physicians towards patients. The earliest consideration is found in Hippocratic ethics: physicians should "perform [their duties] calmly and adroitly, concealing most things from the patient … revealing nothing of the patient's future or present condition" [3]. The notion that patients should be shielded from their prognosis and be divorced from decision making persisted for several centuries and was reiterated by the American

D.S. Tichansky, J. Morton, and D.B. Jones (eds.), *The SAGES Manual* of Quality, Outcomes and Patient Safety, DOI 10.1007/978-1-4419-7901-8_53, © Springer Science+Business Media, LLC 2012

Medical Association in its Code of Ethics in 1847, which suggested that patients should remain obedient to the prescriptions of their physicians, and not be allowed their own "crude opinions" [4]. It was not until the events and trials of Nuremberg in the 1940s that biomedical ethicists began to seriously consider the importance of consent [5]. Individual legal cases (the common law) have centered on the requirements to obtain consent and provide adequate information for the consent to be considered informed. A few trials addressed cases of gross misconduct prior to the trials of Nuremberg (notably *Pratt v. Davis* in 1905 and *Schloendorff v. The Society of New York Hospitals* in 1914), which emphasized the concept that an adult of sound mind has a right to determine what is done to his/her own body [4]. Both decisions suggested that a surgeon who does not respect this tenant was committing assault, thus setting the precedent that breaches of consent were tried under assault and battery. This interpretation persisted for the first half of the twentieth century, and due to the seriousness of the crime, few cases were tried.

This shifted after *Salgo v. Leland Stanford Jr. University Board of Trustees* in 1957, whereby the term "informed consent" was first utilized in a medical malpractice case [1]. The patient Salgo was described to have a possible abdominal aortic obstruction, for which a trans-lumbar aortogram was recommended for diagnosis. At that time, the use of intravenous contrast dye was not routine for this purpose. Salgo became paralyzed following the procedure. Despite this being a known complication, it was not discussed prior to the procedure. The court in California ruled that the physician violated his duty to the patient in that he withheld facts needed to form "intelligent consent" [4], although they allowed for some discretion. This has been viewed as a half-hearted attempt to encourage open discourse between patients and their physicians without damaging the trusting relationship [4]. On appeal, this lower court decision for the plaintiff was overturned on a technicality, but introduced the phrase of informed consent into case law. Over the next two decades, other cases further refined the nature of this interaction. *Natanson v. Kline* in 1960 suggested that consent language must be "as simple as necessary" and disclose the "nature of the ailment, the nature of the proposed treatment, the probability of success or of alternatives, and perhaps the risks of unfortunate results and unforeseen conditions within the body" [4]. In the early 1970s, both federal and numerous state courts recognized a patient's right to informed consent After Roe v. Wade (410 US 113. 1973), the right to an abortion has evolved from a shared decision-making process between physician and patient, to that of a right held by a woman alone [6].

Legal Issues

The legal conceptualization of informed consent has evolved over time. Initial cases suggested that a lack of informed consent was tantamount to battery, where the only defense was arguing that full disclosure was provided. Over time cases were tried under the tenant of negligence, which is more favorable to physicians because multiple defenses are allowed, and that penalties could be covered by malpractice insurance. Today, the only cases framed as battery are those in which no consent was given at all, where the procedure performed was substantially different than the one agreed upon, or when a different person provides the care than was agreed upon [1]. There has been a suggestion that a "therapeutic privilege" exists, where a physician may not disclose some information s/he deems harmful to the welfare of the patient (or if the information is deemed so upsetting as to render the patient incapable of rational decision making); however, this remains a gray area [4].

Despite these numerous cases, the legal definition of informed consent remains unclear. Most agree that the "informed" aspect addresses a physician's disclosure obligation, while "consent" refers to the patient's response to the information provided [4]. For the most part, informed consent can only be given by competent individuals, which may be assigned in legislation or based on a common law understanding of possessing the ability to understand the nature of the procedure (minors tend to be presumed to be incompetent in this regard). States initially interpreted this concept differently – about half adopt the standard of what a "reasonable patient" would find material in making a healthcare decision, while the other half utilize a "professional standard," which relies on what a reasonable physician would tell a patient regarding a procedure. In practice today these two concepts become similar since most professional associations have adopted ethical standards that dictate physicians must supply patients with enough information to make an intelligent choice [1]. The only federal legislation found is language in three sections of the Medicare requirements from the Centers for Medicare and Medicaid Services (CMS). The first[1] is

---

[1] 42 CFR 482.13(b)(2): "Standard: Exercise of rights. (1) The patient has the right to participate in the development and implementation of his or her plan of care. (2) The patient or his or her representative (as allowed under State law) has the right to make informed decisions regarding his or her care. The patient's rights include being informed of his or her health status, being involved in care planning and treatment, and being able to request or refuse treatment. This right must not be construed as a mechanism to demand the provision of treatment or services deemed medically unnecessary or inappropriate" [7].

found under the patient's rights section, which stipulates the concept of involved decision making, although it specifically notes that a patient may not demand care their physician deems inappropriate. The second[2] outlines proper documentation of the informed consent (notably without mention of the need for a witness or other verification). The third[3] is found in the Surgical Services Condition of Participation code, noting only that a form denoting informed consent must be found in a patient's chart prior to undergoing an operation. While an individual jurisdiction may have more specific requirements, these federal requirements are notably concerned with only specific aspects of informed consent.

Current Definition

Professional bodies such as the American Medical Association (AMA) and the American College of Surgeons (ACS) have taken the lead in guiding physicians in how best to obtain informed consent from their patients. The AMA suggests that complete informed consent contain the following components [8]:

1. The patient's diagnosis, if known.
2. The nature and purpose of a proposed treatment or procedure.
3. The risks and benefits of a proposed treatment or procedure.
4. Alternatives (regardless of their cost or the extent to which the treatment options are covered by health insurance).
5. The risks and benefits of the alternative treatment or procedure.
6. The risks and benefits of not receiving or undergoing a treatment or procedure.
7. Allow the patient to ask questions.

Broadly speaking, a physician must disclose the name and nature of the treatment or procedure, the probability of a bad result, the kind and degree of harm that might follow, and information about alternatives [1]. Some

---

[2] 42 CFR 482.24(c)(2)(v): "All records must document the following, as appropriate: (v) Properly executed informed consent forms for procedures and treatments specified by the medical staff, or by Federal or State law if applicable, to require written patient consent" [7].

[3] 42 CFR 482.51(b)(2): "A properly executed informed consent form for the operation must be in the patient's chart before surgery, except in emergencies" [7].

states also require the physician to inform the patient regarding the risks of refusing treatment. Situations where exceptions to informed consent may be made differ from one jurisdiction to the next, but most include the following three concepts. The primary one is an emergency exception in which a patient is in need of urgent care and is unable to participate in the consent process. Two other commonly cited exceptions include language for common knowledge (information already understood by the patient) and for patients who waive the right to relevant information [1]. Waiving decision-making authority is typically allowed as an aspect of patient autonomy, although some suggest that it is the physician's duty to inquire as to the reasons the patient wants this done [4].

Advice to Practitioners

Physicians should consider four categories of consent when speaking with a patient, which would help decipher what information may be considered material [4]. For acute disorders, disclosure should be limited to only the most essential facts. For elective procedures, a full degree of disclosure is standard, with shared decision making paramount. If a patient's prognosis is dire, the conversation should be performed at a slower pace, with adjustment made to the patient's reaction. Finally, for a minor disorder or procedure, informed consent is not commonly required, if the patient is agreeable.

The AMA suggests several steps that physicians should take to protect themselves from litigation surrounding informed consent [8]. The first is to ensure that they carry adequate liability insurance, which typically covers failure of informed consent (since it falls under negligence). The next is to document the communication process as thoroughly and as timely as possible by placing a note in the patient's chart. This documentation should strike a balance between being overly broad or highly detailed, both of which could be detrimental in court. It should neither appear that the consent was completed simply to satisfy a legal requirement (such as stating that "all material risks have been explained to me") nor should a comprehensive listing of complications be cited. This is not only difficult for patients to understand, but also suggests that any omission from the list is to be presumed undisclosed. Any listing should be prefaced by language that indicates no total exclusivity ("included but not limited to").

The Future

Recent research into informed consent has focused around two areas: the use of advanced technologies in enhancing patient understanding and the inclusion of facility- and/or surgeon-specific performance rates into the process. Groups in Germany [9] and the UK [10] have investigated the use of multimedia-based programs to comprehensively and impartially explain procedures. Bollschweiler et al. [9] found that adding a multimedia program (a computer-based module using information, videos, and animation) improved perceived patient understanding and satisfaction with the consent process. Patel et al. [10] have developed a "virtual hospital" where patients can interact with hospital equipment and allows exploration at the patient's own pace. These techniques are far from being accepted as standards in providing information for consent, but their use is increasing.

The question of whether full informed consent includes a discussion of facility- or surgeon-specific performance rates has been brought before the courts several times. The 1996 case *Johnson v. Kokemoor* in Wisconsin suggested that a surgeon is obliged to inform a patient if a procedure is less likely to result in death or disability if performed by another practitioner with more experience [1]. A New Jersey court in 2002 found that "significant misrepresentations concerning a physician's qualifications can affect the validity of consent obtained" [11]. While the standard of disclosing experience may be considered material, it is not widely followed today [12]. Some legal experts believe we are moving toward full disclosure of other aspects of physician information (such as hours of sleep or difficulties in one's personal life) that may affect outcome, if the patient asks [1]. These questions seem especially pertinent in light of a recent understanding of how surgeon volume (as a representation of ability) relates to patient outcome, as well as the rising interest in policy initiatives aimed at defining and improving quality [13]. Some wonder whether it will ever be possible to obtain statistically significant quality measures for low-risk or low-volume procedures that would allow a generalization for any given physician [14]. Others question how seriously such a disclosure would undermine the trust in any individual physician [13]. In the end, perhaps it is the responsibility of the professional and certifying bodies to ensure proper expertise in a given field or for a particular procedure.

In general, courts have steered the concept of informed consent toward a compromise that balances active patient participation with safeguarding the trust-based physician–patient relationship [1]. While informed consent may originally have come about to address the power imbalance between physicians and patients during the explosion of medical technology and hence choice in care, embracing it may now help "tame the onslaught of commerce" in medicine and rehumanize patients [4]. Physicians must continue to hold themselves to high standards, because patients do.

Selected Readings

1. Dolgin JL. The legal development of the informed consent doctrine: past and present. Camb Q Healthc Ethics. 2010;19(1):97–109.
2. American College of Surgeons: Code of professional conduct, 2008. http://www.facs.org/fellows_info/statements/stonprin.html. Accessed 5 Mar 2010.
3. Hippocrates Decorum. (Jones W, Trans.). Cambridge: Harvard University Press; 1967. p. 297.
4. Katz J. Reflections on informed consent: 40 years after its birth. American College of Surgeons, Committee on Ethics, 1998. http://www.facs.org/education/ethics/katzlect.html. Accessed 5 Mar 2010.
5. Beauchamp TL, Childress JF. Principles of biomedical ethics. New York: Oxford University; 2009. p. 117.
6. Ruger TW. Ruger Health Law's Coherence Anxiety. Georgetown Law J. 2008;96: 625–41.
7. Centers for Medicare and Medicaid Services, Center for Medicaid and State Operations/Survey and Certification Group. Revisions to the Hospital Interpretive Guidelines for Informed Consent. 13 Apr, 2007, Ref: S&C-07-17.
8. American Medical Association: Patient physician relationship topics, informed consent, 2010. http://www.ama-assn.org/ama/pub/physician-resources/legal-topics/patient-physician-relationship-topics/informed-consent.shtml. Accessed 8 Mar 2010.
9. Bollschweiler E, Apitzsch J, Obliers R, Koerfer A, Mönig SP, Metzger R, et al. Improving informed consent of surgical patients using a multimedia-based program? Results of a prospective randomized multicenter study of patients before cholecystectomy. Ann Surg. 2008;248(2):205–11.
10. Patel V, Aggarwal R, Kinross J, Taylor D, Davies R, Darzi A. Improving informed consent of surgical patients using a multimedia-based program? Results of a prospective randomized multicenter study of patients before cholecystectomy. Ann Surg. 2009;249(3):546–7. author reply 547–8.
11. Supreme Court of New Jersey. Howard v. University of Medicine & Dentistry of New Jersey, 800 Atlantic Reporter 2nd 73; 2002.
12. Iheukwumere EO. Doctor, are you experienced? The relevance of disclosure of physician experience to a valid informed consent. J Contemp Health Law Policy. 2002;18(2):373–419.

13. Schwarze ML. The process of informed consent: neither the time nor the place for disclosure of surgeon-specific outcomes. Ann Surg. 2007;245(4):514–5.
14. Burger I, Schill K, Goodman S. Disclosure of individual surgeon's performance rates during informed consent: ethical and epistemological considerations. Ann Surg. 2007;245(4):507–13.

54. Enterprise Risk Management

Jeffrey Driver and Renée Bernard

Risk management is an evolving science. Traditionally, regardless of industry, it has looked at current risks one at a time – on a largely compartmentalized or decentralized basis. Today, the emerging trend in risk management is Enterprise Risk Management (ERM), a proactive, coordinated, enterprise-wide model that assesses and manages all risks together, and uncovers opportunities. In the healthcare field, it promises to drive down losses as identified through deep analysis of patient safety data. With an ERM framework in place, organizations can better identify, measure, manage, and disclose key risks so they can improve patient safety systems and drive down claims costs while increasing value to stakeholders.

The Stanford University Medical Center (SUMC) uses ERM to enhance its ability to make decisions based on defined evidence of risk and to address this risk with specific interventions. SUMC incorporates decision analysis, a process that has been in practice at the Stanford University School of Management Sciences and Engineering for more than 40 years [1]. ERM focuses on data captured through a variety of sources such as patient-initiated complaints, patient feedback through voluntary surveys, quality review processes, and legal claims and malpractice suits. This type of data analysis is the source of truth in risk management, and when supported by top management and shareholders, it can significantly add value to an organization by aligning risk management initiatives with the business strategies and operations of the company. To achieve this goal, institutions like SUMC need to understand their appetite for risk, and then actively mitigate it.

At SUMC, human and financial loss control involves conducting focused risk assessments. These risk assessments incorporate four major "cornerstones" [2]. For loss control, the four cornerstones are as follows: *first*, real-time risk assessment and mitigation of errors, accidents, and near misses; *second*, proactive risk assessment of loss drivers; *third*, management of patient and family expectations through education;

D.S. Tichansky, J. Morton, and D.B. Jones (eds.), *The SAGES Manual of Quality, Outcomes and Patient Safety*, DOI 10.1007/978-1-4419-7901-8_54,
© Springer Science+Business Media, LLC 2012

and *fourth*, advancing healthcare practitioner education. This cornerstone approach is used to embed risk management practice and philosophy throughout the organization, and to effectively drive down losses across the organization as a whole. With this cornerstone approach, organizations can better understand the connection between what drives losses and the risk control programs designed to attack the drivers of these losses.

SUMC's executive team and board members alike have been champions and advocates of this risk management methodology. While buy-in of risk management activities from high-level leadership is critical, and will eventually trickle down throughout the enterprise – by collaborating with the Quality Improvement and Patient Safety Department (QIPS) from the beginning, SUMC ensures that its ERM philosophy will be embedded at local practice levels across the organization. This prevents siloed risk management activity that lessens the positive impact of value-adding strategies for the entire enterprise.

This chapter introduces ERM as the most current trend in healthcare risk management and explains how Stanford University Medical Center uses this innovative model and its "focused risk assessments" to better understand from a very fundamental level what drives human and financial loss. For purposes of this discussion, the focus is on using data compiled from claim files to identify and effectively address areas of vulnerability. We start by discussing Harvard's ground-breaking study, then highlight Stanford ERM innovations, and how we turn the data into actionable and measurable risk management strategies.

The Proof Is in the Data

Data analysis *is* the heart of enterprise risk management. For empirical evidence, all one has to do is review the CRICO/RMF's Malpractice Insurers' Medical Error Surveillance and Prevention Study (MIMESPS) [3]. MIMESPS involved a review of claim files at five participating malpractice insurers, including CRICO/RMF (Harvard-affiliated hospitals), to help analyze medical error. The study covered approximately 33,000 physicians, 61 acute care hospitals (35 academic and 26 non-academic), and 428 outpatient facilities.

The study included a review of claim files at participating insurers by physician reviewers trained to use a specific coding taxonomy. The taxonomy was designed to detect injuries due to the medical care (as opposed to the underlying disease process), to guide the physician reviewers' implicit judgments to determine if the injury was due to treatment or diagnostic error, and to parse out the specific etiology of the errors identified. The participating physicians reviewed 1,452 claims files that spanned over 20 years though most were recent to the study. In fact, 83% of the claims closed between 1995 and 2004.

In terms of injury type, 3% of the claims did not have an adverse outcome (no injury) from medical care; 4% of the claims involved patient-reported psychological or emotional injury with no physical injury; and 1% stemmed from a breach of the duty to obtain informed consent and also did not involve physical injury. The lion's share – 93% of the claims – involved physical injury with 54% of injuries rated as "severe."

What were the key takeaways from the study? This deep dive into the claim files data identified a number of broad themes. For one, errors generally stem from a combination of cognitive and patient safety system errors. Additionally, the study highlighted the role of patient behavior in errors (present in almost a third of all errors detected in MIMESPS), the multifactorial nature of errors, trainee involvement in errors, and the prevalence of frivolous litigation. The study evidenced that the use of this level of data enhances the current gold standard of using medical record review as the process by which to determine the etiology of medical errors in patient safety research.

According to the study, "The findings to date from the MIMESPS project are humbling. They shed light on the tremendous casual complexity that underlie many errors… our results underscore the need for continuing efforts to develop the "basic science" of error prevention in medicine which remains in its infancy" [3].

Building on the MIMESPS Study: SUMC's ERM Approach and "Focused Assessments"

SUMC believes CRICO/RMF has developed the most effective taxonomy for analysis of patient safety data designed to identify risks and implement interventions. SUMC ERM strives to take this data analysis to the next level by utilizing focused risk assessments and cyclic analysis to continually identify risk factors in a particular area, thus prompting opportunities for reassessment of patient safety and intervention.

One such focused assessment was done for perioperative medicine – an area that addresses the medical care of the surgical patient and focuses on the patient's status before, during, and after the actual surgical procedure. While it is common knowledge that surgical specialties carry inherently higher risk than other medical disciplines, the need for data analysis and other considerations convinced SUMC to engage an outside consultant to conduct a full-scale, perioperative-based services risk assessment. The results provided SUMC with tangible opportunities to add value to its perioperative services and the organization as a whole. This led to targeted interventions including team training in improved communication surrounding the consent process, effective utilization of surgical safety checklists, enhancement of timeouts to ensure standardization, and the use of critical language and triggers for better communication between residents and attending physicians.

SUMC leadership also gained an evidentiary basis for funding of simulation programs such as Fundamentals of Laparoscopic Surgery, Team Training, and In-Situ Emergency Recognition Training. Additionally, informed consent processes were enhanced by implementing programs from Emmi Solutions® [4], a Web-based patient expectation management tool. These interventions are proactively monitored on an ongoing basis to ensure improvement in the original data and for further identification of opportunities for improvement.

The Model Methodology: How SUMC Turns Data into Actionable Information

In ERM, analyzing patient safety data is critical to understanding and managing/mitigating enterprise-wide risk. The deeper the dive into the data – the more rich the data source becomes. Boston-based RMF Strategies, a division of the Risk Management Foundation of the Harvard Medical Institutions, has developed a model methodology that recommends a six-step approach to patient safety data analysis [5]. The steps are cyclic and the analysis can begin at any point within the cycle – depending on when the risk is identified. For example, when interventions have already taken place on an identified risk, the risk manager would begin evaluation by considering if vulnerability still exists and measure the effectiveness of the intervention by comparison to more recent data (Fig. 54.1).

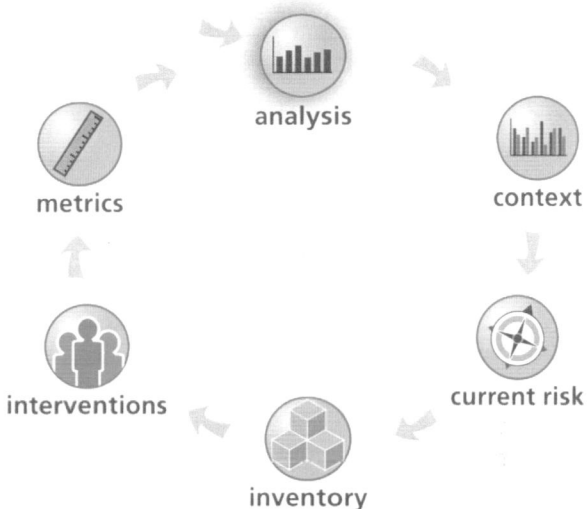

Fig. 54.1. This figure illustrates the six-step approach of CRICO/RMF's model methodology for patient safety data analysis [5].

Model Steps

Here are the six steps to follow with this approach.

Step 1: Capture Vulnerabilities as They Occur

Contemporaneous analysis of malpractice claim files provides immediate notice of potential risk issues. Beyond litigation documents, these claim files are data rich, providing information on internal investigation reports, expert opinions for and against the care provided, and pertinent medical records. Claim files analysis identifies vulnerable areas that may require focused risk intervention and sheds light on causative factors and loss drivers. Typically, the file will reveal at least one if not several loss drivers related to human factors in addition to system issues. The most common human factor risk management categories noted are technical skill, clinical judgment, and breakdowns in communication [2]. These categories can then be broken down even further into subcategories to pinpoint the etiology of vulnerability. The subcategories aim to clarify the exact human behavior contribution that led to the error or perceived error that prompted the claim in the first place.

Referring back to the previous example of surgical services, SUMC data analysis identified many of the common risk management issues related to surgical cases and further identified the percent of occurrence as well as relevant subcategories. The data was first parsed out into areas of specialty and cases within perioperative services. This revealed to SUMC that of the cases identified and assessed, 40% involved technical issues, 35% involved the selection and management of therapy issues, and 25% involved inadequate consent for a surgical procedure and issues with premature discharge, communication breakdowns, and documentation issues. These numbers indicated a need for action, however, such action could not be defined without more information about the numbers, hence a deeper dive.

Step 2: Put the Data in Context

By integrating relevant denominator data and peer comparative data, SUMC was able to add relevant context to the collected claim files data. Springing into action based on mere numbers without further understanding exactly how many occurrences there were in a particular area, how many occurrences involved particular care practices or practitioners, and the details of each is an exercise in futility harkening back to reactionary traditional risk management. SUMC uses a metric-oriented approach to narrow the focus on key risk drivers [6]. The numbers clarify trends vs. clusters or coincidences, or practices unchecked by particular practitioners or teams. Another important step to gaining context is framing the data against that of our peers. Without this context, the data loses its useful meaning and opportunities to drive down losses will likely be missed. And finally, by tying the drivers of risk back to financial metrics, we are creating an analysis that is quantitative. It shows us opportunities for adding value back into patient care safety systems such as in the perioperative and surgical specialties while improving the value added to the organization as a whole.

Step 3: Reassess Identified Vulnerability

ERM promotes a process by which the enterprise assesses current risk – through risk assessments and focus groups. The assessment of present-tense risk reveals whether there is remaining potential for reoccurrence, and considers any value-adding steps taken since the events. Getting at the root of the claim data ensures the true valuation of the potential for a vulnerability to reoccur. SUMC uses a ranking system that establishes priorities on addressing the risks identified, and takes into account the likelihood of reoccurrence, the impact to the organization, and degree of imminent impact.

RISK	TYPE OF RISK	FREQUENCY	SEVERITY
1.	CATASTOPHIC LOSS	SLIGHT	SEVERE
2.	FINANCIAL MARKETS	MODERATE	MANAGEABLE
3.	BRAND EROSION	SLIGHT	MODERATE
4.	HUMAN RESOURCES	PROBABLE	MODERATE
5.	LEGAL/REGULATORY	PROBABLE	MANAGEABLE
6.	REPUTATION	SLIGHT	MODERATE
7.	INFORMATION TECHNOLOGY	PROBABLE	MANAGEABLE
8.	ENVIRONMENTAL, HEALTH, SAFETY	MODERATE	MODERATE

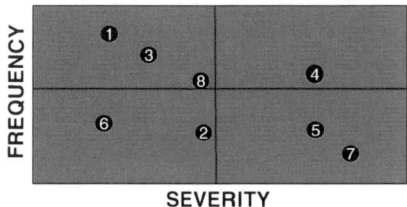

Fig. 54.2. Types of risk vs frequency.

Step 4: Determine Potential Solutions

A number of tools can assist with the data analysis process for identifying potential solutions. Risk maps and influence diagrams are valuable ways to capture the ERM process visually to better see where the organization has been with a risk *and* where it is going [6]. For instance, risk maps graphically depict the impact of the risk or severity on the horizontal axis and frequency of occurrence (or likelihood) on the vertical axis. And influence diagrams can be used to map risk drivers and capture root causes and likely events that lead to this risk [1].

While risk maps and influence diagrams help visually depict data, there is a need for a roadmap for strategic loss control interventions and strategies (Fig. 54.2). Claims analysis can be an effective ERM tool for developing that roadmap. This roadmap must follow an analysis, solution, and impact continuum where reassessment reoccurs on a regular basis. The continuous identification of relevant models, processes, education, and training programs that address key risk areas will enable the enterprise to repeatedly drive down losses.

Step 5: Implement Changes that Are Effective

SUMC takes advantage of several methods of measurable interventions. The following are examples of risk reduction interventions in the area of claims and litigation, patient education, medical staff risk management education, and monitoring of physician behavior (Table. 54.1).

Table 54.1. Risk driver specific interventions.

Identified risk drivers	Intervention
Physician–patient communication	Emmi Solutions®
	For more information visit :www.emmisolutions.com
Claim file volume and closure	Early offer program
	For more information on SUMC's early offer program, Process for the Early Assessment and Resolution of Loss (PEARL) visit: http://src.stanfordhospital.org/
Patient dissatisfaction	Vanderbilt PARS®
	For more information visit: http://www.mc.vanderbilt.edu/centers/cppa/services.htm
Patient safety systems	Simulation-based learning
	For more information visit: http://cape.lpch.org/ and http://cisl.stanford.edu/

Early Offer Programs are quickly being recognized as a way of reducing claim activity. These programs inherently require fastidious investigation and categorization of events resulting in prompt and appropriate intervention. The Stanford University Medical Indemnity and Trust Insurance Company's (SUMIT) Process for the Early Assessment and Resolution of Loss (PEARL) [7] program is a principle-based policy that promotes transparency, integrity, fairness, and healing. Due to a reported lower claim volume and faster claim-closing pattern since implementation of the program, it is also considered smart business practice. SUMIT's approach in PEARL is best described as optimistic and cautious. The approach is heavily influenced by the Stanford research mission – the quest to isolate and determine individual and overall PEARL outcomes and compare those success drivers to partial disclosure programs. Since its implementation, claim volume has dropped precipitously by 87% of the original claim volume. SUMC has also achieved a significantly faster claim-closing pattern.

Since the implementation of PEARL, SUMIT data supports the key trends on the value of an early offer program. The journey to an effective and fast claims closing pattern requires prompt evaluation of patient concerns and appropriate intervention. In order to maintain enterprise-wide participation in the program, education and training is an essential component. Most importantly, early and intensive investigations pay dividends in warding off and defending claims.

EMMI Solutions® [4], an online education tool, enhances communication between patient and physician. This interactive, Web-based tool enhances patient engagement in their healthcare decisions through interactive modules that patients can work through at their own pace and provides patients with an opportunity to send questions to their physician about the information received. Improving patient understanding of their care is value adding because it improves the patients' perception of clinical outcomes, which, in turn, improves financial outcomes. Emmi modules are considered key intervention tools in the surgical and perioperative arena, and offer a wide variety of modules geared toward inherently high-risk areas such as neurosurgery, orthopedics, and obstetrics and gynecology. The modules improve the informed consent process and provider–patient communication because they are patient driven and allow the patient to work through the information and develop questions at their own pace. Providers also have the ability to gather data about the use of the modules such as the number of patients who log in, complete the modules, and the types of questions asked.

Simulation-based education [8], common to many other industries, is a valuable intervention in hospital-patient systems. Since the late 1980s, Stanford University has been at the forefront of simulation techniques, having pioneered immersive and simulation-based learning [9]. SUMC depends on simulation-based education as a method of improving physician clinical judgment and technical skill. Simulation plays a critical role in risk management in education, training, performance assessment, and research because physician competency for a particular care situation or condition can add significant value to SUMC. Simulation programs run the gamut from the use of computerized mannequins to patient actors for role playing, to part task and procedural trainers, to computer-screen simulations and to comprehensive replicas of clinical settings (ER and ICU wards) and even virtual worlds such as those seen in the aviation industry. The most important aspect of a successful simulation program is quality instructors and meaningful investment of time by practitioners. While funding for such a program may pose a daunting hurdle at first, the return on investment via improved patient safety systems and decrease in human and financial loss is extremely attractive.

The Patient Advocacy Reporting System (PARS)® [10] is a risk intervention used by SUMC to improve physician communication and behavior. PARS® analyzes data generated from patient complaints gathered and documented in the patient relations department. Patient dissatisfaction with physician interactions can lead to malpractice suits – the risks are simply higher when physicians cannot establish rapport with their patients, or fail to meet their patient's expectations [11]. Given this causal link, it would be in the best interest of physicians and the organization as a whole to monitor physician behavior complaints in an effort to identify a physician who is at higher risk of being sued than his colleagues. This assessment of physician behavior creates an opportunity to identify physicians with higher risk for litigation prior to a lawsuit, thereby providing the opportunity for an intervention. Interventions involve counseling by superiors with hard data showing the mean of the physician's peers and the degree to which the identified physician is an outlier.

Step 6: Measure and Metrics

The key to any successful ERM program is to measure the impact in the near term with a predictive eye for the long term. Interventions and risk management tools, such as those outlined above, must be evaluated for their effectiveness and impact on both the organization's near-term and longer-term needs on a regular basis.

Conclusion

SUMC's transition to the ERM model will likely provide dividends to the organization or a "risk return" for many years to come. The past, the present, the future – must be evaluated in this new ERM model. In particular, emerging vulnerabilities that could bring future risk of claim activity are just as important to assess as current claims. There is a wealth of data already available within any organization that can serve as a basis or starting point for this particular ERM analytical process. The healthcare industry requires a solid business approach in today's uncertain economic environment, and ERM is a good solution. It provides a framework that healthcare institutions can follow to continuously assess and effectively intervene on loss drivers while adding value appreciated by all stakeholders.

Selected Readings

1. Celona J. Decision analysis for the professional. Menlo Park, CA: SmartOrg, Inc; 2001–2007.
2. Greenwald J. Risk management by the numbers drives down losses. Bus Insur. 2008;2(8):35.
3. Medical Malpractice Insurer's Medical Error Surveillance and Prevention Study, 2001–2005. http://www.rmf.harvard.edu/research-resources/research-studies/MIMESPS-study.aspx. Accessed 21 July 2011.

4. Emmi Solutions®. Patient satisfaction: engaging patients leads to a healthy bottom line, 2008. http://www.emmisolutions.com/downloads/Patient_Satisfaction-Healthy_bottom_line-Emmi_Solutions.pdf. Accessed 21 July 2011.

5. CRICO/RMF strategies. http://www.rmfstrategies.com/. Accessed 21 July 2011.

6. RIMS.org. Accessed 21 July 2011.

7. Stanford University Medical Indemnity and Trust Insurance Company, et al. Process for Early Assessment and Resolution of Loss (PEARL). Stanford, CA. 2007.

8. Halamek LP. Simulation: the new "Triple Threat". Pediatr Res. 2010;67:130–1.

9. cape.lpch.org/. Accessed 21 July 2011.

10. Hickson GB, Pichert JW, Webb LE, Gabbe SG. A complementary approach to promoting professionalism: identifying, measuring, and addressing unprofessional behaviors. Acad Med. 2007;82:1040–8.

11. Hickson GB, Federspiel CF, Pichert JW, Miller CS, Gauld-Jaeger J, Bost P. Patient complaints and malpractice risk. JAMA. 2002;287:2951–7.

55. Surgical Devices: Equipment Malfunction, FDA Reporting, Off-Label Use

Michael Tarnoff, Joe Sapiente, David Olson, and Tracy Palmer Berns

Surgery has never been more technology driven. The utilization of minimally invasive techniques across all surgical disciplines has been the result of stepwise collaboration between healthcare providers and the medical device industry. The presence of medical devices in operating rooms worldwide has never been greater or more relevant to patient care and postoperative outcomes. Accordingly, the regulations under which medical device manufacturers must operate and the standards to which they must comply have taken on greater significance to physicians and their patients. This chapter presents an overview of a few of the more salient policies that govern the use of medical devices in surgery and that serve to enhance patient safety.

Industry Requirements for Reporting of Perceived Surgical Device Malfunctions

The Food and Drug Administration's (FDA or Agency) Quality System Regulation (QSR) and international standards promulgated by the International Organization for Standardization (ISO) require medical device manufacturers to implement procedures and processes to monitor and control customer complaints. An effective complaint-handling process provides firms with valuable postmarket data that can be used to measure product quality and evaluate regulatory risks. The chain of regulatory requirements in the United States also extends to mandatory reporting of serious adverse events. As surgery has become more device

D.S. Tichansky, J. Morton, and D.B. Jones (eds.), *The SAGES Manual of Quality, Outcomes and Patient Safety*, DOI 10.1007/978-1-4419-7901-8_55, © Springer Science+Business Media, LLC 2012

intensive and technology driven, the relevance of these regulations to practicing clinicians and their patients has never been greater.

Medical devices risk management and Quality Assurance (QA) has been evolving for nearly a half a century. Not forgotten from the early days of "Good Manufacturing Practices (GMP)" are the routine QA tasks such as material and product inspection techniques, capability and reliability, supplier quality management, and continuous improvement. However, in today's highly regulated medical device manufacturing industry, QA has incorporated a risk management system that requires the manufacturer to focus on ensuring product performance and patient safety. This is done through risk analysis, hazard analysis, user interface, and human factors assessments.

Today's harmonized standards are essential requirements of a medical device manufacturer's quality system and include:

- *FDA's Quality System Regulations (QSR) (21 CFR pt. 820).* The FDA has defined the quality system as "the organizational structure, responsibilities, procedures, processes, and resources for implementing quality management" 21 CFR §820.3(v). A medical device manufacturer's goal is to implement a quality system that achieves desired outcomes and insures consistent high-quality final products.

- *Medical Device Reporting (MDR) (21 CFR pt. 803).* FDA's regulations also impose reporting requirements on manufacturers when the manufacturer receives information that reasonably suggests that one or more of its devices has (or may have) caused or contributed to a serious injury or death or has malfunctioned and the malfunction is likely to cause or contribute to a death or serious injury if the malfunction recurred. Determining whether a complaint triggers the filing of a Medical Device Report (MDR) is always a challenge for device manufacturers and also a concern of the Agency. In addition, user facilities, such as hospitals and nursing homes, are also legally required to report suspected medical device-related deaths to both FDA and the manufacturer, and serious injuries to the manufacturer or to FDA if the manufacturer is unknown. Serious injury is defined by the Agency as an injury or illness that:

- Is life-threatening; or

- Results in permanent impairment of a body function or permanent damage to a body structure; or

- Requires medical or surgical intervention to prevent permanent impairment of a body function or permanent damage to a body structure.

Depending on the nature of the adverse event, firms have between 5 and 30 calendar days from becoming aware of the event to report the incident to FDA. The goal of the regulation is to require manufacturers to detect and correct potential device issues in a timely manner. Manufacturer and user facility reports sent to FDA are entered in a database and reviewed by Agency staff to identify device issues and potential trends. In some cases, FDA will contact the user facility or manufacturer for more information about the adverse event. At other times, FDA will initiate an inspection of the manufacturer to assess the firm's compliance with the QSR.

FDA is currently implementing improvements in the MDR system through the development of electronic reporting tools, making it easier for manufacturers to relay information to FDA.

- *ISO 13485:2003 Medical Devices; Quality Management System:* assures the documented requirements for risk management are met throughout product realization or manufacturing and introduction.
- *ISO 14971:2007 Application of Risk Management to Medical Devices*: requires a documented, maintained process for identifying hazards associated with a medical device, estimating and evaluating associated risks, controlling these risks, and monitoring the effectiveness of the controls. The process includes the following elements: risk analysis, risk evaluation, risk control, production and postproduction information.

Product performance is monitored and patient safety is ensured using these and other harmonized standards. As an example, the perceived malfunction of a surgical device that results in a serious injury or death should trigger an MDR report by the user facility. This report is typically initiated by a clinician and serves as the primary mechanism by which healthcare professionals should notify a company of an incident in which one or more of its devices has (or may have) caused or contributed to a serious injury or death. Upon receipt of such a report or of a complaint, the manufacturer may perform a health hazard evaluation (HHE). This internal postmarket risk analysis process is an important tool in a manufacturer's risk management and quality system. It relies on input from product complaints, manufacturing data and controls, internal observations and postmarket surveillance, and clinicians having advanced knowledge of the particular patient or population, anatomy, and physiology. This process is utilized during root cause investigation of complaints to support corrective and preventive actions and continuous improvement and may be used in cases where additional remedial field action may be necessary.

In certain instances, a company's complaint investigation, HHE, and/ or risk assessment may reveal that a device could pose a patient risk. When this occurs, the manufacturer conducts a field action or recall to remove the device from the market or correct the device. Reaching a decision to correct or remove a product involves careful evaluation, including identification of the specific products or lots of products to be recalled, execution of an HHE, and implementation of a Corrective and Preventive Action (CAPA) plan, including root cause analysis.

There are several misconceptions regarding the term recall. FDA defines recall as a firm's removal or correction of a marketed product that the Agency considers to be in violation of the laws it administers and that may pose a risk to health (21 CFR pt. 806). Products that may be violative in some way are not always removed from the market. In fact, a recall notice might be for a change in instructions for a product's use, or to recommend additional training to assure safer product use, or the recall might consist of a software revision to ensure safe operation of a device.

A second misconception is that the FDA initiates all recalls. In most cases, the manufacturer recalls a device on its own, or conducts what is termed a "voluntary" recall. Once a firm initiates a recall it has 10 working days to notify FDA of the action. Information provided to FDA includes:

- Identity of the product involved
- Reason for the recall
- Evaluation of the risk associated with problem
- Estimated amount of product in distribution
- A copy of the recall communication
- Proposed strategy for conducting the recall

FDA reviews the information submitted and classifies the recall into one of three categories depending on the potential risk the device poses: from Class I representing high risk to Class III representing low risk. This classification process normally occurs after the firm has issued its recall.

The classification determines the number of checks a firm has to make and the number of audits FDA will conduct to ensure a recall is effective.

Off-Label Use

Another area of Agency concern involves so-called off-label marketing. Device manufacturers receive clearance or approval from the FDA for their products' specific "intended uses," supported by way of regulatory premarket submissions. Once an FDA-regulated product, whether device or drug, gets on the market, clinicians may realize new uses for that product that may be outside of the intended use(s) approved by the Agency. These new uses are considered "off label" and FDA does not regulate such uses because they are within the scope of the practice of medicine, which is specifically excluded from FDA's jurisdiction. However, FDA does regulate companies' manufacturing, as well as the promotion and sale of devices and drugs and requires all such activities to be clearly within the scope of the approved intended uses or "on label."

In addition to promoting a device for an unapproved use, another way a manufacturer can run into issues would be if it promotes the product for a specific claim that is not approved even if the intended use is approved (e.g., a product might be approved for treatment of a disease but the manufacturer makes claims about lowering incidence of certain adverse effects). Off-label promotion, as opposed to off-label use, is a violation of the Federal Food, Drug, and Cosmetic Act (Act) and may subject the responsible company and individuals at those companies to a full range of enforcement actions from the FDA. Promotions of devices for off-label uses that do not involve harm to patients might result in a Warning Letter from the FDA to the president of the responsible company. In such letters, which are widely publicized, FDA typically states that off-label promotions are a demonstration of a company's intent to market the product for that unapproved used, which adulterates and misbrands the subject device because introduction of devices into interstate commence without proper premarket authorization is violation of the Act. Other situations might result in additional enforcement activities by the FDA ranging from an injunction to force the manufacturer to stop selling the product to actions for civil penalties and even criminal prosecution of the company or its executives.

In recent years, FDA and the Department of Justice (DOJ) have been particularly vigilant about the off-label promotional activities of the manufacturers of device and pharmaceutical products. Government officials have also expressed interest in the connection between promotional practices and healthcare practitioners. Some of the largest settlements in the healthcare industry have involved claims of off-label promotion and activities designed to influence use or prescribing practices. For example, in 2010, record settlements included a $2.3 billion fine to Pfizer related to its promotional practices of Bextra and a $1.4 billion settlement by Eli Lilly for its promotion of Zyprexa. While medical device manufacturers have not been subject to fines of this magnitude, they have also been the subject of legal actions and settlements with the government. FDA and DOJ officials have repeatedly stated that they have the healthcare industry, including medical device manufacturers, under scrutiny, and as a result of whistleblower bounty provisions, they do not lack for cases to pursue.

Selected Readings

1. 21 CFR pt. 820 Quality System Regulation
2. 21 CFR pt. 803 Medical Device Reporting
3. 21 CFR pt. 806 Reports of Corrections and Removals
4. ISO 13485: 2003 Medical Device: Quality Management System
5. ISO 14971: 2007 Application of Risk Management to Medical Devices
6. Federal Food, Drug, and Cosmetic Act, 21 USC Section 301 et seq.

56. Video Recording: Responsibility and Liability

Minhao Zhou and John J. Kelly

Introduction

The use of photography and video recording is common in healthcare. Before and after photos are necessities and required in plastic surgery, intraoperative videos of laparoscopic procedures are routinely used for teaching and seminars, families often record the birth of a child. These recordings can be considered as part of the medical record, and federal and state regulations must be observed to avoid any potential liability. Liabilities include invasion of privacy especially if images are exploited for commercial benefit (such as before and after photos), or under the type of invasion of privacy known as disclosure of embarrassing private facts. Before patient photography is taken, consideration must be made as to why and how the images will be used.

Federal Regulation

Health Insurance Portability and Accountability Act (HIPAA) of 1996 is the federal regulation for privacy of individually identifiable health information which includes photographs and videos [1]. Section 160.103 defines health information as follows:

Health information means any information, whether oral or recorded in any form or medium, that

1. Is created or received by a health care provider, health plan, public health authority, employer, life insurer, school or university, or healthcare clearinghouse; and

D.S. Tichansky, J. Morton, and D.B. Jones (eds.), *The SAGES Manual of Quality, Outcomes and Patient Safety*, DOI 10.1007/978-1-4419-7901-8_56, © Springer Science+Business Media, LLC 2012

2. Relates to the past, present, or future physical or mental health or condition of an individual; the provision or health care to an individual; or the past, present, or future payment for the provision of healthcare to an individual.

This definition implies the inclusion of patient photography and video. Furthermore, requirements for de-identification of protected health information in order for records to avoid the protected health information status and fall outside the regulations are specified in Section 164.514(b):

Implementation specifications: requirements for de-identification of protected health information. A covered entity may determine that health information is not individually identifiable health information only if:

(2)(i) the following identifiers of the individual or the relatives, employers, or household members of the individual, are removed:

(A) Names;

(C) All elements of dates (except year) for dates directly related to an individual, including birth date, admission date, discharge date, date of death; and all ages over 89 and all elements of dates (including year) indicative of such age, except that such ages and elements may be aggregated into a single category of age 90 or older;

(H) Medical record numbers;

(Q) Full face photographic images and any comparable images

(R) Any other unique identifying number, characteristic, or code...

HIPAA makes the distinction that medical records under its regulation contain identifiable information that can be tracked to an individual patient. Intraoperative videos of laparoscopic procedures that do not include identifiable information specified by HIPAA including images of the face and potentially unique body tattoos does not violate a patient's privacy rights. If identifiable information is included, then the photograph or video falls under HIPAA and should be handled as such which include the following: (1) Storing the images with the patient's medical record and the issues of patient privacy and confidentiality needs to be addressed when maintaining them and protected from unauthorized viewing. (2) They should be stored in a manner that ensure timely retrieval if requested by the patient. (3) Because they are part of the patient's record, they should be kept for the same time period that state law requires medical records be kept.

State Regulation

In addition to Federal regulations under HIPAA, States may have additional requirements that can be more stringent than what is required under federal law. An example is a recent California law in effect as of January 1, 2009 [2]. The California law goes beyond HIPAA in significant ways. For example:

1. Individuals have a private cause of actions for violations. Under HIPAA, the most you can do is file a complaint with the Health and Human Services Office of Civil Rights who regulate HIPAA covered entities.
2. It is a misdemeanor to unlawfully access, use, or disclose protected information.
3. Disclosures for the purpose of financial gain can bring a fine of up to $250,000. There are no defined fines under HIPAA.
4. Fundraising is not allowed without an individual's consent. This is in contrast to HIPAA which allows for fundraising as a healthcare operations function.

HIPAA Privacy rules do not specify medical record retention requirements. Rather, State laws generally govern how long medical records are to be retained. For the state of Illinois, records must be kept for at least 10 years, for Massachusetts, the requirement is 20 years.

Clinicians must be familiar with the regulations specific to the State they practice. As a general rule, clinicians should adhere to the more stringent rules so as to assure all regulations whether federal or local are not violated.

Informed Consent

The Joint Commission on Accreditation of Healthcare Organizations (JCAHO) advises organizations to obtain informed consent when photography or video are taken during the care of a patient. For intraoperative video recording, this can be easily achieved by incorporating the consent into the operative consent. The following is an example from the operative consent from our institution (UMass Memorial Medical center, Worcester, MA):

I understand that my procedure may be observed, recorded or videotaped for medical education or consultation purposes. Efforts will be made to protect my confidentiality and privacy during my recording, videotaping process, or distribution of tissues. I understand I have the right to refuse such observation, recording, videotaping or use of tissues… I understand that the quality of care I receive at this hospital will not be affected in any way if I decided not to participate.

Patients should be made aware that images may be taken and offered the right to refuse without affecting their quality of care. For image recording outside of the operating room, a separate consent should be obtained. This can either be standalone consent or be incorporated into the generic consent for medical care.

If any photograph or video with any identifiable information as defined under HIPAA is used publicly and not related to patient care, a separate authorization form should be signed by the patient or legal representative for the specific images being used. Any additional images to be used should be covered under a new authorization form specifying those images. These authorizations remains valid unless and until the patient or their legal representative withdraws or restricts the authorization.

Research

Video or photographs taken as part of a research protocol should be approved by an institutional review board (IRB). Consent should be incorporated into the research protocol consent to participate. The IRB should be directly involved in the decisions related to practices regarding the collection and release of patient video and or photography.

Data Integrity

In 2005, a malpractice claim was filed in NY against an orthopedic surgeon [3]. The surgeon provided the patient with a copy of his spine operation. Unfortunately, the patient had poor outcome after his surgery and sued the surgeon for malpractice. The key to the prosecution's case was a discrepancy between the identification number on two implanted titanium fusion cages on the video and what was documented in the medical record. The prosecution challenged the surgeon's credibility and questioned the authenticity of the video. The court ruled for the surgeon because the prosecution failed to prove medical malpractice and did not present any evidence to indicate misinterpretation of the videotape rather than an honest error in the medical chart.

As image recording become part of the medical record, care must be taken to ensure the integrity and maintenance of these records. Just as the written medical cannot be altered without documentation to the reason and circumstance, the same applies to photographs and videos. With the availability of easy to use image and video editing software, the original recording must always be maintained in the original unaltered format to ensure integrity of the medical record.

Possible Future Legislation and Regulation

January 2007, Massachusetts state representative Martin J. Walsh a Democrat, introduced a bill that would require licensed hospitals in Massachusetts to make video and audio recordings of all surgeries. Failure to do so would result in a substantial fine. The rationale for this bill is to protect patients and "shed light on medical errors." Fortunately, the Massachusetts bill did not pass into law.

November 2009, Rhode Island Department of Health mandated Rhode Island hospital to video and audiotape all surgeries at the facility after the hospital had its fifth wrong-site surgery in 3 years [4]. Currently, Rhode Island hospital is in the process of preparing to video and audio tape all patients in the operating room up until the surgical time out is performed. Recordings of the actual operation are not currently required. Some logistics of these recordings before full implementation have yet to be worked out such as (1) How long should they keep these recordings? (2) Will patients have the right to request these recordings as part of their medical record? (3) Privacy concerns such as patient's as well as medical staff's faces will be readily identifiable in these video recordings. (4) How will it affect the working environment and morale of the operating room? etc. This experiment at Rhode Island hospital will raise some interesting questions in the future. If wrong site surgery is prevented in the next 1, 3, 5 years, etc., will it be attributed to the video recording policy vs. proper adherence to surgical site marking and time out procedure? Will other departments of health adopt this policy? Is video recording or proper adherence to the surgical pause and effective operation room communication the best way to prevent wrong site surgery? With the current economic climate, the cost of implementing, maintaining, and securing an audio and video recording system must also be considered.

Such mandates on video and audio recordings have far reaching consequences on physician patient relationships, medical legal ramifications, medical cost and logistics, patient and medical staff privacy, etc. As video and photography become easier and more common, clinicians who utilize this medium need to be aware of the current federal and state regulations and be involved in any future legislation or regulation to protect the privacy of both the patient and medical staff involved. Clinicians should not hesitate to consult the hospital legal staff whenever there is uncertainty to the current state or federal regulation.

Conclusion

As photography and video become easily available with new laparoscopic operating theaters all equipped with video recording, cell phones with the ability to take still photos and or video, easily assessable and easy to use video editing software, recording and manipulation of surgical videos have become common. As laparoscopic surgeons, we routinely record our operations for either our personal archive, teaching purposes, and or for presentations at professional meetings or publications. With the introduction of HIPAA and increasing concern for patient and medical staff privacy, the clinician needs to be aware of their responsibility and possible liability in making these recordings. Consent should always be obtained and an option to opt out should be given. To avoid privacy regulations, recordings must be stripped of all identifying information including but not exclusive of names, dates, ID numbers, faces, and even something as innocuous as a serial number on an implanted prosthesis. If identifying information is included with the recording then it must be treated and protected as mandated by Federal and State law.

Selected Readings

1. http://www.dhhs.gov/ocr/privacy/hipaa/understanding/summary/index.html.
2. http://www.ohi.ca.gov/calohi/MedicalPrivacyEnforcement.aspx.
3. http://www.thefreelibrary.com/NY%3a+was+surgery+patient+depicted+in+videotape%3f%3a+court+upholds+jury...-a0135000036.
4. http://www.medpagetoday.com/HospitalBasedMedicine/Hospitalists/16788.

57. Minimizing Medical Malpractice Exposure

Robert W. Bailey, Andrew Jay McClurg, and Philip M. Gerson

Socioeconomic and Psychological Impact

Claims related to alleged medical malpractice continue to represent a substantial burden upon the healthcare system [1]. Medical malpractice claims comprise the majority of all reports to the National Practitioner Database [2]. Medical negligence claims affect healthcare costs, utilization of resources, patient access to care, and provider well-being. Not surprisingly, awards related to medical malpractice actions continue to increase. The median jury verdict in medical liability cases increased from $157,000 in 1997 to $487,500 in 2006, a more than threefold increase [3]. The average award increased from $347,134 in 1997 to $637,134 in 2006 [3]. But, malpractice verdicts don't tell the entire story.

As a result of the threat of malpractice claims and the financial and emotional toll they impose, most healthcare providers practice some form of *defensive* medicine [1, 4]. Physicians routinely order diagnostic tests, request consultations, and manage the care of their patients in a manner that may not be medically necessary. This practice of defensive medicine is driven by a perception that the malpractice tort process is unfair and arbitrary [4]. This is true even in states where the physicians' risk of being sued is low [4].

This widespread practice of defensive medicine has an enormous cost implication. While the overall cost of malpractice litigation is estimated to be approximately $55.6 billion a year [1], the cost of practicing defensive medicine is estimated to be $45.59 billion [1] or an amazing 82% of the total costs related to medical malpractice litigation. Further, this estimate does not consider the costs related to the damage to a surgeon's reputation or the emotional ramifications of having to endure a prolonged legal battle [1].

D.S. Tichansky, J. Morton, and D.B. Jones (eds.), *The SAGES Manual*
of Quality, Outcomes and Patient Safety, DOI 10.1007/978-1-4419-7901-8_57,
© Springer Science+Business Media, LLC 2012

Doctors see lawsuits as an attack on their integrity. While malpractice lawsuits may be business as usual for plaintiffs' lawyers, they are intensely personal to physician-defendants [5]. A medical writer explained it this way:

Lawyers, I find, appear to look upon a lawsuit much as the medical profession does a case of chicken pox – unpleasant perhaps, but no cause of shame and certainly not the end of the world. To the lawyer, a malpractice action means another client to be listened to and another set of papers to be filed at the court-house. To the physician, at the very least, a malpractice suit is a personal affront and an attack on perhaps the most vulnerable part of his personality – his sense of personal integrity and professional competence [6].

Committing an error that harms a patient cuts deep into the core of a doctor's self-concept as a helper and healer, the very reasons for his or her existence as a professional. In his candid book, *How Doctors Think*, Jerome Groopman, MD, states that he remembers every error he has made in his 30-year career. He recounts a diagnostic error that led to a patient's death and says he has never forgiven himself for it [7].

In light of these nationwide statistics and personal consequences to surgeons, minimizing medical malpractice liability should be a paramount goal for every surgeon and the surgical community as a whole. A brief review of some of the keys aspects to this important issue follows. More in-depth and well-presented discussions of this topic are available and recommended to the interested reader [8–12].

Preventive Factors

The single most important factor in minimizing medical malpractice exposure is the surgeon. While this seems obvious, as there can be no surgical complication without a surgeon and a surgical procedure, the role of the surgeon in preventing malpractice litigation is far more intricate. While many factors influence potential medical malpractice claims, none is more important that those directly related to the surgeon. These include (1) the overall technical and intellectual competence of the surgeon, (2) the surgeon's ability to recognize potential areas of deficiency in his or her clinical competence, (3) the surgeon's pre-emptive willingness to seek education or assistance in the management of difficult or unusual cases, (4) the surgeon's ability to timely diagnose and treat a postoperative complication, (5) the surgeon's willingness to transfer the care of an injured patient to another surgeon or external medical facility, and (6) the health of the surgeon-patient relationship.

Surgeon Competence

The cornerstone of risk prevention is the surgeon's technical and intellectual competence [8]. Despite a lengthy training period and a rigorous certification and credentialing process, failures to properly diagnose and render appropriate care still account for a substantial portion of medical malpractice claims against surgeons [2].

A surgeon who renders care to a patient without possessing an adequate fund of knowledge and/or the requisite surgical skills necessary to provide the best care to a specific patient represents a serious situation. Fortunately, the rigorous training and credentialing process for general surgeons appears to screen out practitioners with gross deficiencies. However, due to the infinite variations in clinical presentation, even for similar disease processes, it is impossible for a surgeon to be a proverbial master of every clinical scenario.

This dilemma presents two interesting obstacles which the surgeon must overcome in order to avoid a preventable complication. First, the surgeon must recognize that he or she may have a deficiency, be it small or large, in their knowledge base or skill set as it relates to a specific area of clinical interest. Second, once a potential deficiency is identified, the surgeon must take the necessary steps to refresh or increase his or her knowledge and technical skills.

Recognition and Repair of Cognitive or Procedural Deficiencies

Every surgeon should undertake an objective assessment of his or her knowledge and technical experience as it relates to each patient's clinical presentation. If a surgeon identifies potential areas of deficiency, as might be expected with infrequently encountered conditions, the surgeon has several options. Resources available to the surgeon include literature searches, discussion with colleagues, consultation with specialists, use of a mentor or proctor, and referral of a patient to another surgeon or medical center with more expertise. These are all prudent courses of action to a surgeon faced with a unique or unfamiliar clinical scenario.

For patients with straight-forward and frequently encountered conditions, such as appendicitis or gallbladder disease, the surgeon is likely to possess the requisite knowledge and skills that will lead to a safe outcome. It is unlikely that the surgeon will need to seek additional education or consultation under such circumstances. However, as the complexity and challenge of the surgical disease increases, so does the risk that the surgeon may have areas of deficiency in his knowledge or skill base. In some situations, the surgeon may not be aware of a deficiency and therefore, may not know to seek additional assistance. A surgeon should regularly update his knowledge base whenever he or she is faced with an unfamiliar enigmatic or complex surgical patient. A surgeon should maintain a low threshold for requesting additional consultation or assistance in the management of a difficult patient or unfamiliar condition. When faced with a technically challenging procedure or new technology, a surgeon should consider enlisting the assistance of a surgeon with more expertise. This is especially true when the surgeon does not have recent clinical experience with a particular procedure, even though he or she may have privileges to perform the procedure. Under such circumstances, the surgeon should also consider direct referral of the patient to a surgeon with more expertise. The loss of revenue from the referral of a single case is far less than the financial and emotional costs associated with a major complication and any subsequent legal action.

Failure to Properly Diagnose

A substantial portion of lawsuits against general surgeons result from a surgeon's failure to properly and timely diagnose and treat a presenting condition or postoperative complication. Unfortunately, this aspect of patient care has not received much attention in the medical literature. In a recent article addressing this issue, the author points out that misdiagnoses account for nearly 20% of all medical errors [13]. The first decade of the *patient safety* movement was focused on adverse events amenable to system wide solutions, such as infections associated with health care and medication errors [13, 14]. However, diagnostic errors, although often serious, have not received similar attention. The article further states that the field of patient safety has all but ignored this problem [13]. Since diagnostic errors usually result from cognitive mistakes on the part of one or more members of the medical staff, Wachter points out that such errors are "challenging to measure and less amenable to system wide solutions." Wachter postulates that this inattention is driven by the "human nature" of these mistakes and therefore such failures of cognition are less amenable to "systems solutions" such as checklists and standardization. Wachter stresses the importance of integrating the ability to measure, prevent, and mitigate harm from diagnostic errors into policy initiatives to improve patient safety [13].

With this in mind, it is not surprising that medical malpractice claims against surgeons often stem from a surgeon's failure to timely diagnose a postoperative complication. Often, the hallmark features of the complication are present, yet the surgeon, his colleagues, and consultants fail to either consider that a postoperative complication has occurred or fail to order the appropriate diagnostic studies to rule out (or in) the presence of such a complication.

While this failure may be due to innate human nature [13], other factors are also at work. First, when managing difficult and complex patients, many surgeons request consultations from other medical specialties, such as internal medicine, pulmonary medicine, critical care, infectious disease, and nephrology. The surgeon must recognize that these other specialists do not typically possess the same body of knowledge or experience as a practicing general surgeon. The surgeon should not fully abdicate his clinical impressions under such circumstances. Rather, a surgeon needs to continue to (a) properly examine his patient for the presence of a surgical complication, (b) order the diagnostic tests necessary to rule out a potential surgical complication, and (c) properly interpret diagnostic tests from a surgical perspective. The surgeon must remain vigilant and provide sound surgical oversight of the working diagnoses being offered on the patient.

A second factor is that relates to the fact that complications occur infrequently and therefore, the surgeon may have a lack of experience in evaluating and managing such patients. In essence, a deficiency might exist in the ability of the surgeon to diagnose and treat a complication simply due to its infrequent occurrence. To help overcome this pitfall, a surgeon should remain alert to basic surgical premises when evaluating a patient with a potential postoperative complication.

Whenever a patient's expected postoperative course deviates substantially from the norm, a thorough search for a postoperative complication should be sought. One example would be a patient who has had an elective laparoscopic cholecystectomy. If that patient is not ready for discharge by the first postoperative day, the surgeon should be alerted to the presence of a possible intra-abdominal complication. Following any abdominal operation, an untoward clinical symptom or finding, especially if it persists, should prompt the surgeon to rule out exclude an intra-abdominal complication. Symptoms such as severe pain, pain out of proportion to what is expected, pain remote from the surgical site, shortness of breath, persistent nausea, vomiting, or chills and fever should create suspicion. Similarly, findings such as tachycardia, tachypnea, decreased blood pressure, decreased urine output, among others, should prompt further investigation. The surgeon should recognize that these symptoms and findings may wax and wane over time. A patient whose heart goes from 115 to 140 on 1 day back down to 115 the next should not be considered a patient who is improving. A heart rate of 115 still represents significant tachycardia in a postoperative patient. Surgeons should also be hesitant to attribute postoperative findings such as persistent tachycardia to factors such as postoperative pain alone. Tachycardia from postoperative pain should be relatively short-lived and should resolve with the administration of adequate pain medication. The surgeon has a responsibility to exclude other more serious causes of tachycardia before relying, for example, on pain as its cause. Surgeons must also remember that significant intra-abdominal complications often present with nonabdominal manifestations such as shortness of breath, pleural effusions, decreased oxygen saturation, confusion, decreased urine output, or renal insufficiency, to name a few.

Lastly, certain aspects of a surgeon's innate human nature should be emphasized in more detail. A similarity to the proverbial *ostrich with its head in the sand* mentality is seen and most likely will continue to occur. There is an innate tendency for all human beings, including surgeons, to believe that their actions have taken place in an uneventful fashion. After all, this is the predominant result experienced by practicing surgeons. If a surgeon were to become aware of a major complication during a surgical procedure, then he or she would certainly address it immediately. This belief in almost universally good outcomes may on occasion lull a surgeon into a false sense of security. The surgeon must always remain on the alert for a surgical complication, regardless of how well he or she believes the operation went.

The surgeon will also be placed in situations where a complication has occurred, its presence has been recognized, and where treatment has been initiated. However, the surgeon must avoid the tendency to believe that his or her treatment of the complication is certain to be successful. It is human error for the surgeon to steadfastly believe that once a complication is recognized and treated that no further intervention is warranted. The surgeon must continually re-evaluate any such patient to make sure that the nature of the complication has been accurately identified and that the treatment being rendered is effective.

Finally, situations may develop where the surgeon may not appreciate the complete nature or severity of the complication. Under this scenario, there is a tendency for a surgeon to believe that the patient will recover with conservative efforts and without the need for more aggressive surgical intervention. This *wait and see* attitude often serves to only delay the administration of appropriate intervention.

Regardless of the specific scenario, a general surgeon should always consider the possibility of an intra-abdominal complication when a patient is not recovering *on schedule* following a surgical procedure. The surgeon has a responsibility to be aware of the red flags or early warning signs of a complication and to make every reasonable effort to order and properly interpret the diagnostic tests necessary to exclude the presence of a serious complication, especially following intra-abdominal surgery.

Patient-Surgeon Relationship

It is well recognized that a poor surgeon-patient relationship may make it more likely that a medical malpractice claim is filed [8]. Lack of effective communication between the surgeon and the patient is a common theme when evaluating patients who have filed a malpractice action.

It is of the utmost importance that surgeons establish a meaningful relationship with their patients. The first opportunity to do this is at the time of *first contact*. Nothing is more important than first impressions. A surgeon should carefully evaluate the manner in which initial office interviews and hospital room visits are managed [8]. Even though time is a very precious commodity, making a good first impression is of critical importance. Listening is of paramount importance. If a doctor does not listen, he will be making assumptions based upon incomplete information. Dr. Groopman, in his interesting book, "How Doctors Think," notes that, on average, doctors listen to patients relating their stories for only 18 seconds before interrupting [7]. Taking an extra few minutes to listen to a patient's concerns and answering any questions goes a long way to establish a healthy physician-patient relationship [8]. A surgeon should provide the patient with a description of the patient's disease process and discuss the intended course of action, including upcoming diagnostic testing and planned surgical procedures. If the patient's first encounter with a surgeon involves a lengthy waiting room delay, a hurried and brief encounter, a lack of explanation, or a condescending attitude, the patient is likely to leave with a very poor first impression [8]. If a complication is encountered, the patient may allow their poor first impression to influence any subsequent decision to initiate legal action. The surgeon should consider the value of spending a few extra minutes in consultation and contrast this to the enormous time, cost, and emotional toll incurred if a lawsuit is filed.

However, allocating extra time with your patient is easier said than done. A system problem exists that often limits the amount of time a physician can spend with his patients. It is safe to assume that doctors would prefer seeing fewer patients and providing them with better care if they had that option and could earn the same money. Unfortunately, doctors who try to listen and answer every question may get backed up with their office visits and fall far behind on their daily schedule. To those patients waiting to be seen, this can be very frustrating and may negatively impact the patient-surgeon relationship. It is equally frustrating for the physician who may experience stress from not being able to practice medicine as they see fit. After all, there are only so many hours in the day, and with steadily decreasing reimbursement, surgeons must see and treat far more patients to maintain a stable level of income.

One of the most important situations where excellent surgeon communication is required is immediately after a complication has occurred. Effective communication between the surgeon and the patient and his or her family is crucial to maintaining a healthy relationship. Unfortunately, several factors exist that tend to detract from this goal.

Initially, the exact nature and severity of the complication may not be known. As such, a surgeon may be hesitant to discuss a potential complication with a patient until the actual presence of the complication and its severity has been confirmed. It is also human nature to avoid admitting an error, especially with the ever-present threat of costly litigation hanging overhead.

Nonetheless, once a potential complication is on the radar screen, the surgeon should consider setting aside time to explain his or her concerns to the patient. This will help to alleviate the patient's inherent anxiety and foster the patient's belief that all efforts are being expended to assure their well-being. A surgeon should not assume that a complex clinical situation cannot be explained to his patient. It should always be possible to provide a basic, albeit rudimentary, explanation to a patient about his or her clinical condition, the recommended diagnostic interventions, and overall prognosis. The surgeon should avoid responses such as, "it is too hard to explain," "leave the medicine to me," "I don't have time right now," or a terse "don't worry, everything is OK." Such attitudes do not provide the patient or the family with any meaningful reassurance and will likely alienate the surgeon from his patient.

What additional steps may be taken to improve surgeon-patient communications? Surgeons should become familiar with techniques of dealing with difficult clinical situations and also with the difficult patient. Educational material and strategies are readily available to assist the surgeon in such endeavors [15–18]. Difficult and disruptive patients present a particularly stressful situation for the surgeon. If a patient is upset and argumentative, try to respond to the issue or concern of the patient, rather than the anger and demeanor of the patient. If the patient fears or concerns are allayed, the patient's demeanor will improve.

The problems associated with a professional-lay person relationship are not unique to the medical profession. Clients who file a grievance against their attorney with an association to the Florida bar cite poor attorney-client communication as the number one reason for their complaint [19]. What is even more concerning is why this unfortunate set of circumstances has existed for many years, both for physicians and attorneys, and will likely continue into the future.

Surgeons should also be aware that they may not be communicating with their patients as well as they might think. A recent study compared how effectively physicians believed they were communicating with their patients to an actual survey of patients and their impressions of how well their physicians were communicating with them [20]. The surveys indicated a lack of patient awareness of their diagnoses and treatments, yet the majority of physicians reported they effectively communicated with patients. The study suggests that such gaps in understanding and communication could result in decreased quality of care. It recommends that steps be taken to improve patient-physician communication.

Tort Reform and Minimizing Exposure

There is an ongoing and heated debate over tort reform and its potential outcome on medical liability [1, 3, 8, 10, 21]. This is a very complex issue and one which cannot be adequately reviewed in this chapter. There are plausible arguments on both sides of the argument. At one end of the debate, advocates for reform argue that trial lawyers and their lobbyists are preventing meaningful reform due to financial interests. On the other side, plaintiffs' advocates argue for patient safety and are quick to point out that medical malpractice costs are only a small portion (2%) of overall healthcare costs [21]. Physician and insurer groups like to limit conversations about the increase in healthcare costs to malpractice reform, while their attorney-opponents trivialize the role of defensive medicine and reform in reducing healthcare costs. Mello and colleagues argue that both these simplifications are wrong – the amount of defensive medicine is not trivial, but it is unlikely to be a source of significant savings [1].

Other authors point out that capping damages on the back end of litigation does not address all of the factors that lead to litigation on the front end. These groups point out that there is in fact a fundamental dissonance between the medical liability system and the patient safety movement. The latter depends on the transparency of information on which to base improvement; the former drives such information underground. As a result, neither patients nor healthcare providers are well served by the current medical liability system [10]. Regardless of one's viewpoint, the enormous burden ($46 billion) associated with the practice of defensive medicine seems to offer an area ripe for the introduction of cost-saving measures. Unfortunately, substantial cost-savings cannot be expected until the underlying root of the problem, physicians' fear of litigation, is addressed and cured.

A Trial Lawyer's Perspective

After 40 years of reviewing medical malpractice claims, my view is that surgeons often fail to adequately educate patients prior to surgery of

- (a) The severity of the medical condition which requires surgery
- (b) Realistic expectations of what surgery can accomplish
- (c) The inherent risk factors for poor outcomes measured against hopeful expectations from surgical outcomes
- (d) The inherent risk factors for poor outcomes measured by recognized complications which may occur with competent or even extraordinary surgical skill and proper management
- (e) The importance of the patient's participation in their pre- and postsurgical evaluation and care
- (f) Risk avoidance and the availability of alternate or nonsurgical therapies

Defensive Medicine

Some aspects of so-called defensive medicine may be illusory. Requesting unnecessary consults or tests are just two obvious examples. Surgeons should remember that the standard of care for competence is ultimately based on medical not legal standards and that the unreasonable use of diagnostic measures should be controlled by physician consensus based on specialty accepted standardized protocols. Unnecessary or so-called defensive utilization is a self-serving burden on the medical system. Further, so called grey area defensive measures should be disclosed to patients, administrators, and specialty panels for approval. Information technology has changed the rules so that surgeons now instantly have the state-of-the-art knowledge and experience of peers at their fingertips. Ultimately, the exercise of clinical judgment is needed despite peer standards and information technology; surgery must be seen as technique applied to clinical judgment, except for extraordinary or experimental last resort measures.

Tort Reform Issues

Cooperation with, not opposition to, the civil justice system will provide the greatest benefit to both surgeons and patients. The voluntary disclosure of peer review findings will make surgery/medicine more transparent and thus understandable by other professionals and the public. The voluntary acceptance of fault for deviations from the standard of care with an adverse effect will validate competent surgical practice and enhance public confidence in the medical profession. Vigilant self-policing by medical professionals is the most effective method to reduce errors and unacceptable outcomes. Early dialogue with patients and their families and representatives will reduce litigation needed to obtain information necessary for patients to understand the reasons for unexpected or unwanted outcomes.

So long as we have an open judicial system unjust claims will be made and unjust defenses will be asserted. It is in the interests of the medical and legal professions to isolate and expose abuse in litigation.

A Law Professor's Perspective

Practice of Defensive Medicine

The practice of defensive medicine is not a myth. I have experienced it myself. Some time ago I was seen by a physician for evaluation of a small skin lesion. The doctor looked at it and said it was nothing to worry about.

He then took off his gloves, indicating that the examination was over. As he was about to leave the room, he casually asked what I did for a living and I told him I was a law professor. He asked what I taught and I hesitantly muttered "Torts." He responded, "Let me have another look at that spot," and then decided it needed to be biopsied.

However, the extent of the fear of being named in a malpractice lawsuit – the cause of defensive medicine – may not be well-founded. The Harvard Medical Practice Study, an analysis by interdisciplinary researchers of the medical records of a representative sample of more than 30,000 patients hospitalized in 51 New York hospitals in 1984, suggested that "the real tort crisis may consist of *too few* claims" [22]. The study found that the malpractice system is indeed irrational, but that doctors may benefit from the irrationality more than they lose because the vast majority of people injured by medical negligence never pursue claims.

Looking at the correlation between the negligent medical errors they found and subsequent malpractice claims, the researchers concluded that only 2% of medical negligence occurrences – 1 in 50 – led to a claim being filed [23]. The researchers offered several possible explanations for this surprising result, including that patients may have received adequate health and disability benefits, may not want to disrupt their relationships with their physicians, may regard their injuries as minor, may consider the small chance of success to not be worth the cost, may find lawyers repugnant, or may not recognize that they received negligent care [23].

On the other hand, the study also found that only 17% of the claims that *were* filed – fewer than one in five – involved negligent medical injury, a similarly surprising figure. The study did not determine that the other 83% of the claims were "frivolous," as in wholly without substance, but only that the hospital records lacked sufficient proof of negligence to convince the medical researchers, who sometimes disagreed in evaluating the records, that the patients suffered a negligent injury [23].

That statistically sound research yielded such bizarre claims-matching results raises serious questions as to whether the medical liability system efficiently serves the restorative and deterrent functions of tort law, and should cause all interested parties – doctors, lawyers, patients, and legislators – to pause and reassess their positions on reforming the medical injury claims process. In the meantime, the data suggests that doctors may over-estimate the risk of being sued for malpractice.

Cost of Practicing Defensive Medicine

The cost of defensive medicine is no doubt a large sum, but it is a difficult cost to reliably estimate. Lawyers are fond of touting that the overall costs of medical lawsuits, including defensive medicine, make up only 1–2% of overall healthcare costs, putting their emphasis on "only" [5, 24]. But even accepting the lawyers' figure as accurate, 1–2% of our estimated $2.3 trillion dollar annual healthcare bill [25] is between $26 and $46 billion dollars.

But is the practice of defensive medicine, which could just as easily be called "cautious medicine," necessarily a bad thing? In doing a cost-benefit analysis regarding defensive medicine, how does one assign a value to the incidental discovery of a previously occult malignancy as the result of obtaining an "unnecessary" diagnostic test? Even if the probability is small, would not most patients want their doctor to check things out? For the most part, it is probably safe to assume that doctors do not order tests unless there is at least some chance, even if only a small one, of the tests turning up something meaningful. If a doctor thinks there is a 1 in 100 or even 1 in 1,000 chance that a patient has cancer, would not most patients want the test done? In attacking defensive medicine, critics focus on the tests as being costly (which they are) and unnecessary (meaning that the probability of discovering something bad is remote), but an accurate cost-benefit analysis also requires that one consider the gravity of the risk if it does, in fact, manifest itself.

In the end, one step toward minimizing malpractice exposure may be, as I have called for [5], improved relations between doctors and lawyers. Doctors and lawyers both have strong self-interests in reducing their level of conflict. The constant tearing down of each other's professions only increases public distrust of both, to everyone's disadvantage. On the subject of defensive medicine, for example, the more frequently the public hears doctors insisting they have to practice defensive medicine because of lawyers, the more people will distrust not only lawyers for causing the problem, but doctors when they order tests. Patients may begin reacting to every test with the internal question: "Do I really need this expensive, time-consuming, painful, invasive or side effect-fraught test or is my doctor just doing this to protect himself?" Lack of trust also may make patients and clients more likely to resort to legal action when results come out differently from what they had expected or hoped for.

Selected Readings

1. Mello MM, Chandra A, Gawande AA, Studdert DM. National costs of the medical liability system. Health Aff. 2010;29:1569–77.
2. National Practitioner Data Bank 2006 Annual Report. U.S. Department of Health and Human Services. Health Resources and Services Administration. Bureau of Health Professions. Division of Practitioner Data Banks.
3. Medical Liability Reform – NOW! AMA. 2008. http://www.amaassn.org/go/mlrnow.
4. Carrier ER, Reschovsky JD, Mello MM, Mayrell RC, Katz D. Physicians' fear of malpractice lawsuits are not assuaged by tort reforms. Health Aff. 2010;29:1585–92.
5. McClurg AJ. Fight club: doctors vs. lawyers – a peace plan grounded in self-interest, Temple Law Rev. 2011;83:309–67.
6. Gillette RD. Malpractice: why physicians and lawyers differ. J Legal Med. 1976;4(9):9–10.
7. Groopman J. How doctors think. New York: Houghton Mifflin; 2007. p. 24–5.
8. Nora PF, editor. Professional liability/risk management: a manual for surgeons. 2nd ed. Chicago, IL: American College of Surgeons; 1997. p. 137.
9. Kern KA. Medicolegal perspectives on laparoscopic bile duct injuries. Surg Clin North Am. 1994;74:979–84.
10. Joint Commission on Accreditation of Healthcare Organizations (JCAHO. Health care at the crossroads: strategies for improving the medical liability system and preventing patient injury. Washington, DC: JCAHO; 2005.
11. McCarthy ED. The malpractice cure: how to avoid the legal mistakes that doctors make. New York: Kaplan; 2009.
12. Choctaw WT. Avoiding medical malpractice: a physicians' guide to the law. New York: Springer; 2008.
13. Wachter RM. Why diagnostic errors don't get any respect – and what can be done about them. Health Aff. 2010;29:1605–10.
14. Kohn LT, Corrigan JM, Donaldson MS, editors. To err is human: building a safer health system. A report of the Committee on Quality of Health Care in America, Institute of Medicine. Washington, DC: National Academy Press; 2000.
15. McGrath MH. The difficult or disruptive surgical patient: practical strategies for diagnosis and management. Bull Am Coll Surg. 2010;95:10–1.
16. Stevens LA. Responding to the difficult patient. Bull Am Coll Surg. 2010;95:12–5.
17. Dunn GP. Dealing with the difficult family: lessons from palliative care. Bull Am Coll Surg. 2010;95:16–9.
18. Reisman NR. Risk management perspective on the difficult patient and family. Bull Am Coll Surg. 2010;95:20–3.
19. Practicing with professionalism symposium. The Florida Bar, Miami. 20 Aug 2010.
20. Olson DP, Windish DM. Communication discrepancies between physicians and hospitalized patients. Arch Intern Med. 2010;170:1302–7.
21. Limiting tort liability for medical malpractice. Economic and Budget Issue Brief. Congressional Budget Office. 8 Jan 2004.

22. Weiler PC, Hiatt H, Newhouse JP, et al. A measure of malpractice: medical injury, malpractice litigation and patient compensation. Cambridge, MA: Harvard University Press; 1993. p. 62.

23. Localio AR, Lawthers AG, Brennan TA, et al. Relation between malpractice claims and adverse events due to negligence – results of the Harvard Medical Practice Study III. N Engl J Med. 1991;325:245–51.

24. Malpractice a tiny percentage of health care costs. Am Assn Justice. http://www.justice.org/cps/rde/xchg/justice/hs.xsl/8686.htm.

25. National Health Expenditures 2008 Highlights. Centers for Medicare & Medicaid Services. US Department of Health & Human Services. 2008. http://www.cms.hhs.gov/NationalHealthExpendData/downloads/highlights.pdf.

58. The Expert Witness and Tort Reform

Edward Felix

The purpose of this chapter is to look at the relationship between medical liability and the practice of bariatric surgery. We will ask, and I hope answer several questions which will shed light on the complex relationship between medical liability and the manner in which bariatric surgery is practiced. We will make several suggestions both to the bariatric surgeon and the system which may improve the overall environment.

Does Medical Liability Drive up the Cost of Care and if It Does, Who Pays for It?

There are several possible answers to these questions. Costs may be covered by the government, the insurance industry, the patient, or you the provider. As you will see, however, costs are not only financial but sometimes emotional. To determine who is paying these increased costs we must break it down into components.

The first hard cost is malpractice insurance paid for by the practicing bariatric surgeon. The level of the premium paid by the bariatric surgeon varies widely according to the state in which the surgeon practices and even is further modified by the county or city in which the surgeon performs bariatric surgery. From state to state and city to city the premiums can vary as much as 50 to a 100,000 dollars per year. In fact in some localities malpractice coverage has been impossible to obtain at any cost. In addition to the malpractice premium there are other indirect costs which the surgeon may suffer if a law suit occurs. These include, time away from the office and operating room, as well as a decreased ability to see and consult with new patients. If a lawsuit reaches the courtroom, as much as 1–2 weeks of normally productive time can be lost. Unfortunately, office expenses and overheads continue during this period.

D.S. Tichansky, J. Morton, and D.B. Jones (eds.), *The SAGES Manual of Quality, Outcomes and Patient Safety*, DOI 10.1007/978-1-4419-7901-8_58, © Springer Science+Business Media, LLC 2012

Not only is the law suit detrimental to the bariatric surgeon's practice and income, but it usually results in a shift in the manner in which they practice bariatric surgery. Yes, the shift can be beneficial in improving the practice pattern of the bariatric surgeon, but on the other hand the shift may be harmful. It is not unusual for a surgeon who has been sued to begin practicing in a very defensive style. Practice patterns sometimes change dramatically. Unnecessary tests which are costly and sometimes even harmful to patients are ordered indiscriminately to buffer the surgeon. These unnecessary tests increase the cost to the system and patient. In extreme cases can delay or prevent appropriate bariatric treatment. Finally, some patients suffer because bariatric surgeons may no longer take on those cases that are considered high risk. The larger and more severely ill patients, who in fact are in greater need of treatment, are avoided to decrease risk.

Why Does the Cost of Malpractice Insurance Vary so Widely?

The cost between the states varies widely because the rules vary from state to state. What is needed to bring an action against the physician in one state may be very different in another. Some states have a formalized system that requires an educated panel to review cases before they can proceed. While other states allow even the most frivolous suits to take place. On top of this, liability varies widely between states. States such as California have a cap on pain and suffering while others have absolutely no restrictions on the level of liability. Finally, populations of patients vary widely from region to region and the chance of having an action brought against you may vary widely. The type of procedure performed by an individual surgeon also influences to some degree the level of liability. The one thing that can dramatically reduce the chances of being sued, however, unfortunately does not influence the insurance premium. This is the relationship of the doctor to his or her patient. It has been well documented that a good relationship between physician and patient, as well as the patient's family, dramatically reduces the chance of being sued. This, however, is not taken into consideration for each individual surgeon by the malpractice carriers.

There are as just mentioned, some things that the bariatric surgeon can do to decrease his or her risk although they do not decrease the out of pocket premium cost. An improved patient–doctor relationship has been shown to be crucial in decreasing the likelihood of a malpractice law suit. There are now consultants who specialize in improving a physician's ability to relate to his or her patients, in order to decrease the likelihood of a suit. It has been shown that an honest interaction with a patient is extremely important. An honest and compassionate discussion with the patient when a complication has occurred can go a long way in decreasing the chance of litigation.

Patient selection can also decrease the likelihood of litigation. An educated patient and a well-documented informed consent is crucial to preventing litigation. Studies have shown that a patient's memory of what they have been told changes dramatically after the fact. It is therefore crucial to document the patient's and the patient's families understanding of the procedure to be performed and the potential risks and complications. Many surgeons now have the patient's document their understanding of the procedure in their own words in a letter before the procedure takes place.

Proper training of office personnel is essential. Many lawsuits have occurred because of actions taken by the surgeon's office employees. The surgeon is responsible for all actions taken by his or her employees and therefore must train them to be compassionate and understanding to the patients. In addition, meticulous record keeping is crucial to document interactions between office personnel and patients. When and what is told to patients by nurses and secretaries in the office must be part of the record.

How and what you as the surgeon document can be important in avoiding litigation or supporting your case if litigation occurs. Operative notes and patient encounters should be properly dictated and timed when they occur. What is dictated is all important. What you find or do not find at the time of surgery can be as important as the actions which you have taken at the time of surgery. The chart is not a place for confrontation or accusations and one should never vent emotions in the record. Finally, if you order a test, it is crucial you get the results and act timely and appropriately. An abnormal result, whether a lab value or a CT report, must be acted upon when it becomes available. A delay in action may appear to have as much or more consequences than delaying the test itself.

What you do after you are sued can have important financial consequences. Obviously you must not discuss the case with anyone except your lawyer. Anyone other than your lawyer or insurance company with whom you discuss the case can be subpoenaed. When it comes the time for you to be deposed it is essential for you to be prepared. You must review the case and the records before your deposition.

At deposition, it is always important to refer to the records to make sure you are accurate. All of your answers must be honest but brief. You are not there to give expert opinions and you must not get angry and argue with the opposing attorney. You must choose your words well.

Can Rule Changes Improve the System?

There are several measures that if initiated could reduce costs to both physicians and patients. As previously discussed there are some states that have caps on pain and suffering, this would obviously reduce the cost of malpractice insurance as well as the costs to the system if initiated in all states. Some states require cases to be brought before a panel before a law suit can be initiated. If this were done in a fair and proper fashion for the patient, plaintiff, and defendant, it would reduce the overall cost.

Finally, if experts were held to the guidelines and rules set by the American College of Surgeons costs would be reduced. According to the American College of Surgeons an expert must be actively practicing, be an expert in the area of surgery under dispute, and testify according to the standards at the time the care was instituted as well as deliver objective testimony. Following these guidelines for the use of experts, would eliminate the so-called for-hire experts, which are far too common. If a surgeon testifies he knows he is reviewable by the American College of Surgeons. There are severe consequences for his accreditation if an expert violates the rules of the college. Limiting expert testimony in this way would eliminate frivolous law suits, but would also improve the quality of testimony for both the defense and the plaintiff.

Is Litigation Itself Harmful?

Unfortunately, litigation can be detrimental to the surgeon even if he or she prevails. The physician is forced to have multiple days in court or in deposition and is away from their normal practice patterns. Not only is the financial cost high, but the emotional strain on the surgeon, office staff and surgeon's family, can be tremendous. Even when the outcome of the litigation is positive, doubt is left in the mind of the physician. As stated earlier, the experience will result in increased costs for future patients. Surgeons tend to develop new practice patterns which can incorporate unnecessary, costly and sometimes morbid tests in an attempt to act in a more defensive manner. They tend to avoid therapies that may have greater risks but more benefit for patients and limit access for certain types of patients. This change in behavior can seriously increase the overall costs for the system and future patients.

Is there an Answer for the Problems that We Have Outlined?

The answer is that we should have a reform throughout the USA to make the system more fair. If done in a proper fashion, changes would not only lower costs for surgeons, hospitals, and insurance companies, but improve the legal system which ultimately would benefit the patient. Plaintiffs' attorneys have been hesitant to allow reform but if properly done they would actually benefit from this reform. Cases with merit would more easily move through the court system, because of the elimination of the more frivolous suits. Physicians, insurance companies, and lawyers need to work together to reorganize the malpractice system.

Selected Readings

1. Studdert DM et al. Defensive medicine among high-risk specialist physicians in a volatile malpractice environment. J Am Med Assoc. 2005;293(21):2609–17.
2. Brennan TA, Sox CM, Burstin HR. Relation between negligent adverse events and the outcomes of medical-malpractice litigation. N Engl J Med. 1996;335:1963–7.
3. Localio AR, Lawthers AG, Brennan TA, et al. Relation between malpractice claims and adverse events due to negligence: results of the Harvard Medical Practice Study III. N Engl J Med. 1991;325:245–51.
4. Horton JB, Reece E, Janis JE, Broughton II G, Hollier L, Thornton JF, et al. Expert witness reform. Plast Reconstr Surg. 2007;120(7):2095–100.
5. Patient Safety and Professional Liability Committee, American College of Surgery. Statement on the physician acting as an expert witness. Bull Am Coll Surg. 2007;92(12):24–5.

Part IX
Conclusions

59. The Culture of Safety and the Era of Better Practices

Matthew M. Hutter

The SAGES Quality, Outcomes and Safety Manual demonstrates how SAGES members are driving the patient safety/quality improvement movement and promoting a culture of safety and an era of better practices. "Best practices" are our goal, but we realize that only with continuous quality improvement and ongoing initiatives developing "better practices" will we work to optimize the care of the surgical patient. It is this kind of thoughtful effort to promote a culture of safety which sets SAGES members apart as leaders and educators in the field of surgery.

SAGES members are passionate about improving quality, outcomes and safety in the care of their patients. The SAGES Quality, Outcomes and Safety Manual began as a project developed within the SAGES Quality, Outcomes and Safety Committee, and has grown to include the efforts from other SAGES members, and national and international leaders in the field of surgery. Thought leaders, clinical leaders, leaders in innovation and in research, and future leaders who will define the field of surgery for years to come, have all helped create this manual to promote high quality and safe care for our patients.

This manual provides a concise yet comprehensive up-to-date analysis of the patient safety and quality improvement movement in surgery, with a special focus on minimally invasive surgery. It covers topics describing patient safety/quality improvement initiatives, understanding error, preoperative risk assessment, common complications and their management, organizations promoting safety and quality, professional education, simulation and medical legal considerations. Efforts to provide safe care at the patient level, the hospital level, and the national level are all described within. Specific focus is on the processes and systems of care that promote a culture of safety.

The national spotlight – political and economical – is focusing on healthcare and its escalating costs. As advocates for our patients, we, the surgeons, have to continue to help maintain the emphasis on high quality

D.S. Tichansky, J. Morton, and D.B. Jones (eds.), *The SAGES Manual*
of Quality, Outcomes and Patient Safety, DOI 10.1007/978-1-4419-7901-8_59,
© Springer Science+Business Media, LLC 2012

and safe care. Efficiency and cost are critical; however, "value" is the nation's next focus. "Accountable care organizations," "bundled payments," and "care redesign" are the current catch-phrases coming from Washington and hospital boardrooms. Value can be defined as quality divided by cost. Costs are easy to quantify. Quality is harder to define and differentiate among healthcare systems, hospitals and caregivers. The concern is that the easily quantifiable cost metric will overshadow the hard to determine quality metric, and the resulting "value" metric will be driven solely by cost.

We, as healthcare providers, need to maintain the focus on promoting higher quality and safer care. We need to measure the quality of care, continuously examine our processes, and develop and promote better practices. And we need to help minimize cost and maximize efficiency while doing so. We need to continuously advocate for our patients at the individual level, the hospital level, the state level, and especially the national level to determine policy. This SAGES Quality, Outcomes and Safety Manual not only contains the content to develop and maintain a culture of safety and era of better practices, but also demonstrates the passion, prowess and leadership abilities that surgeons possess in the efforts to provide the best possible care for their patients.

Index

D.S. Tichansky, J. Morton, and D.B. Jones (eds.), *The SAGES Manual*
of Quality, Outcomes and Patient Safety, DOI 10.1007/978-1-4419-7901-8,
© Springer Science+Business Media, LLC 2012